# ANESTHESIA AND ORGAN TRANSPLANTATION

*Edited by*

## SIMON GELMAN, M.D., Ph.D.

Professor of Anesthesiology and Vice Chairman for Research,
Department of Anesthesiology,
The University of Alabama at Birmingham
Birmingham, Alabama

1987—W. B. SAUNDERS COMPANY

Philadelphia, London, Toronto, Mexico City, Rio de Janeiro, Sydney, Tokyo, Hong Kong

W. B. Saunders Company: West Washington Square
Philadelphia, PA 19105

**Library of Congress Cataloging-in-Publication Data**

Anesthesia and organ transplantation.

   1. Transplantation of organs, tissues, etc.
2. Anesthesia.  I. Gelman, Simon.  [DNLM: 1. Anesthesia.
2. Transplantation.  WO 660 A579]
RD87.3.T7A54  1987    617'.95    86-20285
ISBN 0-03-0-11504-3

Acquisition Editor:  Dean Manke

Developmental Editor:  Carol Morrison

Production Manager:  Frank Polizzano

Manuscript Editor:  Agnes Kelly

Illustration Coordinator:  Kenneth Green

Indexer:  Nancy Guenther

Anesthesia and Organ Transplantation          ISBN   0-03-0-11504-3

Last digit is the print number:    9    8    7    6    5    4    3    2    1

To our students and colleagues who stimulated us with thought-provoking questions, to our surgeons who presented us with challenging patients, and especially to our patients who exemplified courage and a never-ending hope for life.

# Contributors

JOHN P. EBERT, D.O.

Associate Professor of Anesthesiology, Department of Anesthesiology, University of Alabama at Birmingham; Staff Anesthesiologist, University Hospital, Birmingham, Alabama.

*Replantation of Severed Limbs; Blood Transplantation–Blood Transfusion*

ELLEN L. FINCH, M.D.

Acting Assistant Professor, Department of Anesthesia, Stanford University School of Medicine; Staff Physician, Stanford University Hospital, Stanford, California.

*Heart and Heart-Lung Transplantation*

BRUCE A. FREEMAN, Ph.D.

Associate Professor of Anesthesiology and Biochemistry, University of Alabama at Birmingham, Birmingham, Alabama.

*Organ Preservation*

SIMON GELMAN, M.D., Ph.D.

Professor of Anesthesiology and Vice Chairman for Research, Department of Anesthesiology, University of Alabama at Birmingham; Staff Anesthesiologist, University Hospital, Birmingham, Alabama.

*Liver Transplantation; Conclusions and Future Trends*

GWENDOLYN B. GRAYBAR, M.D.

Professor of Anesthesiology, Department of Anesthesiology, University of Alabama at Birmingham; Staff Anesthesiologist, University Hospital, Birmingham, Alabama.

*Kidney Transplantation*

MONTO HO, M.D.

Professor of Medicine, Microbiology, and Pathology, School of Medicine and Graduate School of Public Health, University of Pittsburgh; Chief, Division of Infectious Diseases, and Director of Clinical Microbiology, Presbyterian-University Hospital, Pittsburgh, Pennsylvania.

*Infection and Organ Transplantation*

YOO GOO KANG, M.D.

Assistant Professor of Anesthesiology, University of Pittsburgh School of Medicine; Director, Liver Transplantation Anesthesia, Presbyterian-University Hospital, Pittsburgh, Pennsylvania.

*Liver Transplantation*

J. A. JEEVENDRA MARTYN, M.D.

Associate Professor of Anesthesia, Harvard Medical School; Associate Anesthetist, Massachusetts General Hospital; Associate Director of Anesthesia, Shriners Burns Institute, Boston, Massachusetts.

*Skin Transplantation*

ROBERT D. McKAY, M.D.

Associate Professor of Anesthesiology, Department of Anesthesiology, University of Alabama at Birmingham; Staff Anesthesiologist, University Hospital, Birmingham, Alabama.

*Brain Death and Ethics of Organ Transplantation*

DALE A. PARKS, Ph.D.

Assistant Professor of Anesthesiology and Physiology, University of Alabama at Birmingham, Birmingham, Alabama.

*Organ Preservation*

JAMES D. PEARSON, M.D.

Assistant Professor of Anesthesiology, Department of Anesthesiology, University of Alabama at Birmingham; Staff Anesthesiologist, University Hospital, Birmingham, Alabama.

*Skin Transplantation*

BRUCE S. RABIN, M.D., Ph.D.

Professor of Pathology, University of Pittsburgh School of Medicine, Pittsburgh, Pennsylvania.

*Immunological Aspects of Tissue Transplantation*

BYERS W. SHAW, JR., M.D.

Associate Professor of Surgery and Chief of Transplantation, University of Nebraska Medical Center, Omaha, Nebraska.

*Immunosuppressive Therapy in Organ Transplantation*

NEELAKANTAN SUNDER, B.S., M.B.

Assistant Professor of Anesthesia, Harvard Medical School; Assistant Anesthetist, Massachusetts General Hospital, Boston, Massachusetts.

*Skin Transplantation*

MARGARET TARPEY, M.D.

Fellow, Department of Anesthesiology, University of Alabama at Birmingham, Birmingham, Alabama.

*Kidney Transplantation*

PAM DUNCAN VARNER, M.D.

Assistant Professor of Anesthesiology, Department of Anesthesiology, University of Alabama at Birmingham; Staff Anesthesiologist, University Hospital, Birmingham, Alabama.

*Brain Death and Ethics of Organ Transplantation*

R. PATRICK WOOD, M.D.

Assistant Professor of Surgery, University of Nebraska Medical Center, Omaha, Nebraska.

*Immunosuppressive Therapy in Organ Transplantation*


JANET WYNER, M.B., Ch.B.

Associate Professor, Department of Anesthesia, Stanford University School of Medicine; Staff Physician, Stanford University Hospital, Stanford, California.

*Heart and Heart-Lung Transplantation*

# Preface

Organ transplantation, once an uncommon, often extraordinary event, has rightfully assumed a prominent position among routine procedures performed at most centers. Few endeavors in medicine enable the physician to so profoundly influence change in a patient's physiology and thereby improve the quality of life. Rapid expansion of the scientific foundations of immunology and surgery, as they apply to transplantation, has contributed to the accelerated growth in this field; however, like so many other provinces of surgery, ultimate success of the project has been founded on the dedicated support of members of other specialty groups such as cardiologists, hepatologists, internists, and, of course, anesthesiologists. Growth in knowledge and experience in organ transplantation is so explosive that in the near future almost every center, large or small, will undoubtedly be involved in the transplantation of at least one organ on a regular basis. Because of this, acquisition of the data base and understanding of the nuances of organ transplantation will be essential for specialists whose contributions to this undertaking are so vital. Patients in need of organ transplantation have, by definition, functional failure of one organ, and in some circumstances, more than one. Therefore, knowledge of normal organ function, as well as the physiological consequences of organ failure, are the cornerstones of management for these patients.

The proliferation of both the type and quantity of transplantation procedures is welcome and inevitable. It is imperative that those caring for transplant recipients fully appreciate all factors on which survival and longevity depend. Although successful anesthetic management depends on complete understanding of the physiology of organ failure as well as the technical aspects of the operation itself, the story does not end here. For instance, the impact of aggressive immunosuppressive therapy on the eventual outcome and biological responses to injury in the face of underlying immunological compromise should not be underestimated. Furthermore, organ transplantation procedures are often lengthy and are uniquely composed of three separate phases, each of which is distinguished by its own nuances. The first is that of organectomy, characterized by the medical features of chronic organ failure and in many circumstances, surgical encumbrances common to the extraction of a diseased part. Second is the "an-organ" phase, in which global bodily functions are profoundly influenced by the complete absence of physiological services usually provided to some extent by the failing organ. Last, there is the stage of post–organ implantation, typified by the welcome addition of sound organ services but often complicated by insults related to the release from this same organ of potentially harmful substances associated with organ preservation. Successful completion of these stages authorizes entrance into the challenging arena of the postoperative period, encompassing all of the features of the healing process in a critically ill patient and complicated by the ever-present double-edged sword of organ rejection and infection. The therapeutic balance is delicate.

With these considerations in mind, it seems logical that a book devoted to the anesthesiological problems encountered in organ transplantation would be a valuable source of information, not only for anesthesiologists, but for any physician involved in the complex struggle of helping patients undergoing these surgical procedures. The text focuses on general topics, including immunological problems and immunosuppressive therapy related to organ transplantation, organ preservation, and specific complications of organ transplantation such as rejection and infection. A lion's share of the book is devoted to specific anesthesiological problems occurring during transplantation of organs such as the heart, heart–lung, liver, kidneys, and a few others. Certain organs are not discussed. For example, there are no chapters related to corneal, pancreatic, or intestinal transplantation. The reason for these omissions is that there are not enough specific anesthesiological problems related to these particular operations clearly identified in the literature. However, one chapter is devoted to tissue transplantation that anesthesiologists perform routinely; namely, blood transplantation–blood transfusion. Even though organ replantation is not actually organ transplantation from one human to another, there are certain problems important to anesthesiologists. Therefore, a chapter is devoted to this topic.

This book is an attempt to help us better execute our roles in the process of organ transplantation when one human donates the gift of life to another.

SIMON GELMAN

# Acknowledgments

Writing absorbs an immense amount of time and eventually involves an entire department, including the chairman, physicians, nurses, technicians, and secretaries. It involves time away from families, as well as time away from the operating room and other duties. Because of this, I am indebted to all who shared in the workload. I especially want to thank staff members who covered in the operating rooms and performed other duties in the absence of the contributors so that they could spend their time writing.

I am especially grateful to all the authors. Without them, this book would not have been possible. To each one individually, I owe a debt of gratitude for their time and efforts, for their knowledge, and for their willingness to share that knowledge.

The secretarial and administrative support was a major undertaking. I appreciate the efforts of everyone at the University of Alabama at Birmingham, the University of Pittsburgh, Harvard Medical School, Stanford University, and the University of Nebraska Medical Center who assisted in the tedious task of preparing manuscripts.

To my assistant, Rae Kerutis, I owe a special note of gratitude. She helped in the preparation of manuscripts, tolerated my revisions, and worked very closely with me in the editing and organization of this book.

Finally, I would like to share with you, the reader, my personal and professional satisfaction at having the privilege of touching the edges of a relatively new field of medicine which will continue to save lives through the dedicated endeavors of many physicians such as the authors of this book.

SIMON GELMAN

# Foreword

No other development in the history of medicine has had the conceptual and philosophic implications of organ transplantation. In all past times, the objective of physicians and surgeons faced with diseases of specific organ systems was to extract the last grudging moment of function from a failing heart, lung, liver, or kidney using medicines or with operative procedures that often were poorly conceived but brilliantly executed. When the function of a vital organ system reached a certain level, the whole body died even though all the other organ systems were without defect.

It is breathtaking to contemplate the departure from this rear-guard approach which has been made possible with transplantation. With one bold stroke, health and life can be restored, and with considerable reliability and safety. The ability to provide these services has descended like magic into the consciousness of a new generation of social observers, physicians, and patients.

The history has been so short that most of the workers present at the beginning of this new field are still alive, and many are still active professionally. Yet, less than 25 years ago, Nobel Laureate Frank MacFaralane Burnet reviewed the field of transplantation in the *New England Journal of Medicine* and wrote that ". . . much thought has been given to ways by which tissues or organs not genetically and antigenically identical with the patient might be made to survive and function in the alien environment. On the whole, the present outlook is highly unfavorable to success . . . ."

Only a few months after the publication of this pessimistic view, the avalanche of successful renal transplantations began which definitively opened the modern era of transplantation, made possible by combination drug therapy with azathioprine and steroids. Many improvements have been introduced since that time, but the most practical and therefore the most important have been made possible by the new drug cyclosporine.

The boldness and effectiveness with which these improvements in immunosuppression, and collateral improvements in tissue procurement and preservation, have been applied would have been thought to be pure fantasy if they had been predicted only a few years ago. Even multiple organ transplantation has been feasible. It has become commonplace to transplant the lung plus heart, a kidney plus pancreas, a liver plus heart, a liver and pancreas, or various other combinations of organs.

Application of these wonderful new therapeutic tools has provided the ultimate challenge to a new breed of anesthesiologists whose skill has become legendary in monitoring moment-to-moment physiologic changes and in making adjustments in pharmacologic therapy. No surgeon who works in the difficult field of organ transplantation can fail to view his colleagues in anesthesiology with anything but awe.

In this book, these warriors at the head of the table have revealed their secrets against a background provided in the other chapters by bright young immunologists, internists, and surgeons. The result is a lively and informative book that should find its way to anesthesia preparation rooms throughout the world, thereby providing a great service both to anesthesiology and to surgery.

THOMAS E. STARZL, M.D., PH.D.

Professor of Surgery
University of Pittsburgh School of Medicine

# Contents

**11**

John P. Ebert

**12**

Simon Gelman

# 1

# Immunological Aspects of Tissue Transplantation

BRUCE S. RABIN

## DESCRIPTION OF THE IMMUNE SYSTEM

The immune system is a multifaceted structure designed to protect against the development of infectious and malignant diseases. In this regard the immune system has been capable of responding to the presence of specific infectious agents and developing specific reactions to eliminate them. For example, the elimination of pyogenic organisms requires that the immune system produce antibody that will combine with the bacterium and eventually destroy the organism either by direct killing or by phagocytosis. Viral infection is primarily resisted by the cellular immune system, which functions independently of antibody.

On occasion the immune system has been known to make a mistake. When it does so it begins to react against self-tissue and produces diseases that are termed autoimmune. Examples of such diseases are insulin-dependent diabetes, thyroiditis, adrenalitis, hemolytic anemia, thrombocytopenia, and pemphigus vulgaris. Autoimmune responses directed against liver, kidney, and heart also

occur. Such autoimmune responses lead to damage of these organs. Thus it is not surprising that when an organ is transplanted from one individual to another, the immune system will look upon the transplanted organ as foreign and produce an immune response against it. The manifestation of the immune response to the transplanted organ is transplant rejection.

Transplant rejection occurs because the immune system of the recipient looks at antigens of the transplanted tissue and recognizes them as foreign. When transplantation occurs between identical twins there is no problem of transplant rejection. This suggests that the antigens on the transplant that stimulate the immune response are determined by genetic factors. It is important to understand the genetic factors that may be responsible for rejection and the immunological components that may bring about rejection. An understanding of these factors may suggest ways in which the immune system can be altered or tissue matching may occur to reduce the severity of the rejection response.

1

It is important to note that transplant failure can occur for reasons other than immunological rejection. For example, if excessive time elapses between harvesting of the organ and transplantation, and there is enzymatic degradation with alteration of the physiological activity of the transplanted tissue, the organ may fail to function. Complications may occur during surgery leading to impairment of an adequate blood supply to the organ. Organs harvested for transplantation may be damaged prior to transplantation. However, assuming that the organ being transplanted is healthy and all of the harvesting and surgical procedures are performed in an optimum fashion, the major reason for transplant failure is immunological rejection. The following will review the various components of the immune system that are factors in rejection, the mechanisms of immunological rejection, and various immunological assays that should be considered when transplantation takes place.

## CELLULAR COMPONENTS OF THE IMMUNE SYSTEM

**Macrophages.** There are both specific and nonspecific cellular components of the immune system. An example of a nonspecific cell is the macrophage.

Macrophages are capable of attacking and ingesting foreign microorganisms or foreign tissue when present in an individual. The macrophage is not specifically sensitized (immunologically reactive) to the substance it attacks. Rather, the macrophage possesses receptors on its surface for immunoglobulin that has been bound to an antigen. Thus, when a bacterium is coated with antibody it will be ingested by a macrophage (Fig. 1–1). Similarly, tissue antigens that are coated with antibody may be attacked by macrophages.

Macrophages also participate by contributing to activation of lymphocytes. In this regard macrophages have the capability of concentrating antigen on their surface, allowing lymphocytes to react with the antigen. In addition, a soluble material termed interleukin-1 is released by macrophages when they interact with an antigen. Interleukin-1 activates the T helper population of lymphocytes, which then induces specific immunological reactions.

**Lymphocytes.** There are two major populations of lymphocytes. One population produces antibody and is termed B lymphocytes.

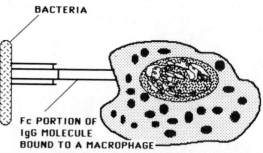

**Figure 1–1.** When an infectious agent, such as bacteria, is exposed to an antibody reactive to those bacteria, the antibody will bind and the Fc portion of the immunoglobulin molecule will be exposed. Phagocytic cells (macrophages, monocytes, and polymorphonuclear leukocytes) have a receptor for the Fc portion of immunoglobulin on their surface. When the immunoglobulin molecule is bound to the phagocytic cell Fc receptor, the infectious agent will be ingested and degraded. In this manner the immune system is capable of resisting infectious disease.

The other population (T lymphocytes) is involved in immunological regulation and reactions of cell-mediated immunity.

Following exposure to antigen (for example, immunization with tetanus toxoid) the immune system responds by producing antibody to the antigen. The antibody may neutralize the antigen by combining with a toxic site on the antigen molecule or cause its removal by the phagocytic cells of the body. Thus antibody production is generally beneficial. However, if antibody is produced to self-antigens (for example, erythrocytes) a disease process may result. If antibody is produced to transplanted tissue, rapid rejection of the transplanted tissue may occur. An example is transplantation of a blood group A kidney into a blood group O recipient. The blood group O recipient has antibody to blood group A antigen. Thus, once blood circulation occurs in the transplanted kidney, the antibody to the A antigen will combine with antigens on the endothelial cells of the transplant, activate the complement system, and lead to immediate rejection of the kidney (Fig. 1–2).

To become functionally active the T lymphocyte population of cells is dependent upon hormones released by the thymus gland. There are at least three different cell populations, with different functional activities, that are known as T lymphocytes. These are generally termed the T helper cell, the T suppressor cell, and the T cytotoxic cell. In addition to being functionally different the three populations of cells have different sur-

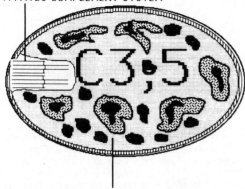

ANTIBODY BOUND TO BLOOD VESSEL WALL
ACTIVATES COMPLEMENT SYSTEM

COMPLEMENT ATTRACTS PHAGOCYTIC CELLS
AND PLATELETS. FIBRIN DEPOSITS IN BLOOD
VESSEL LUMEN. PHAGOCYTIC CELLS
DEGRANULATE RELEASING HYDROLYTIC
ENZYMES. LUMEN IS OCCLUDED AND DISTAL
TISSUE BECOMES ANOXIC.

**Figure 1–2.** When antibody interacts with an antigen, it is capable of activating the complement system. Two components of the complement system (C3 and C5) mediate an inflammatory response. Activated C5 attracts phagocytic cells to the site of antibody binding, and C3 helps to adhere the phagocytic cells to the site of bound antibody. Platelets are attracted and fibrin deposition occurs. This leads to localized anoxia, and the phagocytic cells degranulate, releasing hydrolytic enzymes. The enzymes and anoxia lead to tissue destruction.

face antigens that can be detected by the use of monoclonal antibody (Table 1–1 and Fig. 1–3).

All T lymphocytes have a surface marker that can be identified by the antibody termed OKT 3 or Leu 4. The T helper population of lymphocytes has a surface antigen detected by the monoclonal antibody OKT 4 or Leu 3. The suppressor and cytotoxic lymphocyte populations have surface markers detected by the OKT 8 and Leu 2 monoclonal antibodies. There is a marker present on the suppressor population termed Leu 15 that is not present on the cytotoxic cell population.

Monoclonal antibody is also useful to detect lymphocytes that are activated, i.e., engaged in an immunological reaction. Such antibody detects surface structures that are present on cells only when they are activated. These monoclonal antibodies are directed either to the receptor for interleukin-2 or to a framework structure of the DR antigen on T lymphocytes.

The T helper cell is a lymphocyte that drives immunological reactions. Although the B lymphocyte can produce antibody to

some antigens by directly interacting with the antigen on the surface of a macrophage, most antigens additionally require a T helper cell to assist the B lymphocyte in producing antibody. A deficiency of T helper cells can lead to impairment of antibody production.

The T helper cell is also necessary for reactions of cell-mediated immunity (delayed hypersensitivity). This type of reaction may be a factor in rejection of transplanted tissue. The delayed hypersensitivity reaction evolves through the interaction of different cell populations with soluble mediators released by T helper lymphocytes (Fig. 1–4).

An example of how the delayed hypersensitivity reaction may occur follows: After exposure of T helper lymphocytes to an antigen, cellular lymphocytes become sensitized (reactive) to the antigen. When this occurs the sensitized lymphocytes undergo a series of changes that primarily involve the release of soluble mediators (lymphokines). One mediator that is released from the sensitized cell has the property of inducing lymphocytes

**TABLE 1–1. Monoclonal Antibodies Available for Testing of Human Peripheral Blood Lymphocytes**

| Antibody | | Population Detected |
|---|---|---|
| Leu 2a, 2b* | OKT 8† | 20–40% mature T cells Suppressor/cytotoxic cells |
| Leu 3a, 3b | OKT 4 | 40–65% mature T cells Helper/inducer subset |
| Leu 4 | OKT 3 | 90–95% mature T cells Peripheral T lymphocytes |
| Leu 5 | OKT 11 | 95% E rosette positive cells |
| Leu 7 | | 5–20% peripheral mononuclear cells Large granular lymphocytes, including natural killer cells |
| Leu 11a, 11b | | 5–20% peripheral mononuclear cells, natural killer cells |
| Leu HLA-DR | OKT Ial | 5–25% peripheral lymphocytes B cells, monocytes, not most T cells |

\* Leu antibodies are produced by Becton-Dickinson, Mountain View, California.
† OKT series of monoclonal antibodies are produced by Ortho Pharmaceuticals, Raritan, New Jersey.

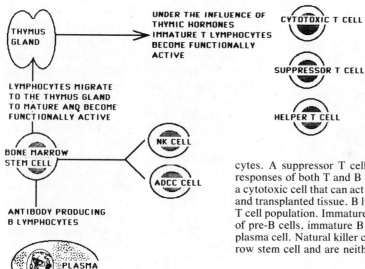

**Figure 1–3.** A bone marrow stem cell is acted upon by hormone-like substances that can influence it along pathways to mature into a T or a B lymphocyte. The T-cell pathway is influenced by hormones released by the thymus gland. As T lymphocytes mature they develop functional activities. One activity of T lymphocytes is a helper cell. The helper cell promotes functional activity of other T lymphocytes and B lymphocytes. A suppressor T cell develops which impedes immunologic responses of both T and B lymphocytes. The third T lymphocyte is a cytotoxic cell that can act against invading foreign microorganisms and transplanted tissue. B lymphocytes are influenced by the helper T cell population. Immature B lymphocytes mature along a pathway of pre-B cells, immature B cells, mature B cells, and the end-stage plasma cell. Natural killer cells and K cells arise from the bone marrow stem cell and are neither T nor B lymphocytes.

that are not reactive to the antigen into mitotic division. This soluble factor may be called blastogenic factor. Blastogenic factor induces nonsensitized lymphocytes into mitosis, increasing the number of lymphocytes accumulated at the site of antigen reaction. An additional factor released from the sensitized lymphocytes is called transfer factor. Transfer factor is capable of converting lymphocytes that are not reactive to an antigen to lymphocytes that are reactive to the antigen. Thus, while lymphocytes are accumulating, they are being converted to lymphocytes that are reactive to the specific foreign antigen. In this way there is an increase in lymphocytes responding to the antigen, all of which are releasing soluble mediators.

Further factors released from the sensitized lymphocytes have the capability of attracting phagocytic cells to the site of reaction. Such cells include polymorphonuclear leukocytes, eosinophils, and macrophages. Other factors activate the phagocytic cells, particularly the macrophages, producing a cell population capable of ingesting and eliminating the foreign antigen. To keep the cells at the site of reaction, factors that are inhibitory to cell migration, such as leukocyte migration inhibition factor and macrophage migration inhibition factor, are released by the T cells.

To allow the accumulating cells out of the vasculature and into the tissue, a substance called skin reactive factor, which has the capability of releasing histamine from mast cells, is released. This results in increased vascular permeability and migration of the various cell populations into the tissue in an attempt to eliminate the foreign antigen. If this reaction is occurring in transplanted tissue, a chronic type of rejection may occur,

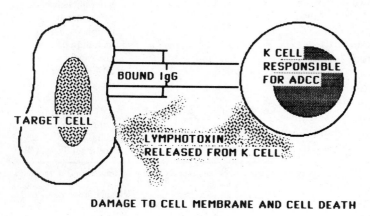

**Figure 1–4.** Antibody-dependent cellular cytotoxicity occurs when a K lymphocyte (which is not sensitized to target antigen) binds to immunoglobulin that is attached to a target cell. The K cell releases a toxin that degrades the membrane of the target cell and leads to cell death.

which over the course of many months may lead to complete destruction of the tissue.

The other T lymphocyte population of major concern in transplant rejection is the cytotoxic T lymphocyte. This population of cells can bind directly to antigens of the transplant. When the cytotoxic T cell binds to transplant antigens, it releases a soluble substance termed lymphotoxin, which can lead to lytic destruction of the tissue cells to which the cytotoxic T cell is bound. The cytotoxic T lymphocyte does not have to recruit inflammatory cells to the site of binding as does the T helper cell. Rather, the cytotoxic T cell acts directly on the transplanted tissue.

There are, in addition, lymphocytes that cannot be classified as either T or B lymphocytes. These cells are classified as belonging to the null lymphocyte population. There are primarily two types of lymphocytes in the null cell population. One cell is termed a K lymphocyte and is responsible for the phenomenon known as antibody-dependent cellular cytotoxicity (Fig. 1–5).

The K cell has a receptor for the Fc portion of IgG on its surface. When circulating in plasma, IgG does not have its Fc receptor exposed. However, when IgG binds to an antigen, the Fc portion of the immunoglobulin molecule is exposed. When this occurs the K lymphocyte can bind to the Fc portion, and although the K cell is not sensitized to the antigen the antibody is bound to, the K cell will release a lymphotoxin that causes destruction of the immunoglobulin-binding antigen. If an immunoglobulin is not capable of activating the complement system and producing inflammation and tissue damage by complement activation, it may still be effective in producing tissue damage if it can bind the K lymphocyte.

The other lymphocyte of the null cell population is the NK or natural killer cell. This lymphocyte population is believed capable of eliminating tissue cells that spontaneously undergo malignant transformation. The mechanism by which the NK cell functions is currently unknown. The cells can be morphologically differentiated as they appear as large granular lymphocytes. In addition, the NK cell has an antigen on its surface that can be recognized by a monoclonal antibody termed Leu 11.

## COMMUNICATION BETWEEN COMPONENTS OF THE IMMUNE SYSTEM

Lymphocytes communicate between each other by producing and releasing soluble factors called interleukins (Fig. 1–6). Interleukins are signals that one population of cells gives to another to initiate specific immunological reactions. When a monocyte encounters an antigen, the monocyte synthesizes and releases a soluble factor termed interleukin-1. The receptor for interleukin-1 is on the surface of T helper lymphocytes. When a T helper lymphocyte binds interleukin-1, the T helper cell begins to synthesize and release interleukin-2. The receptor for interleukin-2 is on T helper cells and T cytotoxic cells. Thus, once a T helper cell begins to release interleukin-2 as a result of interleukin-1 stimulation, the interleukin-2 feeds back on the T helper cell, resulting in increased synthesis of interleukin-2 and also increased generation of receptors for interleukin-2 on the T helper cell surface. There is also an interleukin-3, which may be involved in stimulation of B lymphocytes to synthesize antibody.

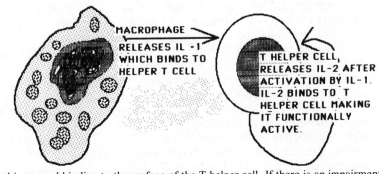

**Figure 1–5.** Release of soluble factors between cells of the immune system influences the activity of the immune system. When a macrophage interacts with an antigen, a substance termed interleukin-1 is released. Interleukin-1 has a receptor on T helper cells. When interleukin-1 is bound by the T helper cell, another substance, interleukin-2, is released which binds to a receptor on the T helper cell. This leads to increased synthesis of interleukin-2 and increased binding to the surface of the T helper cell. If there is an impairment of interleukin-2 production, as occurs when cyclosporine is used as an immunologic suppressant, there is decreased activity of the immune system.

MACROPHAGE RELEASES IL -1 WHICH BINDS TO HELPER T CELL

T HELPER CELL, RELEASES IL-2 AFTER ACTIVATION BY IL-1. IL-2 BINDS TO T HELPER CELL MAKING IT FUNCTIONALLY ACTIVE.

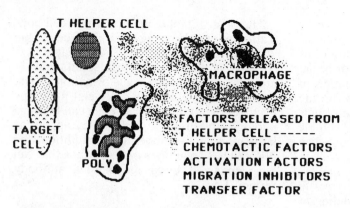

**T HELPER CELL**

**MACROPHAGE**

**TARGET CELL**

**POLY**

**FACTORS RELEASED FROM
T HELPER CELL - - - - - -
CHEMOTACTIC FACTORS
ACTIVATION FACTORS
MIGRATION INHIBITORS
TRANSFER FACTOR**

**Figure 1–6.** The cellular immune response occurs when a T helper cell reacts with an antigen. The T helper cell releases a variety of soluble factors (lymphokines) that are chemotactic for phagocytic cells, activate the phagocytic cells to react against the foreign antigens, and keep the phagocytic cells at the area of reaction. In addition, the T helper cell releases substances that cause lymphocytes, which are not reactive to the antigen, to become antigen-reactive (transfer factor). When this reaction occurs in the skin, it is termed a delayed hypersensitivity reaction.

## IMMUNOLOGICAL ASPECTS OF TRANSPLANTATION

The major immunological reactions responsible for transplant rejection have been mentioned. These include antibody directed to antigens present on the surface of transplanted cells and cell-mediated immune mechanisms of delayed hypersensitivity or direct cytotoxicity. More information in regard to each of these mechanisms will now be given.

**Antibody-Mediated Rejection.** The clearest example of antibody-mediated transplant rejection is that of a kidney transplant that is mismatched for the ABO blood group. The transplant is immediately rejected by the reaction of hyperacute rejection (see Fig. 1–2). The actual rejection process occurs by activation of the serum complement system when antibody binds to antigen. When activated, the complement system is chemotactic for phagocytic cells and induces fibrin deposition. The phagocytic cells occlude blood vessels, leading to anoxia. The phagocytic cells degranulate and release hydrolytic enzymes. Tissue destruction occurs secondary to the local effect of the enzymes and anoxia.

In both heart and kidney transplantation, compatibility for the ABO blood group antigens between donor and recipient is a necessity. However, liver transplants do not have to be matched for ABO compatibility. This is unique to the liver, and the mechanism is not fully understood. It can be speculated that the liver, having an enormous cell mass, can absorb antibody from the circulation without fully losing its functional capacity. The liver can then regenerate because the immunological suppression being used to prevent rejection will suppress the continued formation of high levels of antibody.

Antibody to transplant antigens (histocompatibility antigens) can develop in recipients who have received transfusions or had multiple pregnancies. Also, a patient in whom transplant rejection has occurred, and who is a candidate for a second transplant, may have developed antibody to histocompatibility antigens.

The presence of antibody to histocompatibility antigens may lead to hyperacute rejection in a manner identical to ABO blood group mismatching. To prevent this from occurring, laboratory testing is done (the crossmatch procedure) to determine if a recipient has antibody directed to donor histocompatibility antigens. It is important that the recipient of a kidney or heart transplant does not have antibody to donor histocompatibility antigens. However, similar to the ABO blood group system, liver transplantation is not contraindicated if the recipient has antibody to donor histocompatibility antigens.

Another group of antigens, present on vascular endothelial cells, may also stimulate antibody production and be responsible for hyperacute rejection. The endothelial antigens are shared with peripheral blood monocytes. It is likely that individuals become sensitized to endothelial antigens by monocytes in transfused blood or prior rejection of a transplant.

The endothelial antigens are not present on lymphocytes. In most procedures to detect recipient antibody to donor antigens, donor lymphocytes are used as the target tissue. Thus, if there is antibody to vascular endothelial antigens, it is not detected by the standard crossmatch procedure.

On occasion a hyperacute rejection occurs when a patient has received a kidney or a heart and no antibody has been detected in the recipient to donor histocompatibility antigens. Such rejection may be due to antibody to the vascular endothelial antigens. Since very few laboratories can detect such antibody, this antigenic system will be a continuing problem with transplant rejection.

**Cellular Reactions.** As previously indicated, T lymphocytes are responsible for chronic rejection that occurs weeks to months to years after transplantation. Both delayed hypersensitivity mechanisms and direct cytotoxicity mechanisms may be responsible for cellular rejection. In experimental systems it is possible to isolate many of the cells responsible for delayed hypersensitivity reactions or direct cytotoxicity. These cell populations can be expanded and their functional activity determined in regard to transplant rejection by infusing them into experimental animals. Cytotoxic lymphocytes, by themselves, are not capable of inducing transplant rejection. This is most likely due to the lack of a T helper cell to drive the cytotoxic lymphocyte response. However, when T helper cells are present, cytotoxic T lymphocytes can produce graft rejection.

A natural development from this observation is the use of monoclonal antibody directed to T lymphocytes as a means of reversing graft rejection. Infusion of such antibody into a patient who is undergoing rejection should lead to elimination of the cells mediating the cellular reaction. Indeed, this does occur, and monoclonal antibody to T lymphocytes has been found to be a highly effective means of reversing transplant rejection. However, monoclonal antibodies produced in mice are a mouse gamma globulin. When injected into humans, they stimulate antibody production to mouse protein. With continued use, the anti-mouse protein antibody neutralizes the monoclonal antibody so that it can be used only for a short course of therapy.

## PRETRANSPLANT EVALUATION (Table 1–2)

**Per Cent Panel Reactive Antibody.** A common term used in regard to transplantation is *PRA*, meaning per cent panel reactive antibody. The PRA provides an indication whether a recipient has developed antibody to histocompatibility antigens and how extensively the recipient is sensitized.

The PRA is determined as follows: Lymphocytes are collected from normal individuals. The individuals are selected so that all of the HLA antigens will be represented. As an example, let us assume that 50 normal in-

**TABLE 1–2.  Standard Immunological Tests Associated with Organ Transplantation**

**Tissue typing.** Used for determination of donor and recipient HLA-A/B/DR antigens.

**Panel reactive antibody.** Performed using serum collected each month from potential recipients. Serum reacted against a panel of normal lymphocytes to determine if recipient is sensitized to histocompatibility antigens.

**Crossmatch.** Recipient's serum is reacted against lymphocytes of the organ donor. Recipient serum reacting to T lymphocytes at 37°C is a contraindication to kidney and heart transplants. Liver transplants can be done with a positive crossmatch.

dividuals are required to compose a panel that will represent all of the known HLA antigens. Serum from a potential recipient is incubated with each of the 50 lymphocytes. After a suitable time, serum complement is added. If the recipient's serum has bound to lymphocytes of one of the panel members, it will fix complement and lead to killing of the lymphocytes (Fig. 1–7).

If the recipient has not previously been sensitized to histocompatibility antigens,

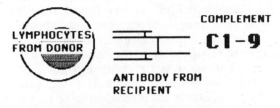

**NEGATIVE CROSSMATCH**

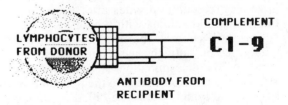

**POSITIVE CROSSMATCH**

**Figure 1–7.** The pretransplantation crossmatch consists of incubating lymphocytes from the donor with serum from the recipient. If the recipient has antibody to antigens on the surface of the donor lymphocytes, the antibody will bind. This will then allow the fixation of normal serum complement. The complement will cause destruction of the donor lymphocytes, indicating that a hyperacute rejection may occur if the transplant is done. A negative crossmatch would indicate that the transplant can be done without risk of a hyperacute rejection.

there will be no antibody in the recipient's serum to bind to lymphocytes of the normal cell panel. This individual will be reported to have 0 per cent PRA. This would indicate that the recipient will not have antibody to lymphocytes of a donor of any tissue that becomes available. Thus, transplantation would be easy in this recipient, as he or she is not sensitized to any histocompatibility antigens.

If the recipient has antibody to lymphocytes of 25 members of the 50-member panel, the recipient would be reported to have 50 per cent PRA. This would indicate that the recipient would have antibody to lymphocytes of approximately 50 per cent of organ donors. Thus, half of the organs available for this donor would not be suitable for transplantation.

A highly sensitized patient, with 100 per cent PRA, would be found to have antibody to lymphocytes from every recipient who can provide an organ. Thus, it would be very difficult to find suitable tissue for such an individual.

Another way in which the PRA can be interpreted is as an indication of the genetic capability of a potential recipient to produce antibody to histocompatibility antigens. For various medical reasons many patients awaiting transplantation receive blood transfusions containing histocompatibility antigens. The immunological capability of making an immune response to histocompatibility antigens is under genetic control. Individuals with a low PRA are less likely to have the genetic capability of responding to histocompatibility antigens than are individuals with a high PRA. Thus, individuals with a low PRA have less rejection episodes after transplantation than individuals with a high PRA.

The PRA can also be used to determine what specific antigens a recipient is sensitized to. By determination of which of the HLA antigens are common to the panel members whose lymphocytes are killed by donor serum, it may be possible to determine if there are specific HLA antigens that the recipient has produced antibody to. When this occurs, organs lacking those antigens can be selected for transplantation to the recipient.

**Pretransplant Crossmatch.** Prior to the actual transplantation of a kidney or heart, it is important to determine whether the recipient has antibody directed to antigens present on lymphocytes of the specific donor (see Fig. 1–6). The reason that lymphocytes from the donor are used is that these cells are easily obtained, and they have the same histocompatibility antigens on their cell surface as those present on the transplanted tissue. Thus they can provide an indication whether a recipient has antibody to donor histocompatibility antigens.

There are four types of reactions one can determine in a crossmatch procedure. There are two different temperatures of incubation and reactivity to either the donor's T or B lymphocytes. Thus there can be a warm reactive antibody (binding at 37°C) to T or B lymphocytes and a cold reactive antibody (binding at 4°C) to T or B lymphocytes.

The antibody that will lead to a hyperacute rejection is the warm reactive antibody to T lymphocytes. Thus, in a patient who has such antibody to a specific donor's lymphocytes, the kidney or heart transplantation should not be done. However, as previously indicated, this is not a contraindication to liver transplantation.

Warm or cold reactive antibody to B lymphocytes and cold reactive antibody to T lymphocytes are controversial in regard to their beneficial or harmful effects. There is evidence that a cold reactive antibody to B lymphocytes may actually be protective and enhance organ survival. This antibody, which is most likely directed to an HLA-DR antigen, may bind to antigens on the vascular endothelium of the transplant and shield the antigen from sensitized lymphocytes. The cold reactive antibody would not activate the complement system or bind K lymphocytes.

If a patient has 0 per cent PRA it is reasonably certain that the crossmatch will be negative. Thus, in patients with a low PRA in whom there is a time constraint on performing the transplantation, particularly in regard to heart transplantation, the transplantation sometimes proceeds simultaneously with carrying out the crossmatch. However, in a patient with a high PRA the transplantation should never be done unless the crossmatch is negative.

Traditionally, when crossmatching was done, each serum specimen, collected monthly from each recipient, was tested. Any specimen showing a positive reaction to donor lymphocytes would indicate that the recipient should not receive that particular organ. The reason for this was that even though reaction of a recent specimen may have been negative, the patient's immune system had been primed at some point in the past to respond to donor antigens. This would lead to rapid rejection of the transplant.

This policy was subsequently modified so that only sera showing a positive response in the PRA test would be tested, and any positive reaction against donor lymphocytes was a contraindication to transplantation. More recently, it has been found, primarily by using cyclosporine immunosuppression, that the transplantation can be done if reaction of the serum specimen obtained just prior to transplantation is negative, regardless whether prior sera specimens may have had antibody reactive to donor lymphocytes. This may reflect that cyclosporine is capable of suppressing the memory phases of the immune response.

**HLA Matching.** The HLA system can be divided into class I and class II antigens. The class I antigens are at the A and B loci on chromosome 6. The class II antigens are located at the HLA-DR locus. All individuals have four class I antigens and two class II antigens. It is well established that the histocompatibility antigens are targets for the immune system to react against and produce tissue rejection. Thus, matching of histocompatibility antigens between donor and recipient should reduce the intensity of the rejection response.

In kidney transplantation using living related donors, there is a correlation between the matching of histocompatibility antigens and graft survival. Thus, transplanting between siblings who share the same HLA antigens produces approximately 90 per cent graft survival after one year. This drops with mismatching for one of the two shared chromosomes and drops further for mismatching of both of the histocompatibility chromosomes.

When kidney transplantation is performed using a cadaver donor, there is a correlation between the number of HLA-A and -B antigens matched and graft survival. However, the number of HLA-DR antigens matched has a greater impact on survival. Thus, matching for two HLA-DR antigens produces significantly greater one- and two-year survival than matching for either one or no HLA-DR antigen. This is particularly true when azathioprine is used as the immunosuppressive agent.

When cyclosporine is used to provide immunological suppression, the benefit of matching for HLA-DR antigens is not as clear as when azathioprine is used. The ben-

efit, if indeed there is one with cyclosporine immunological suppression, is less than with azathioprine. Some data indicate that regardless of the number of HLA-DR antigens matched, graft survival is not affected with cyclosporine. Thus, 90 per cent one-year graft survival can be achieved without matching for HLA antigens. Continuous data collection is needed for better resolution of this point. However, if it can be shown that matching for antigens provides a minor benefit with cyclosporine and potentially newer immunosuppressive agents, then careful consideration will have to be given to the necessity of HLA matching.

It is unlikely that the histocompatibility antigens are the only antigens involved with graft rejection. In this regard each organ has antigens that are unique to it. Thus there are kidney-specific, heart-specific, and liver-specific antigens. Such antigens may have genetic differences between individuals and therefore could be factors in immunological rejection. There has been some initial work in this regard in kidney transplantation and more is needed.

Inadequate information is available in regard to the effect of matching on liver and heart transplants. Preliminary data compiled at the University of Pittsburgh indicate that liver transplantation is not affected by the number of HLA-DR antigens matched when cyclosporine is used as the immunosuppressant agent. Similarly, matching for 0, 1, or 2 HLA-DR antigens in heart transplantation has not had an effect on graft survival. The use of cyclosporine has improved many aspects of kidney transplant graft survival (Table 1–3).

**TABLE 1–3. Comparison of Cyclosporine (CSA) and Conventional Immunosuppression (CI) on Kidney Transplantation One-Year Graft Survival**

| | CSA (%) | CI (%) |
|---|---|---|
| First cadaver transplant | 73 | 62 |
| 1–4 Transfusions | 74 | 61 |
| Percent panel reactive antibody | | |
| <10% | 75 | 65 |
| >50% | 69 | 52 |
| 0 HLA mismatches | 87 | 80 |
| 6 HLA mismatches | 69 | 53 |

## PRETRANSPLANTATION BLOOD TRANSFUSION

In the initial phases of development of transplantation programs, transfusion of blood to a recipient prior to transplantation was contraindicated. Many patients who received transfusion had rapid rejection following kidney transplantation. This may have been due to the use of insensitive crossmatch procedures that did not pick up low levels of antibody produced in response to blood transfusion. Such antibody develops because of lymphocytes or lymphocyte fragments in blood used for transfusion. The individuals who have the genetic capability of responding to histocompatibility antigens can have an immune response to histocompatibility antigens on lymphocytes in the transfused blood products.

However, careful analysis of survival data in patients who had received transfusions indicates that there may be a beneficial effect of transfusion. Indeed, it is now well established that pretransplantation blood transfusion, either with random blood or donor-specific blood, may actually enhance graft survival. The reasons for this are many and not fully understood.

An individual who has the genetic capability of responding to histocompatibility antigens will do so when receiving blood transfusion. Those individuals would be detected by the crossmatch procedure and would not be candidates for receiving a particular donor organ. Thus, transfusion of blood may select out individuals with the genetic capability of responding to histocompatibility antigens, leaving those individuals to receive a transplant who would not respond well. This in itself may lead to enhancement of graft survival.

Transfusion of blood may impair immunological responsiveness by saturating the reticuloendothelial system with particulate matter in the form of degraded red and white blood cells. Such reticuloendothelial blockade may impair the immune system.

It has been shown that following transfusion suppressor lymphocytes develop for histocompatibility antigens in the transfused blood product. Such individuals may have enhancement of graft survival because of the effect of suppressor lymphocytes.

In some transplantation programs blood is specifically transfused prior to transplantation. In others blood is not transfused because of the concern of sensitizing recipients to transplant antigens. There is increased difficulty in finding a suitable donor for a sensitized recipient.

The beneficial effect of transfusion with azathioprine immunological suppression is clearer than with the use of cyclosporine. However, recent data indicate that there is a beneficial effect from using pretransplant blood transfusion with cyclosporine immunological suppression.

## POST-TRANSPLANTATION IMMUNOLOGICAL MONITORING

Ideally the immune system could be monitored to predict when a rejection episode is occurring. Thus, immunological reactivity to either transplant antigens or tissue antigens could be assayed by looking at the functional activity of peripheral blood lymphocytes to these antigens. In this way a noninvasive means of monitoring rejection could be provided.

The primary attempt at immunological monitoring has related to quantitation of the T helper and T suppressor cells in the peripheral blood. An increase in the number of T helper cells in the peripheral blood may indicate that the immune system is being activated to a foreign antigen. There have been reports that this does provide a useful means of monitoring rejection. However, there are many other reports that do not support this. Thus, immunological monitoring of T lymphocyte populations in the peripheral blood has not provided a reliable means of monitoring rejection episodes.

Immunological reactivity to donor-specific antigens may provide a means of determining rejection. When a rejection episode is occurring there would be increased reactivity to antigens on donor tissue. However, although such assays may provide an indication of rejection, they take three to five days to perform and therefore are not clinically useful.

In heart transplantation, sequential monitoring for the appearance of large lymphoblastoid cells in the peripheral blood may provide an indication of an impending rejection phenomenon. This has to be coupled with simultaneous monitoring of the helper-suppressor ratio. If large blast cells are present in the peripheral blood and the helper-suppressor ratio is increased, a rejection episode may be occurring. The appearance of large blast cells in the peripheral blood with a reversal of the helper-suppressor ratio usually indicates that a viral infection is present.

Although there is extensive investigative work being done to determine if rejection phenomena can be monitored by a noninvasive immunological procedure, the most reliable method of determining rejection still remains the biopsy. In the biopsy, the ratio of helper to suppressor T lymphocytes can be determined. However, there is no consistent pattern associated with rejection. Classic histological criteria are still needed to determine rejection.

## SUMMARY AND CONCLUSIONS

Transplantation of human organs presents the recipient with antigens that are looked upon as foreign by the immune system. Such antigens stimulate an immune response directed to them. The immune response is capable of bringing about rejection of the transplanted tissue. The exact mechanism of this rejection is unknown, but it probably involves T lymphocytes, either through a delayed hypersensitivity mechanism or direct cytotoxicity. The histocompatibility antigens are the primary target of rejection although tissue-specific antigens may also be targets of rejection.

Further study of the rejection phenomenon will lead to increased understanding of the nature of the antigens responsible for stimulating the immune response that brings about rejection and for the development of means to control the immune response and inhibit it. This should lead to decreased morbidity in association with tissue transplantation. In the future, many of the negative sequelae of chronic immunosuppressive therapy may be alleviated as better means are developed of matching tissue between recipients and donors and of immunological suppression of the immune system.

## REFERENCES

### Antibody-Mediated Rejection

Cerilli J, Brasile L, Galouzis T, Lempert N, Clarke J: The vascular endothelial cell antigen system. Transplantation 39:286, 1985.

Nunez G, McPhaul JJ Jr, Stastny P: Characterization of B cell antibodies in kidney transplant recipients. Transplantation 35:446, 1983.

Paul LC, van Es LA, van Rood JJ, van Leeuwen A, de la Riviere GB, de Graeff J: Antibodies directed against antigens on the endothelium of peritubular capillaries in patients with rejecting renal allografts. Transplantation 27:175, 1979

### Cellular Rejection

Ascher NL, Hoffman R, Hanto DW, Simmons RL: Cellular events within the rejecting allograft. Transplantation 35:193, 1983.

Bradley JA, Mason DW, Morris PJ: Evidence that rat renal allografts are rejected by cytotoxic T cells and not by nonspecific effectors. Transplantation 39:169, 1985.

Hall BM, Bishop GA, Farnsworth AF, Duggin GG, Horvath JS, Sheil AGR, Tiller DJ: Identification of the cellular subpopulations infiltrating rejecting cadaver renal allografts. Transplantation 37:564, 1984.

Hayry P: Intragraft events in allograft destruction. Transplantation 38:1, 1984.

Loveland BE, McKenzie IFC: Which T cells cause graft rejection? Transplantation 33:217, 1982.

### Crossmatch

D'Apice AJF, Tait BD: Improved survival and function of renal transplants with positive B cell crossmatches. Transplantation 27:324, 1979.

Delmonico FL, Fuller A, Cosimi AB, Tolkoff-Rubin N, Russell PS, Rodey GE, Fuller TC: New approaches to donor crossmatching and successful transplantation of highly sensitized patients. Transplantation 36:629, 1983.

Jeannet M, Benzonana G, Arni I: Donor-specific B and T lymphocyte antibodies and kidney graft survival. Transplantation 31:160, 1981.

Klouda PT, Jeannet M: Cold and warm antibodies and graft survival in kidney allograft recipients. Lancet 1:876, 1976.

Sanfilippo F, Vaughn WK, Spees EK, Bollinger RR: Cadaver renal transplantation ignoring peak-reactive sera in patients with markedly decreasing pretransplant sensitization. Transplantation 38:119, 1984.

Ting A: The lymphocytotoxic crossmatch test in clinical renal transplantation. Transplantation 35:403, 1983.

### HLA Matching

Busson M, Raffoux C, Bouteiller AM, Betuel H, Cambom-Thomsen A, Fizet D, Fauchet R, Mercier P, Seignalet J, Bignon JD, Hors J: Influence of HLA-A, B and DR matching on the outcome of kidney transplant survival in preimmunized patients. Transplantation 38:227, 1984.

Goeken NE, Thompson JS, Corry RJ: A 2-year trial of prospective HLA-DR matching. Transplantation 32:522, 1981.

Moen T, Albrechtsen D, Flatmark A, Jakobsen A, Jervell J, Halvorsen S, Solheim BG, Thorsby E: Importance of HLA-DR matching in cadaveric renal transplantation. N Engl J Med 303:850, 1980.

Sanfilippo F, Vaughn WK, Spees EK, Heise ER, LeFor WM: The effect of HLA-A, -B matching on cadaver renal allograft rejection comparing public and private specificities. Transplantation 38:483, 1984.

Sanfilippo F, Vaughn WK, Spees EK, Light JA, LeFor WM: Benefits of HLA-A and HLA-B matching on graft and patient outcome after cadaveric-donor renal transplantation. N Engl J Med 311:358, 1984.

Taylor RJ, Andrews W, Rosenthal JT, Carpenter B, Hakala TR: Influence of DR matching in cadaveric renal transplants performed with cyclosporine. Transplantation 38:616, 1984.

### Effect of Transfusion

Flechner SM, Kerman RH, Van Buren C, Kahan BD: Successful transplantation of cyclosporine-treated haploidentical living-related renal recipients without blood transfusions. Transplantation 37:73, 1984.

Sanfilippo F, Spees EK, Vaughn WK: The timing of pretransplant transfusions and renal allograft survival. Transplantation 37:344, 1984.

Sanfilippo F, Vaughn WK, Bollinger RR, Spees EK: The influence of pretransplant transfusions, using different blood products, on patient sensitization and renal allograft survival. Transplantation 37:350, 1984.

Smith MD, Williams JD, Coles GA, Salaman JR: Blood transfusions, suppressor T cells, and renal transplant survival. Transplantation 36:647, 1983.

### Post-Transplantation Monitoring

Chatenoud L, Chkoff N, Kreis H, Bach JF: Interest in and limitations of monoclonal anti-T-cell antibodies for the follow-up of renal transplant patients. Transplantation 36:45, 1983.

Cosimi AB, Colvin RB, Burton RC, Rubin RH, Goldstein G, Kung PC, Hansen WP, Delmonico FL, Russell PS: Use of monoclonal antibodies to T-cell subsets for immunologic monitoring and treatment in recipients of renal allografts. N Engl J Med 6:308, 1981.

Severyn W, Flaa C, Fuller L, Kyriakides GK, Esquenazi V, Miller J: The role of immunological monitoring in transplantation. Heart Transplantation 1:222, 1982.

Van Es A, Tanke HG, Baldwin WM, Oljans PJ, Ploem JS, Vanes LA: Ratios of T lymphocytes subpopulations predict survival of cadaveric renal allografts in adult patients on low dose corticosteroid therapy. Clin Exp Immunol 52:13, 1983.

# 2

# Brain Death and Ethics of Organ Transplantation

ROBERT D. MCKAY
PAM DUNCAN VARNER

The initial experience with kidney transplants was with living related donors. The combination of a dramatic increase in the number of potential kidney transplant recipients and advances in surgical technique and immunosuppressive therapy led to kidney transplants from cadavers outnumbering kidney transplants from living related donors. Pioneering efforts were also made to transplant organs that could come only from a cadaver, such as heart, liver, and heart-lung. The function of organs of a cadaver receiving ventilatory support and having a stable circulatory system was far superior to the function of organs removed after blood circulation ceased. The question arises whether someone with adequate cardiovascular function can be pronounced legally dead.

The concept of brain death is an issue of paramount importance in the identification of potential organ donors that raises moral and legal questions that have no easy answers. The diagnosis of death has traditionally been made by the observation of the cessation of respiratory and cardiac activity. However, it

became apparent that despite respiratory arrest resulting from immersion in water, strangulation, or mechanical airway obstruction, recovery was possible as long as the heart continued to beat. The heart then was viewed as the organ essential to life; when the heart no longer functioned, death ensued. Twentieth-century advances in cardiac resuscitation, coupled with the capabilities of modern mechanical ventilators, can often restore and/or support cardiorespiratory function so that the heart beats, oxygenation is provided, and carbon dioxide is eliminated.

The brain, however, is more sensitive to anoxia than the heart and is not as easily resuscitated. Also, the brain can be severely injured by events such as motor vehicle accidents, gunshot wounds, or cerebrovascular accidents that cause neurological catastrophe but minimal damage to the rest of the body. Thus the question, Is someone with a nonfunctioning brain but a beating heart actually dead?

Through the ages it has been feared that death would be prematurely diagnosed and

13

the "deceased" would awaken. There are many reports of exhumations that indicated persons were buried alive.[1] At times precautions were taken either to detect the awakening, if it took place, or to "do something" to the victim to assure that awakening would not take place. Examples of the latter included embalming or the piercing of vital organs, such as thrusting a spear into crucifixion victims. Examples of the former ranged from tying bells to the cadaver that would ring if moved, to an ingenious device patented by Count Karmice-Karmicki in 1897,[1] which upon movement of the chest of the body would trigger a chain of events, resulting in air and light entering the coffin, the raising of a signal flag, and the ringing of a bell. Despite more modern methods of diagnosing death, errors are still being made in the 1980's.[2,3] These errors are most often made in a mass casualty situation, such as war or natural disaster, or when hypothermia or drug intoxication is present, the latter conditions being associated with reductions in cerebral oxygen requirement, prolonging the time that critical levels of blood flow can be tolerated. J. B. Winslow in 1742 stated that "the only satisfactory proof of death is putrefaction."[4] On the other hand, P. R. Medawar concluded in 1957 that a person is legally dead "when he had undergone irreversible changes of a type that made it impossible for him to seek to litigate."[5]

A question arises whether death is a process or an event. Evidence for death as a process includes the series of degenerative and destructive changes such as necrosis of cells, cooling, rigor mortis, dependent lividity, and putrefaction. This series of changes usually begins after the failure of spontaneous ventilation and circulation; it may, however, begin prior to the irreversible cessation of cardiorespiratory function.

A definition of death as an event that occurs at a more or less definite time appears to be preferable to considering death as a process.[6] Under this definition, toward the end of life, the process of dying starts and culminates in death as an event, which is then followed by the process of putrefaction and other postmortem changes. The death of an organism that was a human being must not be confused with the loss of the organism's ability to act like a human being. This latter affliction, unfortunately not uncommon, can be called a vegetative state or neocortical death. Even though it is difficult to treat patients with this condition as if they were alive, declaring them dead could lead to even more difficulties. Who decides exactly how much neurological deficit must be present to declare them dead? What is then to be done with them? Since these patients may have spontaneous respiration and heart beat, it would be difficult simply to bury them or remove vital organs. Certainly most of us would like our bodies to die if we cease to be alive humans,[7,8] but the definition of death (for ethical and legal reasons) must remain distinct and separate from the loss of the ability to act as a human being, particularly if organ donation is considered.

Brain death then is the total and irreversible loss of whole brain functioning. The brain stem is included in this definition; therefore, there will be no spontaneous respiration, and severe cardiovascular instability will eventually develop. Patients with total and irreversible loss of whole brain functioning, even with aggressive cardiorespiratory support and meticulous attention to the details of their management, will suffer untreatable cardiac arrest—adults within one week and children within two weeks.[9] Autolysis of the brain (so-called respirator brain) provides proof that the brain is dead.

Once brain death is diagnosed, one approach is to continue all aggressive measures, knowing the cardiovascular system will fail within two weeks. This approach will enormously inflate medical expenses, dehumanize the victim, provide much anguish to the family, and possibly deprive other patients of the benefits of intensive care. Such an approach is also frustrating and stressful for physicians and nursing staff.

Another approach is to pronounce patients dead when the criteria of total and irreversible loss of brain function are met. Life support can then be discontinued and cardiac arrest will develop shortly thereafter. This approach conserves hospital and economic resources, but results in loss of organs suitable for transplantation.

A third approach is to provide life support to a patient with total and irreversible loss of brain function and to approach the family in an appropriate fashion about organ donation if the victim had not previously given permission for organs to be transplanted. If organ donation is permitted, the victim can be pronounced dead, and life support can be withdrawn after the organs have been removed.

## THEOLOGICAL CONSIDERATIONS

Theological considerations of death have also centered on the cessation of breathing and pulse. In the story of the creation in rabbinical literature, "God breathed life into the nostrils of man." However, rabbinical literature also recognizes that the movements of a body following decapitation are not a sign of life but represent agonal throes. Therefore, if the total and irreversible loss of whole brain function can be construed as a form of a physiological decapitation, Judaism can accept the concept of brain death as synonymous with death of the organism.[1]

Catholicism also has dealt with the difficulty of defining death when cardiorespiratory function is controlled by machines. Pope Pius XII, in addressing a congress of anesthesiologists in 1957, stated that it was not necessary to use extraordinary means to support vital functions when the case is hopeless.[10] Protestant theologians have not taken a consistent stand on the concept of brain death, but individual authors have accepted a similar concept.[1]

## LEGAL CONSIDERATIONS

The legal problem of determination of brain death first arose in criminal law: Did the assault victim die from the assault or when the respirator was turned off? Other legal questions arose later regarding insurance coverage, death benefits, and inheritance disputes. Several model bills have been drafted to help individual state legislatures cope with the concept of brain death. One of the first of these brain death statutes was enacted in Kansas; it provided alternative definitions of death. According to this bill, a person is considered dead if, in the opinion of a physician, based on ordinary standards of medical practice, there is absence of function of the heart *or* the brain, provided that various qualifying criteria have been met. Some states have based statutes on this model.[1] Capron and Kass, as well as others, have criticized this dual definition because of the implication that there were two concepts of death and the physician might choose the criterion arbitrarily. They proposed the following: "A person will be considered dead if, in the announced opinion of a physician, based on ordinary standards of medical practice, he has experienced an irreversible cessation of spontaneous respiratory and circulatory

functions. In the event that artificial means of support preclude a determination that these functions have ceased, a person will be considered dead if, in the announced opinion of a physician, based on ordinary standards of medical practice, he has experienced an irreversible cessation of spontaneous brain function. Death will have occurred at the time when the relevant functions ceased."[11] Some states have based their laws on this definition. The American Bar Association has this definition of death: "For all legal purposes, a human body with irreversible cessation of total brain function, according to the usual and customary standards of medical practice, shall be considered dead."[12]

The National Conference of Commissioners on Uniform State Laws drafted the following statement: "For legal and medical purposes, an individual who has sustained cessation of all functions of the brain, including the brain stem, is dead. A determination of death under this section must be made in accordance with reasonable medical standards." Although this definition does not include cessation of cardiorespiratory function it is understood that a patient who has irreversible cessation of cardiorespiratory function will quickly suffer irreversible loss of whole brain function.

The American Medical Association House of Delegates approved a comprehensive statement for determining death in all situations: "An individual who has sustained either: (1) irreversible cessation of circulatory and respiratory functions, or (2) irreversible cessation of all functions of the entire brain, shall be considered dead. A determination of death shall be made in accordance with accepted medical standards."[13]

One of the first subjects undertaken by the President's Commission for the Study of Ethical Problems in Medicine and Biomedical and Behavioral Research was to establish a definition of death. Representatives from the American Bar Association, the American Medical Association, and the National Conference of Commissioners on Uniform State Laws assisted the President's Commission. The product of their work was the Uniform Determination of Death Act, which is: "An individual who has sustained either: (1) irreversible cessation of circulatory and respiratory functions, or (2) irreversible cessation of all functions of the entire brain, including the brain stem, is dead. A determination of death must be made in accordance with accepted medical standards."[14] This definition is quite similar to that proposed by the American Medical Association; both suffer the same criticisms as the earlier Kansas bill: Two standards of death are listed. In addition, it is difficult, if not impossible, to test all functions of the brain to prove each function had ceased. In actuality, these criticisms have not deterred many states from enacting statutes similar in wording; approximately 40 states have passed laws formally stating that "brain death is death."[15] There have been some fears expressed that such laws may facilitate the introduction of new laws allowing euthanasia.

## MEDICAL CRITERIA FOR BRAIN DEATH

How can the patient with total and irreversible loss of brain function be identified? Mollaret et al., in 1959, described a clinical state characterized by the permanent absence of all neurological responsivity, including respiration but with the preservation of cardiac action; they coined the term *coma depasse*, which means literally "a state beyond coma."[16] In 1968, a report prepared by the *ad hoc* committee of the Harvard Medical School to examine the definition of brain death was published. The report of this committee, chaired by anesthesiologist H. K. Beecher, dealt with the characteristics of irreversible coma.[17] Since then, many others have published their own criteria for brain death, and many institutions have prepared guidelines on brain death for their own use.

### Cause

Perhaps the most crucial criterion for brain death is that the cause of the coma *must* be known, and the patient's physician must be convinced that it is irreversible. If the cause of the coma is unknown, it is difficult to conclude whether it is irreversible or not, since several conditions such as drug intoxication and hypothermia can produce reversible clinical and electroencephalographic signs of brain death.

### Cerebral Unresponsivity

Early diagnosis of brain death required total unresponsiveness to all stimuli, that is, no reflex response at all. However, it became apparent that spinal reflex activity to noxious stimuli can persist from hours to days after all other criteria for brain death are met.[18-20] These spinal reflexes include tendon stretch reflexes and ciliospinal reflex, which can produce eye opening, mediated through the stellate ganglion. Unusual spontaneous movements of the extremities (called Lazarus' sign) have also been described in brain-dead patients, especially upon discontinuation of the ventilator for apnea testing.[21] Perhaps the best way to test cerebral responsiveness without eliciting spinal reflexes is hard rubbing of the supraorbital nerves. Another way is to press the side of a pencil on the fingernail.[22] The stimulation should not leave marks, but must be intense enough to elicit a response to pain.

### Brain Stem Function

Clinical tests examining brain stem function are most useful for diagnosis of brain death.

The Harvard criteria require the pupils to be dilated and unresponsive. Other experts agree with the importance of nonreaction of the pupils to light, but many will accept midposition or even small pupils as long as they are fixed.[1,18] Care must be taken to use a bright light and to ensure that mydriatic agents such as atropine have not been used. Pre-existing ocular or neurological disease, as well as local ocular or nerve damage, may also cause nonreaction of the pupil and therefore must be ruled out.

Testing **corneal reflexes** in patients who are suspected to be brain-dead requires much firmer pressure than is needed for awake patients.[23] Edema or drying of the cornea may attenuate the response.[1]

The **oculocephalic reflex**, also known as doll's eye response, is tested by briskly turning the head to one side for three to four seconds and then 180 degrees to the other side. In a comatose state with intact brain stem, the eyes continually deviate to the opposite side for one to two seconds and then realign with the head. In brain stem death, the eyes remain in the plane of the head. This test requires brisk movement and therefore should not be done in cases of suspected cervical spine injury.

The **oculovestibular reflex** requires patent external auditory foramina and intact tympanic membranes. The head is elevated 30 degrees to the horizontal line, and then at least 10 ml (but not more than 50 ml) of ice water are slowly injected into the ear canal adjacent to the tympanic membrane. The normal response is movement of both eyes toward the side of the ice water injection. In brain stem death there will be no ocular movements. Any ocular movement implies some retained brain stem function. If the tympanic membrane is perforated and the brain stem is intact, the test may elicit bradycardia and hypotension. Pre-existing disease may influence this test.[23]

**Gag and cough reflexes** are tested by introducing suction catheters into the pharynx and trachea. The latter location ordinarily stimulates more response than the former. The use of sedatives, narcotics, muscle relaxants, or topical local anesthetics attenuates the reflexes.

**Apnea testing** should be done carefully to avoid the development of hypoxemia and undesirable hypercarbia and acidosis. The initial approach was to increase the inspired oxygen concentration to 100 per cent for 10 to 60 minutes, disconnect the ventilator, deliver oxygen at 2 to 6 L·min$^{-1}$ via a cannula into the endotracheal tube (this maneuver usually provides $Pa_{O_2}$ greater than 100 mm Hg), and wait 10 to 20 minutes.[24] Arterial blood gases should be obtained at baseline and intermittently during the test. It was felt that the $Pa_{CO_2}$ should exceed 60 mm Hg for the apnea test to be valid.[18] $Pa_{CO_2}$ increases normally during apnea by 3 mm Hg·min$^{-1}$, but the rate of increase is slower in brain-dead patients. If dysrhythmias develop, an arterial blood sample should be drawn for pH and gas tension determinations and ventilation resumed. Recently Ropper et al. reported that preoxygenation is not necessary and that the $Pa_{CO_2}$ has to rise to only 50 mm Hg.[25] The required time for apnea to produce this level of $Pa_{CO_2}$ depends not only on the rate of rise but also on the starting levels of $Pa_{CO_2}$. Patients with suspected increases in intracranial pressure are frequently treated with hyperventilation at a $Pa_{O_2}$ of 25 to 30 mm Hg. Apnea testing in such cases should be done only if other signs of brain death are present, because increases in $Pa_{O_2}$ may be hazardous to viable brain. Of course, this test should not be performed in patients who have pharmacologically induced neuromuscular blockade or respiratory depression. Another potential problem with this test is that patients with chronic lung disease may have respiratory response only to hypoxemia, not to hypercarbia. Thus, apnea testing may be difficult.[22]

Other brain stem tests that are less useful include blood pressure control, heart rate, temperature control, and reflexes such as audio-ocular reflex, snout reflex, and jaw jerk.[1]

Clinical testing for brain death usually consists of two separate examinations. The optimal time interval between examinations has been the subject of much discussion. The longer the time interval, the more assurance the condition is irreversible. However, the longer the interval, the more likely the patient will suffer cardiac arrest during the interval. It is unrealistic to expect a single time interval to be appropriate for all cases. Therefore the time interval is determined by the cause of the brain injury and the judgment of the physician. A patient with complete, visible destruction of the brain may need only one examination. For most patients with a gunshot wound to the head, cerebrovascular accident, or severe closed head injury, the evaluation phase of an irreversible lesion may take at least six hours, and this is the minimum time between examinations.[26] Patients who may be or are definitely intoxicated require longer intervals. Patients who have suffered anoxic brain injury from cardiac arrest or drowning may need observation for 24 hours.[14] Each patient and clinical situation is unique and should be managed accordingly.[27]

In some cases it is desirable or necessary to have a test to confirm brain death. Such tests may involve observations of brain electrical activity, brain blood flow, or neuropathological changes.

**Electroencephalography** is helpful in diagnosing brain death because it provides objective, verifiable hard-copy support to clinical assessments. This objectivity and ability to store the record are especially useful when organ donation is considered. As long as the patient is not hypothermic and is not under the influence of central nervous system depressants, properly done electroencephalography that demonstrates electrocerebral silence for a period of 6 to 12 hours indicates that no recovery of cerebral function is possible and the cerebral cortex is already dead. The EEG will not rule out the possibility of brain stem function and therefore must be correlated with the clinical examination to diagnose total and irreversible loss of whole brain functioning. The EEG is usually obtained in the intensive care unit where the potential organ donor is treated. The intensive care unit environment may have serious electrical interference. An EEG technician experienced at recognizing interferences and artifacts is needed. Also, an EEG that is obtained to support the diagnosis of brain death requires different techniques from the usual diagnostic recording; the technician must be aware that the EEG is requested for diagnosis of brain death. The American EEG Society has developed guidelines for obtaining satisfactory recordings in unshielded areas (Table 2–1). The recommended interelectrode distances of 10 cm are approximately twice the distances in the standard international ten twenty system of electrode placement. Methods of manipulation to test the integrity of the system include inserting ECG into the record, introducing 60-cycle interference, or simply jiggling the wires. Sometimes the recording may be obscured by high amplitude electromyographic potentials from the scalp or neck muscles; eliminating these potentials may require the use of muscle relaxants.[1]

Electrocerebral silence (ECS) does not imply that the cerebral cortex is not generating electrical activity; rather, this activity cannot be distinguished from the background noise of the EEG machine when the calibration is adjusted at 2.0 mV·mm$^{-1}$ or less.

The EEG is not infallible, especially in an-oxic brain injury. Some of these patients may lead a vegetative existence despite an isoelectric EEG early after the insult.[28] This is due to the survival and continued function of the brain stem. Silverman and associates published a survey of 2650 patients with isoelectric EEG's of up to 24 hours' duration; only three patients regained cerebral function. All three had taken large quantities of central nervous system depressant drugs. In some other cases, the diagnosis of ECS could not be supported even though the EEG's were isoelectric, because the techniques were faulty.[29]

The recording of *evoked potentials* may have possible advantages over the usual EEG because evoked potentials may be recorded even during deep levels of drug-induced central nervous system depression. Of the three types of evoked potentials, visual evoked potential, somatosensory evoked potential, and auditory evoked potential, only the last two show promise in the diagnosis of brain death. Somatosensory evoked potential recording in patients with a dead brain will induce only potentials that arise from the cervical spinal cord and dorsal column nuclei. Since somatosensory evoked potentials provide an indication that the impulses are reaching the central nervous system, they may have particular value in the determination of brain death. The absence of somatosensory evoked potential usually precedes other criteria of brain death; their persistence in comatose patients may indicate potential recovery.[30] Auditory evoked potentials have been of considerable value in differentiating coma due to metabolic or toxic causes from coma due to organic brain stem lesions. Wave I of the auditory evoked potential is believed to be derived from eighth nerve potential; therefore its absence is not an absolute indication of brain death. This wave could be absent as a result of trauma or vascular insufficiency to the peripheral auditory structures. When wave I is present, it indicates delivery of the impulse to the central nervous system.[31,32]

Further studies are required to establish the role of evoked potential recording in the diagnosis of brain death.[33]

The absence of **cerebral blood flow** conclusively confirms the diagnosis of brain death. The brain is very intolerant of complete global interruption of its blood supply. There are two potential methods that can lead to cessation of blood flow to the brain: (1) Intracranial pressure may tremendously in-

---

**TABLE 2–1. Guidelines of the American EEG Society for Using the EEG in the Diagnosis of Brain Death***

1. A minimum of eight scalp electrodes and ear reference electrodes
2. Interelectrode resistances under 10,000 ohms, but over 100 ohms
3. Test for integrity of the recording system by deliberate creation of electrode artifact by manipulation
4. Interelectrode distances of at least 10 cm
5. Gains changed during most of the recording from 7.0 mV·mm$^{-1}$ to 2.0 mV·mm$^{-1}$
6. The use of 0.3–0.4 second time constants during part of the recording
7. Recording of an ECG and of extracerebral potentials by a pair of electrodes on the dorsum of the right hand
8. Tests for reactivity to pain, loud noises, and light
9. A 30-minute total recording time

* Data obtained from Plum F, Posner JB: Diagnosis of Stupor and Coma, 3rd ed. Philadelphia, F. A. Davis Company, 1980.

crease and exceed the arterial pressure (this may happen in severe head injury or intracranial hemorrhage) and (2) there may be a progressive reduction in the cross-sectional area of vascular structures, which accompanies death of the brain.

Several methods of testing brain circulation have been evaluated to confirm the diagnosis of brain death. Conventional angiography can be done to examine both the carotid systems and the vertebral system either by selective catheterizations of the vessels or by an ascending aortic injection.[34] In brain death the internal carotid and vertebral arteries fill very slowly, with the dye tapering to a point at variable distances from the base of the skull.[35] Intravenous digital subtraction angiography has also been used to confirm the diagnosis of brain death.[36] Disadvantages of angiography include invasiveness (especially with arterial injections) and the need to transport the critically ill patient (receiving intensive pharmacological and ventilatory support) to and from the radiology suite. If the first attempt to visualize the cerebral circulation fails, methods to reduce intracranial pressure, such as drainage of cerebrospinal fluid via ventriculostomy, may enable repeat attempts of cerebral angiography to be successful.

Another method of studying cerebral circulation involves scanning over the brain for intravenously administered radioactive isotope.[37,38] Scanning is also done over the femoral artery to assure distribution of the indicator. This technique includes minimal invasiveness and can be performed at the bedside by employing portable cameras. The main disadvantage of this method is that scalp blood flow must be distinguished from intracranial blood flow; scalp blood flow is significantly increased with brain death. Another disadvantage is that blood flow to the brain stem often cannot be ruled out.

Other methods that have been applied in the diagnosis of brain death include ultrasound[39,40] and computed tomography with a contrast bolus injection technique.[41]

**Neuropathological studies** have also been proposed to confirm the diagnosis of brain death. Techniques include direct surgical inspection of the brain as well as brain biopsy with microscopic analysis of the tissue. These methods have been criticized as being too invasive and inefficient. The concept of whole brain death requires multiple biopsies of cerebrum as well as brain stem; it is doubt-ful that enough tissue could be obtained and examined ante mortem to conclude that the remaining unbiopsied areas are dead as well.[18] Sayer et al. examined the diagnostic significance of cytological study of nerve cells in cerebrospinal fluid in patients with clinical signs of brain death.[42] This method may demonstrate autolysis.

## Pediatric Considerations of Brain Death

The diagnosis of brain death in children under five years of age can be difficult, especially if the cause of the neurological injury is undetermined. The difficulty is due, in part, to the belief in high recuperative capabilities of the brain in children, especially neonates.[43] That neurological functions may be restored in infants and young children even after they exhibit unresponsiveness for longer periods than adults on neurological examination was reported by the medical consultants on the diagnosis of death to the President's Commission for the Study of Ethical Problems in Medicine and Biomedical and Behavioral Research.[14] The report recommended that physicians be particularly cautious in applying criteria to determine death in children younger than five years. Other requirements suggested for the diagnosis of brain death in this age group have included an interval of at least 24 hours between two clinical examinations, requiring two EEG's indicating brain death,[1] and absence of cerebral blood flow.[44] EEG cortical activity has been demonstrated, despite no measurable cerebral blood flow. The mechanism for this finding is postulated to be extracranial collateral flow supplying isolated small areas of cerebral cortex.[45]

## Relevant Homeostatic Disorders in Brain Death

As mentioned earlier, after total irreversible loss of whole brain function, untreatable cardiovascular failure develops within one week in adults and two weeks in children. Nishimura and Miyata measured cardiovascular parameters in 11 brain-dead patients.[46] They found marked reductions in cardiac output, systemic vascular resistance, and arterial blood pressure. Dysfunction of the left side of the heart was more pronounced than dysfunction of the right side; pulmonary vascular resistance was well maintained and persisted for a much longer period. Logigian and Ropper reported on terminal ECG changes in brain-dead patients following discontinuation of ventilation. They found gradual slowing of the atrial rate with development of atrioventricular block without ventricular escape rhythms. There were three terminal rhythms: (1) atrial activity only, (2) slow sinus or junctional bradycardia, and (3) ventricular tachycardia.[47]

Kolin and Norris studied the effect of intracranial lesions on postmortem myocardial damage. Those patients whose intracranial lesion produced a rapid increase in intracranial pressure were found to be significantly more likely to have transmural myocardial fiber damage. This damage required at least six hours to develop and was not observed after the second week, nor was it seen in victims of sudden death unrelated to intracranial lesions. The postulated mechanism is increased levels of plasma catecholamines secondary to rapidly increasing intracranial pressure.[48] This damage could be important if the victim is a potential donor for heart transplantation. Even though organ donor patients are brain-dead, hemodynamic responses such as tachycardia and hypertension may develop in response to organ(s) removal; these responses to surgical stimulation do not invalidate current criteria for the diagnosis of brain death.[49]

Another common finding in brain-dead patients is diabetes insipidus. Failure to treat the diabetes insipidus results in severe hypovolemia, hyperosmolarity, and hypernatremia. Treatment with fluid replacement alone may result in fluid shifts, interstitial and intracellular edema, and ultimately organ failure. Early administration of vasopressin improves donor management in an animal model.[50]

## ORGAN PROCUREMENT

With the development of immunosuppressive therapy, the demand for cadaveric organs for transplantation has outpaced the supply.[51] Each year approximately 20,000 people suffer brain death from trauma. Only 15 per cent of these patients will become organ donors. The remaining 85 per cent take with them to their final resting place 34,000 kidneys, 17,000 hearts, 17,000 livers, and 34,000 corneas. There are many reasons for this: Individuals fail to bequeath their organs before they die; family members refuse to give permission for organ donation; and physicians and/or hospital staff neglect to approach the family appropriately or at all about organ donation.[52,53]

Many programs have been proposed and in some cases implemented to overcome these difficulties. These programs provide general education, distribution of donor cards, and incorporation of donor permission cards with state drivers' licenses, as well as information aimed at doctors and nurses suggesting appropriate methods of approaching families of victims.[54] A recent survey concluded that the general public is quite supportive of organ transplantation but is not overly enthusiastic about organ donation.[55] Major religions favor donation, and one ethicist, Robert Leach, feels that the concept of donation should not only be supported, it should be considered a moral obligation.[56] There is a proposal for the United States to join with several European countries and enact presumed consent laws. Under this law, a person who does not want to donate organs if brain death should occur has the responsibility of making his or her wishes explicitly known; failure to do so provides presumed consent. Transplant surgeons could act on that presumption without fear of legal reprisals. Experts are divided as to the legality and ethics of such an approach under American law.[56]

The perception of the hospital staff is important in deciding whether or not to approach a victim's family as well as the probable success of such an approach. A survey has shown that while most intensive care unit nurses accept the validity of brain death and approve of organ donation, they find much stress and little reward in treatment of the potential donor.[57,58] Families of brain-dead patients are in a shock phase, with strong feelings of denial, anger, and guilt; they have difficulty accepting the diagnosis because the victim does not look dead. Those staff members experienced in dealing with this situation know when to stay with the family and work through their feelings with them and when to leave the family alone to contemplate in privacy. Clergy may also be very helpful in these times. Many approaches for organ donation have been successful because team members assured the family that other families that have consented to organ donation under similar circumstances were able to take solace in knowing that their loss provided life for someone else. Families who have agreed to organ donation report that after the acute grief they were greatly comforted by their decision.[59]

Ethical considerations for donation of organs for transplantation are not restricted to brain-dead donors. Schneider and Flaherty wrote an investigative reporting series in the *Pittsburgh Press* entitled "The Challenge of a Miracle: Selling the Gift." This series received widespread attention because of some of the practices uncovered by these reporters. They found that wealthy foreign patients were paying donors between $1,000 and $40,000 for one of their kidneys. The surgery was primarily done overseas, but in some cases the recipient and donor came to the United States where the donor indicated a blood relationship to the recipient. Some businessmen set up networks of tissue typing poor people and then connected them with wealthy people with renal failure with a good tissue match. In Japan a loan shark routinely offers debtors the prospect of paying off overdue loans with a kidney. In other countries prison inmates are led to believe that earlier consideration for parole will be given if they donate a kidney. The series also noted that some wealthy foreign patients have been advanced to the top of the lists of recipients, possibly because of their ability to pay well above the usual charges. In other cases, kidneys obtained from American brain-dead donors were exported from the country and sold, with eligible American recipients being bypassed. Kidneys being passed through airports were found repeatedly by dogs trained to sniff drugs.[60]

The Federal Task Force on organ transplantation has issued a statement urging the following: elimination of inappropriate advertising and soliciting of aliens into the United States to receive transplants; elimination of importation and exportation of organs, except when medically justifiable; and elimination of the brokerage for kidneys between living unrelated donors. In addition, aliens entering the United States in need of a kidney transplant should be added to the lists of other waiting recipients in order and their priority determined just like everyone else. Transplant centers should also report organ procurement procedures and transplantations to a national network; failure to do so could result in loss of Medicare payment.[61]

Careful attention must be paid to the ethics of organ donation to facilitate the progress of organ transplantation.

## REFERENCES

1. Walker AE: Cerebral Death, 3rd ed. Baltimore-Munich, Urban and Schwarzenberg, 1985, 206 pp.
2. "Timely Cough Saves Life." Albuquerque Tribune, Feb. 9, 1982.
3. "Woman Believed to Be Dead 'Resurrected' on Autopsy Table." Albuquerque Journal, April 19, 1983.
4. Winslow JB: Dissertation sur L'Incertitude des Signes de la Morte et L'Abus des Enternements et Embaumens Precipites. Paris, 1742.
5. Medawar PB: The Uniqueness of the Individual. New York, Basic Books, 1957, p 19.
6. Bernat JL, Culver CM, Gert B: On the definition and criterion of death. Ann Intern Med 94:389–394, 1981.
7. Youngner SJ, Bartlett ET: Human death and high technology: The failure of the whole-brain formulations. Ann Intern Med 99:252–258, 1983.
8. Veatch RM: The whole-brain-oriented concept of death: An outmoded philosophical formulation. J Thanatol 3:13–30, 1975.
9. Ingvar DH, Brun A, Johansson L, et al: Survival after severe cerebral anoxia with destruction of the cerebral cortex: The appallic syndrome. Ann NY Acad Sci 315:184–214, 1978.
10. Pope Pius XII: The Prolongation of Life (address of Pope Pius XII to an international congress of anesthesiologists). Pope Speaks 4:393–398, 1958. Acta Apostolicae Sedia 49:17, 1957.
11. Capron AM, Kass LR: A statuatory definition of the standards for determining human death: An appraisal and a proposal. Univ Penn Law Rev 121:87–118, 1972.
12. American Bar Association, Insurance, Negligence and Compensation Law Section: Euthanasia-Symposium Issue. 27 Baylor Law Rev 1:1–198, 1975.
13. American Medical Association, House of Delegates Report, 1979.
14. Guidelines for the Determination of Death: Report of the Medical Consultants on the Diagnosis of Death to the President's Commission for the Study of Ethical Problems in Medicine and Biomedical and Behavioral Research. JAMA 246:2184–2186, 1981.
15. Zisfein J: Brain Death in Perspective. Hosp Physician 22:11–16, 1986.
16. Mollaret P, Bertrand I, Mollaret H: Coma de passe et necroses nerveuses centrales massives. Rev Neurol 101:116–139, 1959.
17. A Definition of Irreversible Coma: Report of the Ad Hoc Committee of the Harvard Medical School to Examine the Definition of Brain Death. JAMA 205:337–340, 1968.
18. Plum F, Posner JB: Diagnosis of Stupor and Coma, 3rd ed. Philadelphia, F A Davis Company, 1980.
19. Pallis C: ABC of brain stem death: From brain death to brain stem death. Br Med J 285:1487–1490, 1982.
20. Ivan LP: Spinal reflexes in cerebral death. Neurology 23:650–652, 1973.
21. Ropper AH: Unusual spontaneous movements in brain dead patients. Neurology 34:1089–1092, 1984.
22. Pallis C: ABC of brain stem death: Diagnosis of

brain stem death—II. Br Med J 285:1641–1644, 1982.

23. Pallis C: ABC of brain stem death: Pitfalls and safeguards. Br Med J 285:1720–1722, 1982.

24. Milhaud A, Riboulot M, Gayet H: Disconnecting tests and oxygen uptake in the diagnosis of total brain death. Ann NY Acad Sci 315:241–251, 1978.

25. Ropper AH, Kennedy SK, Russell L: Apnea testing in the diagnosis of brain death. J Neurosurg 55:942–946, 1981.

26. Pallis C: ABC of brain stem death. Br Med J 285:1558–1560, 1982.

27. Crone RK: Brain death. Am J Dis Child 137:545–546, 1983.

28. Brierly JB, Adams JH, Graham DI, et al: Neocortical death after cardiac arrest. Lancet 2:560–565, 1971.

29. Silverman D, Masland RL, Saunders MG, et al: Irreversible coma associated with electrocerebral silence. Neurology 20:525–533, 1970.

30. de La Torre JC: Evaluation of brain death using somatosensory evoked potentials. Biol Psychiatry 16:931–935, 1981.

31. Goldie WD, Chiappa KH, Young RR, et al: Brain stem auditory and short-latency somatosensory evoked responses in brain death. Neurology 31:248–256, 1981.

32. Klug N: Brain stem auditory evoked potentials in syndromes of decerebration, the bulbar syndrome and in central death. J Neurol 227:219–228, 1982.

33. Pfurtscheller G, Schwarz G, List W: Brain death and bioelectrical brain activity. Intensive Care Med 11:149–153, 1985.

34. Riishede J, Ethelberg S: Angiographic changes in sudden and severe herniation of brain stem through tentorial incisure—Report of five cases. AMA Arch Neurol Psychiatry 70:399–409, 1953.

35. Hazratji SM, Singh BM, Strobos RJ: Angiography in brain death. NY State J Med 81:82–83, 1981.

36. Vatne K, Nakstad P, Lundart T: Digital subtraction angiography in the evaluation of brain death. Neuroradiology 27:155–157, 1985.

37. Schwartz JA, Baxter J, Brill D, et al: Radionuclide cerebral imaging confirming brain death. JAMA 249:246–247, 1983.

38. Goodman JM, Heck LL, Moore BD: Confirmation of brain death with portable isotope angiography: A review of 204 consecutive cases. Neurosurgery 16:492–497, 1985.

39. Furgiuele TL, Frank M, Riegle C, et al: Prediction of cerebral death by cranial sector scan. Crit Care Med 12:1–3, 1984.

40. Kreutzer EW, Rutherford RB, Lehman RAW: Diagnosis of brain death by common carotid artery velocity waveform analysis. Arch Neurol 39:136–139, 1982.

41. Arnold H, Kuhne D, Rohr W, et al: Contrast bolus technique with rapid CT scanning, a reliable diagnostic tool for the determination of brain death. Neuroradiology 22:129–132, 1981.

42. Sayer H, Wietholter H, Oehmichen M, et al: Diagnostic significance of nerve cells in human CSF with particular reference to CSF cytology in the brain death syndrome. J Neurol 225:109–117, 1981.

43. Bruce DA, Raphaely RC, Goldberg AI, et al: Pathophysiology, treatment and outcome following severe head injury in children. Childs Brain 5:174–191, 1979.

44. Ashwal S, Smith AJK, Torres F, et al: Radionuclide bolus angiography: A technique for verification of brain death in infants and children. J Pediatr 91:722–728, 1977.

45. Ashwal S, Schneider S: Failure of electroencephalography to diagnose brain death in comatose children. Ann Neurol 6:512–517, 1979.

46. Nishimura N, Miyata Y: Cardiovascular changes in the terminal stage of disease. Resuscitation 12:175–180, 1984.

47. Logigian EL, Ropper AH: Terminal electrocardiographic changes in brain dead patients. Neurology 35:915–918, 1985.

48. Kolin A, Norris JW: Myocardial damage from acute cerebral lesions. Stroke 15:990–993, 1984.

49. Wetzel RC, Setzer N, Stiff JL, et al: Hemodynamic responses in brain dead organ donor patients. Anesth Analg 64:125–128, 1985.

50. Blaine EM, Tallman RD, Frolicher D, et al: Vasopressin supplementation in a porcine model of brain dead organ donors. Transplantation 38:459–464, 1984.

51. Youngner SJ, Allen M, Bartlett ET, et al: Psychosocial and ethical implications of organ retrieval. N Engl J Med 313:321–324, 1985.

52. Caplan AL: Ethical and policy issues in the procurement of cadaver organs for transplantation. N Engl J Med 311:981–983, 1984.

53. Merz B: The organ procurement problem: Many causes, no easy solutions. JAMA 254:3285–3288, 1985.

54. Rosenberg JC, Krome RL, McDonald FD, et al: Identifying and managing the potential transplant donor in the emergency department. JACEP 4:328–332, 1975.

55. Manninen DL, Evans RW: Public attitudes and behavior regarding organ donation. JAMA 253:3111–3115, 1985.

56. Kolata G: Organ shortage clouds new transplant era. Science 221:32–33, 1983.

57. Sophie LR, Salloway JC, Sorock G, et al: Intensive care nurses' perceptions of cadaver organ procurement. Heart Lung 12:261–267, 1983.

58. Pinkus RL: Families, brain death, and traditional medical excellence. J Neurosurg 60:1192–1194, 1984.

59. Montefusco CM, Levine S, Goldsmith J, et al: Obtaining consent for organ donation. Hosp Physician 21:46–50, 1985.

60. Schneider A, Flaherty MP: "The Challenge of a Miracle, Selling the Gift." Reprinted from The Pittsburgh Press, 1985, 55 pp.

61. Krieger L: Overseas transplant market a concern for MDs. American Medical News, December 13, 1985, p 7.

# 3

# *Organ Preservation*

DALE A. PARKS
BRUCE A. FREEMAN

The ability to transplant organs and tissue provides alternative options for treatment of organ failure. Often the major factors in successful outcome of transplantation efforts are the availability of donor organs and viability of tissue once it is implanted in recipients. As more effective techniques of tissue and organ preservation are developed, better functional characteristics of donor organs following implantation will result. In this chapter we will discuss recent strategies for enhancing donor organ viability prior to and immediately following transplantation of heart, kidney, and liver. Preservation techniques are extremely important for these organs, because alternative long-term artificial methods of support for them do not exist, with the exception of the kidney whose function may often be circumvented by dialysis. Optimization of organ preservation conditions will promote life-sustaining organ functional characteristics after transplantation.

At present, the supply of organs for renal, hepatic, pancreatic, cardiac, and pulmonary transplantation is limited. Technical developments and improvements in immunosuppression are leading to increased frequency of transplantation, thereby increasing the need for donor organs. The development and implementation of techniques for multiple organ procurement can help meet the increasing need for cadaveric organs. Ischemic damage to donor organs can be minimized in one of two ways: Efforts can be made to maintain an acceptable blood supply during the entire harvesting period with *in situ* flushing of the procured organs.[1] Alternatively, total body hypothermia can be established for rapid *in vivo* multiple organ cooling prior to harvesting.[2] The rapid and consistent cooling of donor organs prior to procurement minimizes the period of warm ischemia (time between cardiac arrest and perfusion of the organ with cold solution) and the associated compromise of organ viability. When cardiovascular integrity is maintained and the period of warm ischemia minimized, a variety of combinations of donor organs can be removed. For multiple organ procurement the aorta is crossclamped at a level that will allow intra-aortic infusion of cold electrolyte solution into the organs to be removed. In the case of the liver the organ can be infused through both the aorta and portal vein. The kidneys are cooled by aortic infusion only. With minor modifications, the heart can also be removed.[3] This procurement technique requires "brain death" conditions and stable cardiovascular function. An alternative technique can be performed in donors who have had cardiac arrest. In the so-called fast method a crossclamp is placed on the aorta near the diaphragm and cold solutions rapidly infused.

## METABOLISM OF ORGANS TARGETED FOR TRANSPLANTATION

Often brain-dead organ donors have tissue viability maintained by ventilatory support. Cessation of organ blood flow upon removal for transplantation induces tissue hypoxia and ischemia. This leads to several pathological sequelae that ultimately result in loss of organ viability.

The major biological changes occurring during the first hour of tissue ischemia are summarized in Figure 3–1. Within 10 seconds, even after cooling and immersion of the isolated organ in transportation solutions, the tissue demand for oxygen exceeds the supply available, and thus intracellular oxygen tension decreases greatly. Simultaneously with the onset of hypoxia, energy metabolism converts from mitochondrial oxidative metabolism to anaerobic glycolysis.[4] The quantities of ATP generated by anaerobic glycolysis and creatine phosphate, maintained in equilibrium with ATP, are inadequate to maintain the energy charge within the ischemic tissue.

Alterations in ion homeostasis during tissue ischemia are significant and ultimately yield extracellular release of potassium and intracellular calcium overload.[5] There is decreased mitochondrial (and in heart, endoplasmic reticular) calcium uptake due to ATP depletion, loss of $Na^+,K^+$-ATPase activity, and uncoupling of calcium transport from $Na^+,K^+$-ATPase.[6] The lactic acidosis that occurs in ischemic tissue undergoing anaerobic glycolysis has also been implicated in inhibition of tissue $Na^+,K^+$-ATPase activity and ultimate loss of cation concentration gradients. Since maintenance of action potentials of excitable tissues and transmembrane transport of diverse macromolecules are dependent upon sodium gradients, inhibition of sodium and potassium transport will severely compromise cell and organ survival. $Ca^{2+}$-ATPases are also inhibited during ischemia. Calcium has a central role in regulation of numerous tissue metabolic processes. A number of observations have supported the concept that calcium channel blockers such as verapamil protect against ischemic tissue injury.[7]

Recent evidence from a variety of animal models suggests that ischemia leads to oxygen-derived free radical injury and accounts for at least part, if not most, of the damage that occurs following reperfusion of an is-

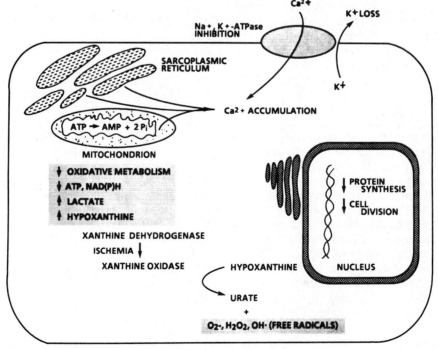

**Figure 3–1.** Major biologic changes occurring in the first hour of tissue ischemia in a cell.

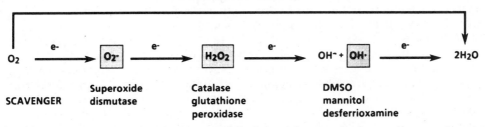

**Figure 3–2.** Univalent reduction of molecular oxygen, depicting defense mechanisms to bypass and prevent accumulation of reactive intermediates. DMSO-dimethylsulfoxide.

chemic region or organ. Free radicals are chemically reactive species that contain an odd number of electrons (Fig. 3–2). When a free radical reacts with a non-radical molecule, another free radical can be produced, which often yields toxic chain reactions thousands of events long. An example of this phenomenon would include lipid peroxidation, which leads to the release of lipid peroxides, free fatty acids, and prostaglandins observed after reperfusion of ischemic tissues.[8]

A recently described mechanism involving the conversion of tissue xanthine dehydrogenase to xanthine oxidase and accumulation of the ATP metabolite hypoxanthine is thought to be the major source of free radicals generated during reperfusion of ischemic tissue[3] (Fig. 3–1). Importantly, this mechanism is thought to be a significant factor in determining the ultimate viability of transplanted organs that have suffered temporary ischemia prior to implantation and reperfusion.[9]

Xanthine oxidase is widely distributed among tissues and appears to be in part concentrated in the vascular endothelium while present in other cell types as well. The enzyme is endogenously present as xanthine dehydrogenase, which, during its catalytic conversion of hypoxanthine to urate, reduces $NAD^+$:

$$\text{XANTHINE} \xrightarrow{\text{xanthine dehydrogenase}} \text{URATE}$$
$$NAD^+ \quad\quad NADH^+ \; H^+$$

After an ischemic phase, xanthine dehydrogenase is modified by sulfhydryl oxidation or limited proteolysis to yield the oxidase form of the enzyme. The oxidase reduces molecular oxygen rather than $NAD^+$, producing superoxide, hydrogen peroxide, and hydroxyl radical (see also Fig. 3–2):

$$\text{XANTHINE} \xrightarrow{\text{xanthine oxidase}} \text{URATE}$$
$$O_2 \quad\quad O_2{}^-, H_2O_2, OH\cdot$$

The conversion of xanthine dehydrogenase to oxidase occurs *in vivo* in ischemic tissues and has been described in heart,[10] intestine,[11] liver,[12] kidney,[13] and isolated skin flaps,[14] in addition to other organs and tissues.[9]

The conversion of xanthine dehydrogenase to oxidase has been most completely studied in liver, intestine, and heart. In these organs, loss of blood flow is responsible for ATP depletion and loss of calcium ion homeostasis as previously mentioned. In heart, sulfhydryl oxidation is the primary mechanism for formation of xanthine oxidase.[15] In other tissues, an elevated cytoplasmic calcium concentration is believed to activate a protease capable of converting xanthine dehydrogenase to xanthine oxidase.[16] Calcium activation of tissue proteases and ultimate generation of xanthine oxidase activity can be inhibited by calcium channel blockers and protease inhibitors.[11]

It is interesting to note that depletion of tissue ATP during ischemia results in hypoxanthine accumulation,[17] thereby providing a substrate pool for xanthine dehydrogenase or oxidase. Thus, during ischemia, xanthine oxidase activity can appear in concert with a required substrate. Upon reperfusion, molecular oxygen is supplied, which is the remaining substrate required for xanthine oxidase activity (Fig. 3–1, Equation 3–2).

Support for the concept that oxygen radicals are critical for loss of ischemic organ viability after reperfusion is extensive and includes the observation that the superoxide scavenger superoxide dismutase, the hydrogen peroxide scavengers catalase and glutathione peroxidase, the xanthine oxidase inhibitor allopurinol, and mannitol or dimethylsulfoxide, scavengers of hydroxyl radical, are all protective against ischemia-reperfusion damage.[18-20] These data are encouraging in that they suggest future pharmacological interventions that can be employed to enhance the viability of organs obtained and intended for transplantation. Depending on the rate of organ conversion of xanthine dehydrogenase to xanthine oxidase, the strategy for protecting tissues would differ. For example, in tissues that have rapid dehydrogenase to oxidase conversion, one would want to pretreat tissues with free radical scavengers before inadvertent induction of ischemia. This would include the heart.[21] In contrast, liver, spleen, lungs, and kidney have a much slower rate of xanthine dehydrogenase to oxidase conversion and may be amenable to later treatment with free radical scavengers.[9] In any event, it would be critical to provide free radical scavengers at or close to the time of reperfusion of tissue with oxygenated solutions or blood. Superoxide dismutase and catalase are extremely efficient scavengers of these reactive oxygen species. Future pharmacological schemes using enzymes will need to employ the human form of the enzyme to prevent host defense reactions, modification of the enzyme to increase its circulating half-life, and inclusion of enzymes in drug delivery systems to effect intracellular delivery. This will permit closer apposition of enhanced antioxidant molecules with tissue free radical-producing systems.[22] Currently, protection against ischemia-reperfusion injury from xanthine oxidase has been observed using extracellularly provided superoxide dismutase and catalase. One may expect greater protection from the enzyme delivered to intracellular spaces, but this phenomenon would have to be examined in a variety of experimental models.

## PRESERVATION OF THE HEART

Low cardiac output and death are sometimes the result of technically successful cardiac operations and can often be attributed to suboptimal myocardial preservation. Unfortunately it is difficult to obtain sensitive

and specific markers of myocardial damage; thus cardiac function and circulating heart-specific isoenzymes serve as the best markers of myocardial preservation. Preservation of cardiac tissue for transplantation, particularly when donor hearts must be excised at locations other than transplant centers, involves infusion of cold (4°C) cardioplegic solution. After establishment of inflow occlusion via ligation of the superior vena cava and ligation and division of the inferior vena cava, the aorta is clamped. Then, cardioplegic solution is infused into the root of the aorta. Once metabolic arrest and perfusion cooling occur, the donor heart is excised and either transferred to the recipient or wrapped in sterile bags and placed in a saline-filled canister packed in ice for transportation. Hearts have been successfully preserved for transplantation for three to four hours using this technique. Optimization of the composition of the cold cardioplegic solution to limit cardiac tissue injury and enhance organ function is currently a subject of intensive examination, in light of the previously discussed data.

Acute myocardial ischemia produces a rapid decline in developed tension and a subsequent increase in resting tension. During prolonged ischemia there is a loss of viable myocardial tissue, the developed tension remains depressed, and resting tension further increases. These phenomena are probably due to the breakdown of cell membrane barriers to calcium and monovalent cations, resulting in an intracellular overload of calcium.[23] Ischemic myocardial tissue also becomes acidotic, which results in proton-mediated depression of sarcoplasmic reticular calcium transport by uncoupling calcium transport from ATP hydrolysis.[24] It has recently been proposed that with more prolonged periods of acidosis, oxygen free radical generation in cardiac tissue is more likely to occur, especially during reperfusion. This, in combination with acidosis, directly leads to the increase in resting tension and decreased cardiac output observed following reperfusion.[25]

In 1971 investigators inadvertently tested the free radical concept of cardiac ischemic injury by evaluating the effect of the xanthine oxidase inhibitor allopurinol on myocardial function and metabolism following global myocardial ischemia.[26] The investigators hypothesized that maintenance of the cardiac pool of functional purine bases would be obtained by blocking the action of the enzyme xanthine oxidase. Allopurinol prevented the usual hemodynamic consequences of diminished myocardial contractility and subsequent development of arrhythmias. Later studies examining the contractile and metabolic characteristics of globally ischemic and reperfused isolated hearts following hypothermic cardioplegia show that myocardial ischemic injury can be similarly reduced with oxygen-derived free radical scavengers, in addition to allopurinol.[9] These studies have been performed in rabbits,[27] cats,[28] and pigs.[29] It was initially observed that addition of superoxide dismutase and catalase to cardioplegic solution enhanced cardiac function upon reperfusion of globally ischemic parts.[27] Decreases in left ventricular pressure, compliance, coronary blood flow, mitochondrial oxygen consumption, and respiratory control ratio following reperfusion can all be attentuated by antioxidant supplementation of cardioplegic solution. In addition, there was inhibition of LDH release by the reperfused part in antioxidant-treated groups.[27–30] The protective effect of antioxidant-supplemented hypothermic cardioplegic solution has been further examined by inclusion of allopurinol and desferrioxamine in cardioplegic solutions.[30] After examination of postreperfusion contractile parameters, including left ventricular pressure development and its first derivative, left ventricular compliance, spontaneous heart rate, and coronary vascular resistance, it was observed that catalase supplementation provided statistically significant improvement of most functional parameters. Somewhat less protection was obtained with allopurinol, little added protection with desferrioxamine, and no evidence of added protection by superoxide dismutase. In these experiments, desferrioxamine is intended to selectively chelate ferric iron, which catalyzes the production of the extremely toxic and reactive hydroxyl radical from hydrogen peroxide. The data suggest that an important component of ischemia-induced cell damage in an asanguineous setting is hydrogen peroxide–dependent, and interventions that either inhibit production of superoxide anion or degrade hydrogen peroxide offer the best protection. Superoxide dismutase may be relatively less effective than catalase because the intracellularly generated and highly reactive superoxide anion may not be accessible to an exogenously added scavenging en-

zyme for detoxification, before superoxide exerts tissue-damaging reactions.

Other markers of myocardial ischemic injury, including leakage of creatine kinase activity, edema, lipid peroxidation, free fatty acid release, and histochemical changes, have also been reduced following treatment with free radical scavenging systems.[30–32] An important control experiment showed that providing exogenous generation of free radical species (produced by addition of purine plus xanthine oxidase to physiological cardiac perfusion solutions) caused degenerative myocardial alterations.[33] These experiments confirm that oxygen-derived free radicals, when generated in the heart, are capable of causing significant injury. Future investigations in this area should involve attempts to directly measure production of reactive oxygen species following reperfusion of ischemic myocardium. Also, pharmacological modification of free radical injury using scavenging enzymes or low molecular weight antioxidant molecules must involve attempts to achieve site-specific delivery of antioxidants so that free radical scavengers are provided in sufficient concentrations near sites of free radical generation. More effective scavenging of toxic species can then occur, thereby circumventing a potentially harmful reaction with target molecules within the organ.

## PRESERVATION OF THE KIDNEYS

Numerous studies have reviewed the relative contribution of a variety of factors to the outcome of renal transplantation. A number of recent advances have had dramatic influence on the success rate of renal transplantation in humans. These advances include (1) a better understanding of the effects of blood transfusion, including donor-specific transfusions; (2) further understanding of the immunogenetics of the HLA system, particularly the HLA-D and -DR regions of the HLA supergene; (3) the advent of new approaches to immunosuppression of transplant recipients; (4) the marked improvement of methods of renal preservation; and (5) further characterization of the effects of age, race, sex, frequency and duration of dialysis, diabetes mellitus in the recipient, and donor and recipient pretreatment. This section will examine the preservation of donor kidneys prior to transplantation.

**Preservation Techniques.** There are two

methods currently used to preserve donor kidneys prior to transplantation: flushing and storage in hypothermic solutions and continuous hypothermic pulsatile perfusion. A considerable amount of controversy exists as to which method should be routinely utilized. Hypothermic storage has many advantages over hypothermic pulsatile perfusion. Hypothermic storage is relatively simple, does not require special equipment or highly trained technicians, and is approximately one quarter of the cost of hypothermic perfused renal storage. The potential for endothelial damage due to cannulation, mechanical problems, air emboli, and defects in refrigeration systems is eliminated. Problems with bacterial contamination are minimal. However, reliability of hypothermic storage is limited to less than 24 hours, while pulsatile perfusion is reliable for longer periods of preservation—24 to 72 hours—especially after a period of warm ischemia. Hypothermic storage is associated with severe damage to the mitochondria, which occurs during prolonged anaerobic conditions. There is less mitochondrial damage associated with pulsatile perfusion. Pulsatile perfusion offers the advantage of the ability to assess viability and function of the kidney during the preservation period.[34]

**Viability Assessment.** Currently both noninvasive and invasive methods exist for the assessment of viability of donor kidneys. In perfused kidneys it is possible to monitor perfusion characteristics, most commonly blood flow, vascular resistance, and urine output; metabolites, enzyme markers, electrolyte profiles, pH, and redox potential can also be determined. Edema formation can also be used as a tool for assessment of kidney viability, although it lacks the required sensitivity.[35] Biopsies of the organ can be used for invasive viability assessment in both cold-stored and perfused kidneys. There appears to be a correlation between the levels of ATP, or the sum of the different nucleotides, and post-transplantation viability.[36] Unfortunately, most of the current methods for assessment of organ viability have not proven to be predictive of renal function following transplantation and are thereby of limited use. Several possible future approaches for viability assessment have been proposed, which include measurement of key metabolites in tissues via nuclear magnetic resonance imaging and nuclear magnetic resonance biochemistry, positron emission tomography, redox imaging, and general biochemistry characterization. Also, contrast agents and nuclear magnetic resonance can be used to perform vascular imaging and vascular characterization.[36]

**Preservation Solutions.** Currently, the solutions used for perfusion and storage are nearly isotonic (e.g., Collins) or hypertonic (e.g., Sacks), with ionic concentrations similar to those of the intracellular fluid (intracellular-like solutions). Perfusion of the kidneys with cold solutions has been routine at many transplant centers, primarily to cool the kidneys rapidly and replace the blood with a more ideal preserving solution. Most perfusates have been shown to be better than blood as a storage solution, although both albumin-Ringer's lactate and invert sugar are inferior to blood left in the kidney.[37] Both direct and indirect evidence may explain why cold perfusion could be detrimental. Cold-stored kidney slices gain water and sodium and lose potassium when deprived of oxygen or nutrients, and whole kidneys lose much of their potassium and magnesium when perfused with cold saline.[37] A substantial proportion of cell energy production is required to provide high-energy phosphate for the $Na^+,K^+$-ATPase. Respiration of kidney cortical slices can be decreased by one third by reduction of extracellular sodium from normal levels to 10 mM,[38] the concentration of sodium in Collin's solution. In addition, cooling alone reduces tissue energy requirements, although significant active transport persists even at $0°C$.[39] The decreased efficiency of the active transport system for sodium and potassium results in distribution of sodium, chloride, and potassium according to a Donnan equilibrium. As a result, cells gain water because of the additional osmotic forces resulting from impermeant intracellular proteins. Cell rupture, which is the ultimate consequence of cell swelling, may result from failure of active transport mechanisms in the cold environment, a situation that might be offset by storage in an intracellular-like perfusate. Although the precise mechanism by which hypothermic perfusates are beneficial is not completely understood, several hypotheses are currently under investigation. It is possible that cellular energy required by the ion pumps during anoxic hypothermic storage is conserved as a result of reduction in transmembrane cation gradients. A second possibility is that the perfusates decrease cell swelling. It is consistent with the first hypothesis that solutions with ionic concentrations similar to intracellular fluid should be utilized, while hyperosmotic solutions (i.e., Sacks, 430 mOsm) have been advocated to prevent cell swelling.

The first isotonic intracellular flushing solution described by Collins et al.[37] contained the pharmacological additives heparin, phenoxybenzamine, and procaine. The role of these components is now questionable. Heparin anticoagulation is unnecessary in the presence of phosphate ions that chelate calcium, while phenoxybenzamine rapidly forms a precipitate in solution and loses its activity. The original Collins solution (C1) contained 0.01 gm of procaine per dl.[37] Procaine content was increased 10-fold in subsequent solutions (C3 and C4) in hope that the agonal vasospasm in cadaver kidneys could be overcome. However, procaine (0.1 gm per dl) was subsequently found to be detrimental in hypothermic storage,[40] presumably owing to its conversion to *p*-amino benzoic acid.[41] Some studies have suggested that hypertonic (e.g., Sack's, 410 to 430 mOsm) intracellular solutions are superior to isotonic intracellular-like solutions in the hypothermic preservation of kidneys.[42] The rationale for using hypertonic preservation solutions, as opposed to isotonic solutions, is to reduce the cell swelling that accompanies hypothermic storage of kidneys. The superiority of the hyperosmotic preservation solution can be attributed, at least in part, to the fact that isotonic solution contains procaine (C3), which is detrimental in hypothermic storage. Coffey and Andrews have reported that there is little difference observed in the kidney ultrastructure between kidneys stored in isotonic (300 mOsm) or hypertonic (400 mOsm) solutions.[43] The most widely used flushing solution in the United States and Europe is a modified Collins solution termed Euro-Collins. Euro-Collins is slightly hyperosmotic (355 mOsm) and does not contain the pharmacological additives mentioned above.

Despite contemporary methods of organ preservation, including flush solutions and cold perfusion techniques, centers continue to report a significant incidence of primary graft nonfunction. It is possible, at least in theory, that pharmacological agents can be used as additives to the flush and storage solutions to improve organ preservation and decrease the incidence of graft nonfunction. Since ischemia-reperfusion is an inevitable consequence of renal transplantation and cytotoxic oxygen radicals have been implicated in ischemia-reperfusion injury in a variety of tissues, it is likely that the transplantation may be amenable to improvement by modification of oxygen free radical metabolism.[19] The mechanism proposed by Parks et al. was first applied to the small intestine and has been subsequently applied to numerous other organs.[44] Highly reactive and cytotoxic oxygen radicals (see Fig. 3–2) can damage renal tubular epithelial cells, glomerular mesangial cells, and arteriolar endothelial cells, as well as structural components of the basement membrane and interstitium.[45]

There is a growing body of evidence to implicate oxygen radicals in the reperfusion injury associated with transplanted kidneys. Superoxide dismutase (SOD), a specific scavenger of superoxide anion, and allopurinol, an inhibitor of xanthine oxidase, provided significant protection following temporary ischemia. This conclusion is based on improved survival, reduced renal dysfunction, and improved renal tubular morphology.[45] Another study reported that a significant protective effect was provided by either allopurinol in the preservation media or by SOD given intravenously at reperfusion.[46] Other investigators have found that addition of antioxidants to the hypothermic perfusate results in minimal damage occurring during the preservation period and marked improvement in post-transplant renal function.[47,48] These studies suggest that oxygen radical scavengers and antioxidants added to the perfusion media and administered intravenously may be promising in current clinical practices.

## PRESERVATION OF THE LIVER

Current procurement techniques extend hypothermic preservation of donor livers *ex vivo* for up to ten hours, although great efforts are made to work within a five- to six-hour time frame. Current methods involve flushing the organ free of blood with cold (4°C) lactated Ringer's solution. Next, the liver is perfused with cold Collins solution and placed in a bag to help prevent evaporative loss and maintain temperature. More cold Collins solution is poured over the liver and low temperature maintained by packing the bag in ice. A variation in the liver preservation technique has been described[49] advocating that the liver be perfused with a cold solution of pasteurized plasma protein fraction. It is possible that intermittent hypothermic perfusion may have some future use in liver preservation.[49] Following transplantation, the donor organs provide relief of jaundice and generate clotting factors.[50]

The liver is extremely vulnerable to ischemic injury because of its high metabolic rate. Athough hypothermia can partially protect the liver from ischemic injury, the size and bulk of this organ create difficulties in achieving rapid and uniform temperature reduction during attempts at *ex vivo* preservation. As with other transplants, the ultimate test of efficacy of donor liver preservation is survival of the transplant recipient. One of the most urgent needs in liver transplantation is the development of better preservation methods that would extend the limits for safe preservation of the liver. A decrease in blood flow to the liver decreases tissue $Po_2$ and results in a shift to anaerobic metabolism. ATP production decreases, and ATP stores become depleted.[51]

There are several reports in the literature that demonstrate a beneficial effect of allopurinol, a competitive inhibitor of xanthine oxidase, in ischemia-induced hepatocellular injury. Allopurinol improves *in vitro* function (using perfusion rate, weight gain, bile flow, and enzyme release as criteria) and posttransplant survival of allotransplanted dog livers.[52] It has also been demonstrated that allopurinol improves restitution of protein synthesis and reduces tissue water following reperfusion of ischemic liver.[53] In addition, allopurinol increased mean survival rate following 60 minutes of normothermic ischemia.[54,55] Other evidence supporting a role of xanthine oxidase in the production of oxygen radicals in postischemic liver includes the observation that the liver has tremendously high xanthine oxidase activity.[56] It has been demonstrated in the liver that the normally occurring xanthine dehydrogenase is converted to xanthine oxidase by a variety of conditions, including hypoxia and proteolysis. The rate of conversion of xanthine dehydrogenase to oxidase is less than 10 minutes in normothermic liver[56] and just under 30 minutes in hypothermic liver.[21]

There is considerable additional evidence implicating oxygen radicals in ischemic injury to the liver. Reduced glutathione (GSH) is an important endogenous scavenger of oxygen radicals in liver, serving as both a scavenger of electrons and a cofactor for glutathione peroxidase, which is responsible for

scavenging of hydrogen peroxide. Hepatocytes contain a large amount of GSH, which forms glutathione disulfide (GSSG) upon oxidation. A significant increase in the ratio of GSSG:GSH has been reported when the liver is subjected to three to four hours of ischemia.[19] Formate, a lipid-soluble hydroxyl radical scavenger, prevented the increase in GSSG:GSH ratio.[57]

Lipid peroxidation is believed to play an important role in the cellular injury produced by ischemia.[58] In support of this contention, pretreatment of rats with coenzyme $Q_{10}$, a potent antioxidant, completely suppressed the increased lipid peroxidation accompanying ischemia-reperfusion in the liver[59,60] and increased survival. The increased lipid peroxidation was observed only when the ischemic tissue was reperfused. Further support for involvement of oxygen radicals in hepatic ischemia was provided by studies with disulfiram, a potent inhibitor of enzymatically and nonenzymatically induced lipid peroxidation.[61] Rats pretreated with disulfiram display significantly reduced hepatocellular injury.[62] Finally, evidence of lipid peroxidation resulting from normothermic and hypothermic hepatic ischemia has been provided using detection of thiobarbituric acid–reacting substances and diene conjugates as indicators of lipid peroxidation.[63]

## SUMMARY AND CONCLUSIONS

Studies in past years have resulted in optimization of the ionic and carbohydrate composition of organ perfusion and storage solutions for tissues targeted for transplantation. Recent observations summarized herein have demonstrated an important role for oxygen-centered free radical injury to tissues undergoing ischemia and reperfusion. Future advances in organ preservation and transplantation will likely involve the incorporation of oxygen radical scavengers in the preservation solution for ameliorating the ischemic injury experienced during the transplantation process.

## REFERENCES

1. Rosenthal JT, Shaw BW, Hardesty RL, Griffith BP, Starzl TE, Hakala TR: Principles of multiple organ procurement from cadaver organs. Ann Surg 198:617, 1983.
2. Toledo-Pereyra LH: Rapid in vivo multiple organ cooling prior to harvesting. Ann Surg 50:493, 1984.

3. Starzl TI, Iwatsuki S, Shaw BW, Gordon RD, Esquivel C, Todd S, Kam I, Lynch S: Factors in the development of liver transplantation. Transplant Proc 17:107, 1985.

4. Jennings RB, Reiner KA: Lethal myocardial ischemic injury. Am J Pathol 102:241, 1981.

5. Hess ML, Warner MF, Robbins AD, Crute S, Greenfield LF: Characterization of the excitation-contraction coupling system of the hypothermic myocardium following ischemia and reperfusion. Cardiovasc Res 15:390, 1981.

6. Jones DP: The role of oxygen concentration in oxidative stress: Hypoxic and hyperoxic models. In Seis H (ed): Oxidative Stress. London, Academic Press, 1985, p 152.

7. Hess ML, Manson NH, Okabe E: Involvement of free radicals in the pathophysiology of ischemic heart disease. Can J Physiol Pharmacol 60:1382, 1982.

8. Corr PB, Sobel BE: Arrhythmogenic properties of phospholipid metabolites associated with myocardial ischemia. Fed Proc 42:2454, 1983.

9. McCord JM: Oxygen-derived free radicals in postischemic tissue injury. N Engl J Med 312:159, 1985.

10. Shlafer M, Kane PF, Wiggins VY, Kirsh MM: Possible role for cytotoxic oxygen metabolites in the pathogenesis of cardiac ischemic injury. Circulation 66:1-85, 1982.

11. Parks DA, Bulkley BG, Granger DN, Hamilton ST, McCord JM: Ischemic injury in the cat small intestine: Role of superoxide radicals. Gastroenterology 82:9, 1982.

12. Atalla SL, Toledo-Pereyra LH, MacKenzie GH, Cederna JP: Influence of oxygen-derived free radical scavengers on ischemic livers. Transplantation 40:584, 1985.

13. Owens ML, Lazarus HM, Wolcott MW, Maxwell JG, Taylor B: Allopurinol and hypoxanthine pretreatment of canine kidney donors. Transplantation 17:424, 1974.

14. Manson PN, Anthenelli RM, Im MJ, Bulkley GB, Hoopes JE: The role of oxygen-free radicals in ischemic tissue injury in island skin flaps. Ann Surg 198:87, 1983.

15. Battelli MG, Della Corte E, Stirpe F: Xanthine oxidase type D (dehydrogenase) in the intestine and other organs of the rat. Biochem J 126:747, 1971.

16. Della Corte E, Stirpe F: The regulation of rat liver xanthine oxidase: Involvement of thiol groups in the conversion of the enzyme activity from dehydrogenase (type D) into oxidase (type O) and purification of the enzyme. Biochem J 126:739, 1972.

17. Imai S, Riley AL, Berne RM: Effect of ischemia on adenine nucleotides in cardiac and skeletal muscle. Circ Res 15:443, 1964.

18. Granger DN, Rutili G, McCord JM: Superoxide radicals in feline intestinal ischemia. Gastroenterology 81:22, 1981.

19. Parks DA, Bulkley GB, Granger DN: Role of oxygen-derived free radicals in digestive tract diseases. Surgery 94:415, 1983.

20. Grogaard B, Parks DA, Granger DN, McCord JM, Forsberg JO: Effects of ischemia and oxygen radicals on mucosal albumin clearance in intestine. Am J Physiol 242:G448, 1982.

21. Roy RA, McCord JM: Superoxide and ischemia: Conversion of xanthine dehydrogenase to xanthine oxidase. In Greenwald R, Cohen G, (eds): Oxy Radicals and Their Scavenger Systems. Vol 2: Cellular and Molecular Aspects. New York, Elsevier Science, 1983, p 145.

22. Freeman BA, Turrens JF, Mirza Z, Crapo JD, Young SL: Modulation of oxidant lung injury by using liposome-entrapped superoxide dismutase and catalase. Fed Proc 44:2591, 1985.

23. Okabe E, Hess ML, Oyama M, Ito H: Characterization of free radical-mediated damage of canine cardiac sarcoplasmic reticulum. Arch Biochem Biophys 225:164, 1983.

24. Krause S, Hess ML: Characterization of cardiac sarcoplasmic reticulum dysfunction during short-term, normothermic, global ischemia. Circ Res 55:176, 1984.

25. Garlick PA, Radda GK, Seeley JP: Studies of acidosis in the ischemic heart by phosphorus nuclear magnetic resonance. Biochem J 184:547, 1979.

26. DeWall RA, Vasko KA, Stanley EL, Kezdi P: Responses of the ischemic myocardium to allopurinol. Am Heart J 82:362, 1971.

27. Shlafer M, Kane PF, Kirsh MM: Superoxide dismutase plus catalase enhances the efficacy of hypothermic cardioplegia to protect the globally ischemic, reperfused heart. J Thorac Cardiovasc Surg 83:830, 1982.

28. Gardner TJ, Stewart JR, Casale AS, Downey JM, Chambers DE: Reduction of myocardial ischemic injury with oxygen-derived free radical scavengers. Surgery 94:423, 1983.

29. Otani H, Engelman RM, Rousou JA, Breyer RH, Lemeshow S, Das DK: Cardiac performance during reperfusion improved by pretreatment with oxygen free-radical scavengers. J Thorac Cardiovasc Surg 91:290, 1986.

30. Myers CL, Weiss SJ, Kirsh MM, Shepard BM, Shlafer M: Effects of supplementing hypothermic crystalloid cardioplegic solution with catalase, superoxide dismutase, allopurinol, or deferroxamine on functional recovery of globally ischemic and reperfused isolated hearts. J Thorac Cardiovasc Surg 91:281, 1986.

31. Lefer AM, Araki H, Okamatsu S: Beneficial actions of a free radical scavenger in traumatic shock and myocardial ischemia. Circ Shock 8:273, 1981.

32. Casale AS, Bulkley GB, Bulkley BH, Flaherty JT, Gott VL, Gardner TJ: Oxygen free-radical scavengers protect the arrested, globally ischemic heart upon reperfusion. Surg Forum 34:313, 1983.

33. Burton KP, McCord JM, Ghai G: Myocardial alterations due to free-radical generation. Am J Physiol 246:H776, 1984.

34. Montefusco CM, Veith FJ: Organ selection and preservation for transplantation: II. Liver, pancreas, skin, and bone marrow. Hosp Phys 21:29, 1985.

35. Grundmann R, Stumper R, Eichmann J, Pichlmaier H: The immediate function of the kidney after 24- to 72-hr preservation. Transplantation 23:437, 1977.

36. Toledo-Pereyra LH: New horizons in kidney harvesting and preservation. Dial Transplant 14:131, 1985.

37. Collins GM, Bravo-Shuarman M, Teraskai PI: Kidney preservation for transplantation. Initial per-

fusion and 30 hours ice storage. Lancet 2:1219, 1969.

38. Reichmann K, Hardie IR, Clunie GJA: In vitro analysis of the cation concentration of solutions for kidney storage. Cryobiology 9:296, 1972.

39. Burg MB, Orloff J: Active cation transport by kidney tubules at 0°C. Am J Physiol 207:983, 1964.

40. Collins GM, Halasz NA: Forty-eight hour ice storage of kidneys: Importance of cation content. Surgery 79:432, 1976.

41. Watkins GM, Prentiss NA, Couch NP: Successful 24 hour kidney preservation with simplified hyperosmolar hyperkalemic perfusate. Transplant Proc 111:612, 1971.

42. Sacks SA, Petritsch PH, Kaufman JJ: Canine kidney preservation using a new perfusate. Lancet 1:1024, 1973.

43. Coffey AK, Andrews PM: Ultrastructure of kidney preservation: Varying the amount of an effective osmotic agent in isotonic and hypertonic preservation solutions. Transplant 35:136, 1983.

44. Parks DA, Bulkley GB, Granger DN: Role of oxygen free radicals in shock, ischemia, and organ preservation. Surgery 94:428, 1983.

45. Baker GL, Corry RJ, Autor AP: Oxygen free radical induced damage in kidneys subjected to warm ischemia and reperfusion. Protective effect of superoxide dismutase. Ann Surg 202:628, 1985.

46. Koyama I, Bulkley GB, Williams GM, Im MJ: The role of oxygen free radicals in mediating the reperfusion injury of cold-perfused ischemic kidneys. Transplantation 40:590, 1985.

47. Bry WI, Collins GM, Halasz HA, Jellinek M: Improved function of perfused rabbit kidneys by prevention of oxidative injury. Transplantation 38:579, 1984.

48. Belzer FO, Hoffmann RM, Rice MJ, Southard JH: Combination perfusion-cold storage for optimum cadaver kidney function and utilization. Transplantation 39:118, 1985.

49. Calne RY, Williams R, Lindop M, et al: Improved survival after orthotopic liver grafting. Br Med J 283:115, 1981.

50. Toledo-Pereyra LH: Organ preservation: II. Liver, heart, lung and small intestine. J Surg Res 30:181, 1981.

51. Hems DA, Brosnam JT: Effects of ischemia on content of metabolites in rat liver and kidney in vivo. Biochem J 120:105, 1970.

52. Toledo-Pereyra LH, Simmons RL, Najarian JS: Factors determining successful liver preservation for transplantation. Ann Surg 181:289, 1975.

53. Nordstrom G, Seeman T, Hasselgren PO: Beneficial effect of allopurinol in liver ischemia. Surgery 97:679, 1985.

54. Kupsculik P, Kokas P: Ischemic damage of the liver: *In vitro* investigation of the prevention of the ischemic lesion in the liver. Acta Hepatogastroenterol 26:279, 1979a.

55. Kupsculik P, Kokas P: Ischemic damage of the liver: *In vitro* investigation of the prevention of the ischemic lesion in the liver. Acta Hepatogastroenterol 26:284, 1979b.

56. Stirpe F, Della Corte E: The regulation of rat liver xanthine oxidase: Conversion *in vitro* of the enzyme activity from dehydrogenase (type D) to oxidase (type O). J Biol Chem 244:3855, 1969.

57. Siems W, Mielki B, Muller M, Heumann C, Rader L, Gerber G: Status of glutathione in the rat liver. Enhanced formation of oxygen radicals at low oxygen tension. Biomed Biochim Acta 42:1079, 1983.

58. Delmaestro RF, Thaw HH, Bjork J, Planker M, Arfors KE: Free radicals as mediators of tissue injury. Acta Physiol Scand 492(Suppl):43, 1980.

59. Marubayashi S, Dohi K, Ezaki H, Yamada K, Kawasaki T: Preservation of ischemic liver cell—Prevention of damage by coenzyme $Q_{10}$. Transplant Proc 15:1297, 1983.

60. Marubayashi S, Dohi K, Ezaki H, Yamada K, Kawasaki T: Changes in the levels of endogenous coenzyme Q homologs, α-tocopherol, and glutathione in the rat liver after hepatic ischemia and reperfusion, and effect of pretreatment with coenzyme Q. Biochim Biophys Acta 797:1, 1984.

61. Freundt KJ, Romer KG, Kamal AM: The inhibitory action of dithiocarbamates and carbon disulphide on malondialdehyde formation resulting from lipid peroxidation in rat liver microsomes. J Appl Toxicol 1:215, 1981.

62. Jennische E, Hansson H: Disulfiram is protective against postischemic cell death in liver. Acta Physiol Scand 122:199, 1984.

63. Koslov AV, Skinkaren KL, Valdimirov YA, Assisova OA: Role of endogenous free iron in activation of lipid peroxidation during ischemia. Bull Exp Biol Med 99:47, 1985.

# 4

# *Immunosuppressive Therapy in Organ Transplantation*

BYERS W. SHAW, JR.
R. PATRICK WOOD

An ancient Chinese legend tells of the exploits of one of China's most famous physicians, Pien Chiao. Sometime around the fifth century B.C. two men became ill and sought treatment from Pien Chiao. After examining the two, Pien Chiao concluded that one man's will was strong but his spirit weak, while the other's will was weak but his spirit strong. He convinced them that if their hearts were exchanged "there would be an equilibrium and the results would be good."[1] When the two men agreed to this treatment, Pien Chiao gave them both a drugged wine "which made them insensible, as if dead, for three days." During that time, he is purported to have "cut open their chests, investigated and exchanged their hearts, replacing them. He then gave them a wonderful drug and sent them both home recovered."

Although in all probability mythological, the legend is interesting in its conceptualization of general anesthesia, organ transplantation, and the need for immmunosuppression, herein referred to as "a wonderful drug." Since there is no mention of the two men having to continue taking any drugs, we must presume, in addition, that Pien Chiao was able to achieve complete tolerance, although we cannot be sure that it was indeed donor specific.

Even though in the last 25 years significant strides have been made in the advancement of transplantation, over 2000 years after Pien Chiao we are still searching for his "wonderful drug." The present chapter will serve as a brief guide to the principles of modern immunosuppressive therapy. Since protocols of immunosuppression are as varied as the personalities of transplant surgeons, the details of different protocols are less important to understand than the individual philosophies behind those differences.

## HISTORICAL BACKGROUND

The earliest solid organ transplants in experimental animals were done without any understanding of the immunological phenomenon of rejection. Ullmann, in 1902, reported the transplantation of kidneys into the necks of dogs (using magnesium tubes as stents for the vascular connections) with function of the organs for several days.[2] The same year, Alexis Carrel reported his technique of vascular anastomosis using fine silk sutures.[3] Eight years later, in 1910, he stated that when a functioning organ failed to continue to function when he transplanted it into another animal using these techniques of vascular anastomosis, "the physiological disturbance could not be considered as brought about by the surgical factors but rather because of the influence of the host, that is, the biological factors."[4]

The elucidation of the "biological factors" has continued to be a major challenge to transplant immunologists even to this day. Although in the 1940's Gibson and Medawar[5–7] described the rejection of skin grafts and the so-called second set phenomenon, which had been reported by Holman as early as 1924,[8] the recognition that solid, vascularized organ grafts were rejected by cell-mediated events followed the work by Billingham et al. in 1954.[9] They demonstrated the phenomenon that they called adoptively transferred immunity when they showed that the ability of mice to reject skin and organ grafts could be transferred between individuals with viable lymphocytes.

The first clinical attempts at renal transplantation between nonrelated individuals took place in the late 1940's and early 1950's and were done without any immunosuppression.[10,11] These early attempts often proved to be technical successes, but the grafts all eventually failed, again because of biological factors in the hosts. The observation that these grafts sometimes worked for longer periods than did similar transplants in experimental animals led Hume and Merrill et al. at the Peter Bent Brigham Hospital to propose that chronic uremia depressed the immune system.[11,12] Furthermore, the success that the group had in transplanting kidneys between identical twins confirmed the concept that biological factors related to genetic dissimilarity were responsible for the phenomenon that would come to be called **rejection**.[12,13]

Once it was recognized that an immune response was responsible for the failure of transplanted allografts, attention was directed toward modifying the immune system. In experimental animals, whole-body irradiation had prevented rejection and, in some models, had even achieved specific tolerance.[14,15] When this technique was used clinically, however, even near-lethal doses failed to reliably prevent allograft rejection.[16] In fact, the only two patients who did obtain long-term graft function were nonidentical twins and probably full HLA matches.

The first drugs that were used as immunosuppressants were antimetabolites originally designed for treatment of malignant neoplasms. Schwartz and Damashek reported in 1959 that one of the antipurines, 6-mercaptopurine, prevented the synthesis of anti-human albumin antibody in rabbits.[17] They called this drug-induced immunological tolerance because the lack of response to human protein persisted even after discontinuation of the drug. The treated rabbits could respond, however, to other foreign proteins, such as bovine gamma globulin. In 1960, Calne[18] and Zukowski et al.[19] independently reported prolongation of canine renal allograft survival using this agent. Hitchings and Elion of the Burroughs Wellcome Laboratories had developed a number of other agents. Among the different compounds tested, azathioprine, an imidazole derivative, proved particularly promising.[20] Calne et al., in Boston at the time working in the laboratory of Dr. Joseph Murray, demonstrated the safety and effectiveness of this drug in the canine renal allograft model.[21] In 1962, Murray et al.[22] reported some initial clinical experiences with the drug and concluded that the dose extrapolated from canine experiments was toxic to humans.

Used alone however, azathioprine was not entirely satisfactory, and the modern era of transplantation awaited the addition of adrenocorticosteroids to the regimen. As early as 1950, steroids had been shown to be effective in the treatment of a number of immunopathological disorders. In 1963, Goodwin et al.[23] reported the results of using cyclophosphamide and corticosteroids in six human kidney recipients. In the same year, Starzl et al.[24] and Hume et al.[25] independently reported improved results in clinical trials using azathioprine and steroids. The same year, one of Starzl's colleagues, Marchioro, and his associates, submitted a paper (published the following year) reporting the successful reversal of the manifestations of allograft rejection with the use of increased steroid dosing.[26] And, in 1967, Starzl's group[27] reported the clinical use of an antilymphocyte serum, a technique based on work reported in 1963 by Woodruff and Anderson using the rat skin graft model.[28]

The combination of azathioprine and prednisone remained the basis of immunosuppression for all solid organ transplantation for nearly 20 years. Various antilymphocyte and antithymocyte (T-lymphocyte directed) preparations were used during this era by a number of centers. These sera and their globulin derivatives were cultivated in a menagerie of sources, including rabbit, horse, pig, cow, goat, and sheep. Many such preparations were effective in reversing acute rejection episodes, but improvements in long-term (two- and five-year) graft survival rates for recipients of cadaver organs have been equivocal. The problems with all of these preparations are severalfold: (1) They must be given parenterally; (2) their effect is mainly upon circulating lymphocytes so that they probably do not induce any long-term adaptation in the host; and (3) often the host rapidly develops antibodies to the foreign protein, thus diminishing their clinical usefulness and raising the specter of serum sickness.

The cyclosporine era had its beginnings in 1972 when Borel, a chemist working in Basel in the laboratories of Sandoz and performing routine screening for immunosuppressive properties of fungal products with antibiotic potential, discovered a cyclic endecapeptide, metabolite 24-556, with great potential.[29] The structural formula of the compound, elucidated soon thereafter by the Sandoz chemists, was found to have a unique amino acid at the $C_9$ position on the ring. Borel's experiments included both *in vitro* and *in vivo* trials of immunosuppressive activity, the latter employing the rat skin graft model.[30] Dr. David White of Cambridge reputedly[31] heard Borel's presentation of these results at the 1976 meeting of the British Society of Immunology and suggested the experimental trial of the drug in solid organ transplants that Kostakis et al. reported in 1977.[32] Using the rat heart allograft model, Kostakis was able to achieve specific tolerance after only a short period of treatment. Further animal work was the source of a great deal of excitement during the next few years. Green and Allison[33] and Dunn et al.,[34] using a rabbit kidney allograft model, demonstrated the development of donor-specific tolerance that lasted indefinitely after withdrawal of the agent. Similar results were obtained occasionally with pig cardiac transplants by Calne et al.,[35] but most of these animals and all dogs with renal allografts were found to experience acute rejection of their grafts upon withdrawal from the drug.[36]

Calne and associates reported clinical success with cyclosporin A for kidney recipients in 1978[37] and for recipients of a variety of other solid organs in 1979.[38] Calne's initial clinical experience with the drug revealed a number of hazards that had not arisen in animals. Among these was the potential for toxicity to the kidney, liver, and heart and the danger of severe overimmunosuppression when the agent was added to the existing drug regimen. Because of the alarming development of lymphomas (thought to be associated primarily with Epstein-Barr virus infection) in a number of Calne's first patients, his group recommended the use of the drug as the sole immunosuppressive agent, with steroids given only for the treatment of acute rejection episodes.[39] In part, this was the basis for using cyclosporine alone in the European Multicentre Study.[40] However, the first American trials with the drug suggested the ineffectiveness of this regimen, and Starzl et al.[41] added steroids to the baseline immunosuppression, much as he had done in 1963 with azathioprine. In the years that followed, clinical trials of cyclosporin A for kidney allograft recipients were carried out in Europe, Canada, and Australia and at five centers in the United States. An objective comparison of the results of these trials reveals not only the inherent difficulties in using this new drug and the natural difficulties of developing standard treatment schedules for its use, but also points out the danger of comparing apples to oranges. Some centers were able to show tremendous improvements in one-year graft survival rates in trials, some randomized, against azathioprine-prednisone therapy,[40-45] while others claimed very little advantage, especially in light of the potential side effects of the new drug.[46-48] The latter centers were largely those involved in the use of a variety of methods of immune preparation of recipients, including routine use of antilymphocyte preparations, deliberate transfusion protocols, routine splenectomy, and obtaining the best HLA matches between donor and recipient. In addition, in some of the comparisons, diabetic recipients were not included, and in others, recipients of kidneys from living related donors were.[47] The most impressive improvements in results were obtained at centers that were not involved in routine use of any of these aforementioned techniques, but were transplanting cadaveric donor kidneys into large numbers of recipients without regard to HLA matching or previous transfusion history and without the use of antilymphocyte preparations or splenectomy.[43,48] At several centers one-year graft survival in such patients increased from 50 per cent to more than 80 per cent. In addition, the drug was attributed to be the single most important reason for improvements during the 1980's in liver transplantation by Starzl et al.[49] and in heart transplantation by Oyer et al.[50] and by Shumway.[51]

Clinical trials of cyclosporin A in the United States ended in the autumn of 1983 when the drug was approved for clinical use by the FDA and released for sale by Sandoz under the generic name cyclosporine. Although its final place in the history of organ transplantation will be determined by its track record over the ensuing years of use in a large number of centers, cyclosporine undoubtedly will be recognized as one of the most important immunosuppressive agents to come along in nearly 20 years of clinical transplantation of solid organs. As will be discussed, much has been learned in the last few years about how to optimize its use. Standard treatment schedules are undergoing rapid evolution fully 6 years after the first clinical trials of the drug.

Mention should also be made of a variety of other immunosuppressive agents and techniques that were employed over the years before the introduction of cyclosporine. These include the use of various alkylating agents (such as cyclophosphamide as a substitute for azathioprine in patients with hepatotoxicity), folic acid antagonists (e.g., methotrexate), pyrimidine analogues (cytosine arabinoside), and antibiotics (chloramphenicol, actinomycin D, mitomycin C, puromycin) in experimental and a few clinical trials. Besides the use of antilymphocyte globulin (or serum), several other lymphoid depletion techniques were tried. Thoracic duct drainage, thymectomy, splenectomy, total lymphoid irradiation, and even lymph node excision have all had (or may still have) their proponents as well as certain degrees of success. But none of these drugs or techniques has become as widely adopted for routine immunosuppression as has the use of steroids, azathioprine, antilymphocyte preparations, and, now, cyclosporine.

## MODERN PROTOCOLS OF IMMUNOSUPPRESSION

Elsewhere in this book is a chapter dealing with details of the immunology of transplantation. Understanding the present discussion requires at least rudimentary familiarity with the principles outlined in that chapter. The present chapter will provide a brief description of the basic principles of all immunosuppressive therapy, the potential harmful effects of that therapy, and a sampling of various strategies of drug therapy that are now popular for kidney, liver, pancreas, and heart transplantation.

### Basic Tenets of Immunosuppression

The armamentarium of immunosuppressive agents available to the modern transplanter is vast enough that the host's immune system can be rendered entirely incapable of responding to the foreign tissue of the grafted organ. Unfortunately, such aggressive immunosuppressive therapy is, for the most part, nonspecific, and it can lead to the development of sepsis, since the host simultaneously has been rendered incapable of responding to other foreign agents such as bacteria, fungi, protozoa, and viruses. Immunosuppression also carries an increased risk (estimated to be as much as 30 times that of the general population) of developing *de novo* malignant tumors, mainly of lymphoid or epithelial origin. Optimum immunosuppression, then, is defined as that level of suppression at which the risk of developing both rejection and complications of immunotherapy (the risk-benefit ratio) is lowest.

Although modern immunosuppressive strategies are more specifically oriented toward amelioration of graft immunity and thus septic complications have become somewhat less prevalent than in the earliest days of transplantation, most of these modern protocols continue to rely upon the assumption that the host will develop some sort of adaptation to the graft. This adaptation then allows gradual relaxation of the intensity of immunosuppressive therapy. The ultimate form of such adaptation, and the organ transplanter's elusive dream, is the development of specific tolerance, i.e., permanent immunological unresponsiveness to the engrafted organ combined with maintenance of normal immune responses to all other antigens. In clinical practice, donor-specific tolerance has yet to be achieved. But adaptation does occur. It is evidenced by the very fact that the intensity of immunosuppressive therapy can be tapered from high levels to levels more compatible with long-term, complication-free survival of the host. If adaptation does not occur, then the ultimate result of a relaxation in immunotherapy will be destruction of the grafted organ by the rejection process. The consequences of graft loss are obviously quite different if some means of extracorporeal support of the patient for failure of that organ is not available and if orthotopic replacement of the native organ has been carried out. This is, of course, the case in orthotopic liver or heart and heart-lung transplantation. It is not the case in renal transplantation for which dialysis provides the safety of extracorporeal back-up or in pancreas transplantation in which exogenous insulin is available.

A major factor in the improved survival of patients undergoing kidney transplantation has been the adoption of the philosophy that, when a choice must be made, loss of a transplanted organ to rejection is preferable to death of the recipient. Improvement in the effectiveness and safety of various means of dialysis is one reason for this change in attitude. But even more important has been the increased availability of transplantable organs and the recognition that retransplantation is a safe and effective alternative.

A similar attitude can be adopted for liver and heart transplantation as well. Although the natural temptation for the physician caring for these recipients is to exhaust all efforts to save the rejecting graft, the use of early retransplantation, before the host has been hopelessly compromised, has been shown to offer a reasonable chance of full recovery.[52-54] As in renal transplantation, knowledge of these data has had a significant impact upon the philosophy of immunosuppression in these patients.

The final and perhaps most important consideration in the administration of immunosuppression is the individual recipient. An examination of most enlightened protocols of antirejection therapy will reveal an essential degree of flexibility. This is because the immune systems of individual patients are different in their pre-existing state of health, their response to the graft, and their response to various immunosuppressive drugs. Formal protocols are important because of the consistency in therapy that they provide and the greater efficiency with which new knowledge can be accumulated. But the first concern must always be directed toward the care of the individual patient.

## Measurement of Cyclosporine Levels

Daily measurement of circulating cyclosporine levels in recipients is extremely important to ensure that the patient is getting enough drug to provide adequate immunosuppression, but not enough to cause serious toxic effects, particularly nephrotoxicity. The method that is used to measure cyclosporine levels is a subject of a great deal of discussion in the transplantation literature. Kahan advocates the use of radioimmunoassay (RIA) kits to measure trough serum levels. A number of others, including Starzl's group, measure RIA levels in whole blood. Still others recommend that high-performance liquid chromatography (HPLC) be used to measure trough levels. Whereas RIA measures both parent compound and all immunoreactive metabolites, HPLC measures only the parent drug. Proponents of the HPLC method argue that they are interested only in the level of available parent compound. Users of the RIA method point out that HPLC is both time consuming and labor intensive when compared to RIA; in addition, since certain metabolites may be responsible for both toxic and immunosuppressive effects, they feel it is more important to have an idea of the level of both parent drug and its immunoreactive metabolites. A number of other subtleties regarding the technique of measuring cyclosporine levels have been discussed in other publications and are not within the scope of this text.[55-57]

In our experience with both renal and hepatic transplantation, the most important considerations in the measurement of cyclosporine levels are to (1) find a method with which an institution's laboratory is comfortable and with which it can provide consistent results; (2) follow levels of all inpatients on a frequent (daily) basis; and (3) learn which levels at the institution are commonly associated with either inadequate immunosuppression or toxic side effects.

## Popular Protocols for Renal Transplantation

Several protocols of immunosuppression for kidney recipients, which differ in their use of cyclosporine, have become popular recently. Their use of cyclosporine differs because of different approaches to the problem of nephrotoxicity of the drug.

The first protocol to be discussed is one used extensively by Starzl and colleagues at Pittsburgh[42,58] and by Kahan et al. at Houston.[44] Cyclosporine is used with steroids from the onset. The initial dose of cyclosporine is given immediately before the transplantation procedure, usually as soon as the recipient is admitted to the hospital for the transplant. For scheduled, living related-donor transplants, Kahan's group gives cyclosporine 5 to 6 mg·kg$^{-1}$ per day by constant intravenous infusion starting five days before the date of the procedure to obtain information about the kinetics and distribution of the drug in the particular individual.[59] Steroids, usually in a large dose (500 mg to 1000 mg methylprednisolone sodium succinate), are administered at the time of revascularization of the graft in the recipient. Postoperatively, steroids are tapered on a daily basis so that maintenance level doses of prednisone are reached within 6 to 8 days after surgery.

Ferguson[60] and Sommer and Ferguson[61] advocate delaying the use of cyclosporine until after the kidney graft shows evidence of satisfactory function. They use Minnesota antilymphoblast globulin (ALG), prednisone, and azathioprine following transplantation until renal function is satisfactory (serum creatinine less than 2.5 mg·dl$^{-1}$, usually reached at 6 to 10 days) before substituting daily cyclosporine at 10 mg·kg$^{-1}$ for ALG and azathioprine. The argument is made that cyclosporine may significantly prolong recovery from acute tubular necrosis (ATN) in the graft, thus delaying discharge from the hospital, prolonging the period of post-transplant dialysis, and making the diagnosis of rejection all the more difficult by virtue of eliminating the usual means of assessing kidney function (urine output and changes in serum creatinine). Ferguson also has expressed concerns that the potent nephrotoxic effects of cyclosporine might have been responsible for the ultimate failures of some of the kidneys transplanted during his group's initial experience with the drug.

Although Kahan admits that this approach may become popular in the management of patients who typically receive kidneys with a high risk of developing ATN (e.g., kidneys taken from non–heart-beating cadavers, those procured by untrained persons, and/or those preserved for long periods), he goes on to point out that no randomized data have shown a significant impact of delayed cyclosporine use on the incidence of ATN, the eventual outcome, or overall costs. One reason is that the potential savings to be gained from fewer dialysis runs may be offset in these patients by the recognized need to include other forms of therapy (such as ALG) during the interval before cyclosporine is introduced and by a potentially greater risk of developing rejection episodes, which, although ultimately reversible, may lead to increasing the overall costs of therapy. Kahan also warns that the advantage obtained from the use of cyclosporine may be greatest during the so-called induction phase of the host's immune response to the new graft, a phase that occurs during the first five to eight days after transplantation. Delaying the use of the drug may reduce or even eliminate the potential advantages that cyclosporine offers over previous drugs. Furthermore, in many patients, especially those who have not undergone splenectomy, the use of ALG may cause neutropenia or thrombocytopenia severe enough to prohibit the use of azathioprine. And in still other patients, renal function may be delayed for more than 10 to 14 days, in which cases a decision must be made whether to continue ALG and/or azathioprine or start cyclosporine instead.[62]

Still another approach has been advocated by Slapak and his group.[63,64] Based upon his experiences as a participant in the European Multicentre Trial[40] (and his disappointment with cyclosporine-only therapy) Slapak now employs steroids, cyclosporine, and azathioprine during the first six to nine months following transplantation. He attempts to minimize the risk of nephrotoxicity by employing lower doses of cyclosporine, which are bolstered, in theory, by the added immunosuppression of low-dose (1 mg·kg$^{-1}$) azathioprine. In addition, he lowers steroid doses on a monthly basis until they can be discontinued at about six to nine months after the transplantation. Using this regimen, this group has had results that are quite comparable to those obtained with the other regimens that have been described.

## Sample Protocol for Kidney Recipients

Our current protocol of immunosuppression for kidney recipients is outlined in Table 4–1 to give the reader an idea of the approximate dose schedule of various drugs and the factors considered in the modification of the schedule. As stressed previously, the details of the regimen are much less important than the rationale behind it.

*Day 0.* On arrival at the hospital the patient is given an oral dose of cyclosporine, 15 mg·kg$^{-1}$. This will usually be at least four to six hours before the anticipated time of surgery. In the operating room at the time of revascularization of the donor kidney, the recipient is given methylprednisolone sodium succinate, 1 gm intravenously.

### TABLE 4–1. Sample Protocol of Immunosuppression for Renal and Hepatic Transplantation in Adults

Preoperative
  Kidney or liver recipients: Cyclosporine 15 mg·kg$^{-1}$
    PO or 2 mg·kg$^{-1}$ IV as soon as possible
    preoperatively
Intraoperative
  Methylprednisolone 1 gm IV at the time of
    revascularization of the allograft
Days 1–5
  Kidney: Cyclosporine 7–10 mg·kg$^{-1}$ PO bid—
    Adjust for 11-hour trough blood level 800–1000
    ng·ml$^{-1}$ *
  Liver: Cyclosporine 2–5 mg/kg IV bid—Adjust for
    11-hour trough blood level 1000 ng·ml$^{-1}$ *; add
    oral dose 7–10 mg·kg$^{-1}$ after resolution of ileus,
    and taper IV dose according to blood level
  Both: Methylprednisolone or prednisone 200
    mg·day$^{-1}$, divided into 4 equal doses, tapered by
    40 mg·day$^{-1}$
Treatment of rejection
  Steroid "recycle"
                or
  Antithymocyte globulin 15–20 mg·kg$^{-1}$ daily for 10–
    14 days
                or
  Monoclonal OKT3, 5 mg daily for 8–14 days
Long-term maintenance
  Prednisone: Taper to 5 mg daily by 6 months unless
    rejection intercedes
  Cyclosporine: Taper to blood levels in the range of
    500–700 ng·ml$^{-1}$,* depending upon toxicity
    versus immune response
  Azathioprine: Add 1–2 mg·kg$^{-1}$ daily for problem
    cases†

* In whole blood as measured by RIA.
† See text.

*Days 1 to 6.* Approximately 24 hours after the first dose was given, oral cyclosporine 8 to 10 mg·kg$^{-1}$ (rounded off to the nearest 100 mg) every 12 hours is started. If the patient is not able to begin oral intake because of ileus, then intravenous cyclosporine, 2 mg·kg$^{-1}$ every 12 hours, is initiated. In either case, doses are given at 08:00 and 20:00 so that blood for an 11-hour trough level can be drawn at 07:00 and taken to the laboratory in time for running the sample on the same day. Administration of prednisone by mouth or methylprednisolone intravenously is started at a dosage of 200 mg·day$^{-1}$ in four equally divided doses (four times a day) and tapered by 40 mg per day (10 mg per dose) until 20 mg per day is reached by day 6.

Cyclosporine doses are adjusted each afternoon after the drug levels have been obtained. In the first two weeks after transplantation, a trough level at 11 to 12 hours of 800 to 1000 ng·ml$^{-1}$, as measured at room temperature in whole blood by RIA, is maintained. Levels are allowed to fall to 400 to 500 ng·ml$^{-1}$ after the first five days if poor urine output, which is thought to be related to ATN, persists. Azathioprine 1.5 mg·kg$^{-1}$ per day is started in all such patients who require lowering of cyclosporine doses. Higher levels are desirable, however, in those patients in whom there is a decrease in urine output, which is thought to be, on the basis of clinical signs, biopsy, ultrasonic examination, and/or nuclear flow scans, related to acute rejection.

The distinction between rejection and ATN and cyclosporine nephrotoxicity is often difficult to make. The less intense form of rejection that patients treated with cyclosporine experience is less obvious than the clinical syndrome of fever, malaise, myalgias, graft tenderness, fluid retention, and sudden oliguria that patients treated with conventional immunosuppression (azathioprine-prednisone) often exhibit. The loss of some of these important clues and the potential for direct nephrotoxicity from the immunosuppressive agent itself are two of the major reasons that the learning curve associated with the use of cyclosporine is initially so steep.

## Immunosuppression for Liver Recipients

Immunosuppression protocols for liver recipients are probably less varied than those for kidney recipients because liver transplantations have been performed at more than a handful of centers for only a short time. Most protocols are spinoffs from that used by Starzl and his colleagues and described in a number of previous reports.[49,65] The reader must realize that many such protocols undergo frequent modification. Our protocol is presented as one example that may have elements in common with those used by many others, but which is by no means the only approach. The protocol is also outlined in Table 4–1.

*Day 0.* As soon as possible after arrival of the patient, an intravenous dose of 2 mg·kg$^{-1}$ of cyclosporine is ordered and sent with the patient to the operating room. Infusion of the dose is begun as soon as intravenous access has been established and requires two to three hours. An oral dose cannot be given in the usual case because of the short time available between arrival of the recipient at the hospital and the induction of anesthesia. The intraoperative dose of steroids consists of 1000 mg methylprednisolone intravenously for adults and children more than 15 kg in weight and 500 mg for those 15 kg or less.

*Days 1 to 6.* The steroid taper for adults is exactly as outlined for kidney recipients. For children 15 kg or under (for liver or kidney recipients) the taper begins at 100 mg per day (25 mg per dose four times a day) and is tapered by 20 mg per day (5 mg per dose four times a day) until a baseline of 10 or 20 mg per day is reached. In addition, almost all patients will receive a bolus injection of methylprednisolone (500 to 1000 mg) on day 5 or 6 unless sepsis in the recipient is a concern at that point. Cyclosporine doses are given intravenously until ileus has resolved and are continued until adequate levels can be maintained on oral dosing alone. This may require intravenous dosing for several weeks because of the vagaries of cyclosporine absorption and metabolism in liver transplant recipients.[66–68] An 11-hour trough level of 1000 ng·ml$^{-1}$ (as measured in whole blood by RIA) is targeted during the first month following transplantation. But levels may be allowed to drift much lower (400 to 500 ng·ml$^{-1}$) in the face of overt nephrotoxicity unaccompanied by any signs of liver rejection. In our experience, levels greater than 1200 ng·ml$^{-1}$ are almost always associated with hepatic toxicity and, if maintained, with nephrotoxicity. On the other hand, levels maintained below 600 to 700 ng·ml$^{-1}$ appear to carry a greater risk of the patient's developing rejection, especially during the first month following transplantation.

Provided no episodes of rejection occur, the daily dose of steroids is lowered to 15 mg by the end of the third postoperative month and to 10 mg by the end of the sixth.

## Treatment of Rejection Episodes

**Kidney Recipients.** The initial treatment of an obvious acute episode of kidney allograft rejection involves a "recycle" of the prednisone back up to the initial post-transplant levels with a similar taper. A bolus of 500 to 1000 mg methylprednisolone may be given at the start of the recycle if the rejection episode appears particularly severe. More often, a bolus of steroid is given automatically at any time between days 5 and 10 if there is evidence of either worsening of renal function or diminution in the rate of improvement in renal function. The recycle is started thereafter if further developments confirm that the diagnosis of rejection is highly probable. We use kidney biopsy only when confusion persists regarding the diagnosis (for example, because of a lack of response to antirejection therapy) or when looking for signs of irreversible graft destruction as when consideration is being given to abandoning the graft and discontinuing immunosuppression.

Antithymocyte globulin is used whenever the rejection episode recurs after the steroid recycle or when it appears unresponsive to steroids after three days of the recycle. We have some experience with the use of the monoclonal antibody directed against T lymphocytes (OKT 3) and have obtained prompt reversal of severe rejection episodes unresponsive to other therapy.

Others have reported a much more extensive experience with OKT 3 in kidney recipients[69–75] and liver recipients.[76,77] This murine monoclonal antibody reacts with a cell surface molecule found only on circulating thymocytes and mature human T cells. *In vitro*, OKT 3 induces self-limited mitogenesis in human T cells which then leaves the cells unresponsive to other stimuli of T cell activity. It also appears to block the killing action of cytotoxic T cells directed against the major histocompatibility complex. The usual daily dose for adults is 5 mg (2.5 mg for children weighing less than 15 to 20 kg) given as a bolus injection, as compared to 15 to 30 mg·kg$^{-1}$ given over 5 to 8 hours for most antilymphocyte sera or globulin preparations. The length of treatment is usually 10 to 14 days, although most users are reporting the onset of effect by three days and maximum effect within eight days of initiating treatment. This drug, another monoclonal directed at another population of cells, or tailor-made mixtures of monoclonal antibodies may prove to be the treatment of choice either for acute rejection episodes or as routine prophylaxis[75] during the induction phase of the host immune response.

In general, cyclosporine dosing is altered, even during a rejection episode, only as indicated by blood levels. The mechanism of cyclosporine's action and the pharmacokinetics of the drug are such that drug levels are probably more important for the prevention of rejection than for the acute treatment of an episode once underway. Certainly, if an acute rejection episode develops in the face of blood or serum levels of cyclosporine that are considered low, and in the absence of signs of serious toxicity, most physicians would attempt to raise those levels sharply by increasing the dose. But this is secondary to the primary treatment with steroids or antilymphocyte therapy.

**Liver Recipients.** Episodes of rejection of the liver are treated initially in a manner identical to that described for renal recipients. The first signs of early acute rejection are most likely to be evident at about the fifth through tenth day following transplantation. Any time the liver function tests show any tendency toward deterioration, the patient receives a thorough work-up to evaluate the possible causes. A number of tests are performed routinely. Duplex ultrasound of the hepatic hilum is used to document portal vein and hepatic artery patency. Evidence of biliary tract leak or obstruction is sought by T-tube cholangiography, if such a tube is present, or, in its absence, by ultrasound of the hepatic ducts. A thorough search for sepsis is made. If all of these studies fail to demonstrate a problem, and some doubt remains about the diagnosis of rejection, then a biopsy of the liver may prove helpful, although the histological appearance of the liver must be interpreted in light of the clinical and other laboratory findings rather than as the *sine qua non* of tests.

If all evidence (or lack thereof) supports the diagnosis of rejection, the patient is given a recycle of steroids identical to that described previously.

If liver function tests continue to deteriorate while steroids are increased, the patient is observed very carefully for any evidence of an error in diagnosis. Care should be taken to repeat any diagnostic tests, including liver biopsy, that were inconclusive before. When a steroid-resistant rejection is strongly suspected, antilymphocyte therapy is begun immediately. At this stage we use commercially available equine antithymocyte globulin (at 20 mg·kg$^{-1}$ per day). Monoclonal OKT 3 has been reported as highly effective at this stage.[76,77]

Cyclosporine hepatic toxicity is rare in the usual therapeutic range of blood levels of the drug. However, we have seen numerous instances of mild elevations of serum bilirubin and transaminase levels associated with trough levels above 1100 ng·ml$^{-1}$. In the face of such minor alterations of liver function, especially after the first two weeks following transplantation, the physician should allow blood levels of the drug to fall below 900 to 1000 ng·ml$^{-1}$ before suspecting rejection.

As mentioned previously, retransplantation of the liver offers the best chance of continued survival of the patient when rejection proves unresponsive to steroids and one or more antilymphocyte preparations. The decision about retransplantation is a complex subject beyond the scope of the present discussion. However, the key to successful use of this option is proper timing. It should be exercised whenever liver failure develops in spite of optimal immunosuppression. This may be acute, when a rapid rejection process continues to destroy the allograft despite aggressive treatment by the methods described previously, or chronic, wherein liver function deteriorates each time immunosuppression is reduced to maintenance levels. The goal should be to use retransplantation before the recipient is so thoroughly compromised by attempts to save the graft that ultimate survival becomes improbable.

## Immunosuppression for Other Organs

In general, protocols of immunosuppression for pancreas, heart, and heart-lung recipients are similar to those already mentioned, although some important differences are worth noting. The use of cyclosporine has allowed reduction in the amount of steroids needed. Advantage is taken of this for heart-lung and pancreas recipients. In the former, the ability to completely avoid the use of steroids during the first two weeks allows sufficient healing of the tracheal anastomosis, eliminating its disruption as the greatest source of mortality for these patients.[78] In pancreatic transplantation, lower steroid dosage has allowed a return to the use of whole-organ pancreaticoduodenal grafts by several groups[79–82] without the penalty of duodenal disruption, perforation, or necrosis that plagued the initial trials of Lillehei et al.[83] For both heart and heart-lung recipients, levels of cyclosporine lower than those used for liver recipients are usually maintained because of the apparent higher incidence of toxicity in these patients.

The diagnosis of rejection in heart recipients is largely dependent upon frequent use of transvenous endomyocardial biopsies.[84] In pancreas recipients, fasting blood sugar levels are notoriously unreliable for diagnosing malfunction of the organ at an early enough stage to allow successful treatment. Measuring the organ's response to glucose is somewhat more useful, and, when the exocrine portion of the gland has been drained into the urinary bladder, can be combined with frequent measurements of urinary amylase concentrations as useful signs of rejection.[81,82]

As with liver or kidney transplantation, care must be exercised to avoid overimmunosuppression. This is especially true for pancreas recipients in whom the ravages of long-term diabetes may markedly increase the risk of septic complications. The enthusiasm for saving a pancreas allograft from destruction by rejection must be tempered by the realization that as yet there is little evidence that pancreas transplantation significantly alters the progression of or reverses the complications of the original disease. In addition, a means of exogenous support (insulin) is available.

For heart and heart-lung recipients, retransplantation is a viable option, although it has been utilized much less frequently than for liver recipients. The eventual role of the artificial heart as a means of support in a patient with a failing heart, either before transplantation or following failure of an allograft, remains to be determined.

## TRENDS IN IMMUNOSUPPRESSION: SUMMARY AND CONCLUSIONS

During the middle and late 1970's, several advances in the field of transplantation resulted in significant improvements in the rates of survival of kidney grafts. These advances were almost entirely in the direction of preoperative conditioning or selection of recipients. The discovery that patients with a previous history of multiple transfusions of blood obtained greater long-term kidney graft survival rates[85] led to the establishment of protocols of deliberate transfusion of recipients prior to transplantation. The effect was equally impressive with donor-specific blood transfusion, even in cases with HLA identity, and thus led several centers to embark upon programs involving deliberate transfusion of recipients with several units of blood obtained from their intended donor.[86,87] In addition, the identification of the D-related (DR) antigens and the observation that obtaining the best donor-to-recipient match at this location resulted in improvements in graft survival,[88,89] which were more convincing than those obtained from traditional matching at the A and B loci, led to increased enthusiasm for sharing of organs to obtain the best DR match.

Such preparatory efforts have their price. Blood transfusions are not without risks, not the least of which is possible sensitization of potential recipients to such an extent that finding a donor with which the recipient is nonreactive becomes impossible. Donor-specific transfusions result in sensitization of 30 per cent of recipients against their related donor, thus making cadaveric donor transplantation the only option.[86,87] Placing priority on tissue matching complicates transplantation, since obtaining complete matches can become practical only if done between large numbers of donor-recipient pairs, thus necessitating nationwide organ-sharing networks. Such protocols can markedly prolong storage (read *ischemia*) times for kidneys and increase overall costs by requiring the organs to be shipped from center to center.

Many saw very early that the real potential of cyclosporine was the obviation of all of these elaborate, somewhat risky, and expensive measures. Support for this early contention has come from the observation that a number of centers have been able to obtain results in kidney transplantation that equal or even exceed the best results obtained by other centers using these preparatory protocols but not cyclosporine.

At the halfway point in the current decade, transplanters have recovered from their initial excitement over the new drug and have long since concentrated on constantly refining protocols for its use. This chapter has already outlined a number of the approaches that have become popular. The future promises still further developments.

## Refinements in Existing Protocols

Some authors have recommended conversion from treatment with cyclosporine to some other treatment (usually azathioprine) as part of the long-term immunosuppressive regimen.[90–96] They reason that this is safe, in terms of not inducing a late rejection episode, and has the advantage of eliminating long-term side effects of the drug. But in our experience and that of others,[95,97–99] this all too often leads to an episode of acute rejection that, although sometimes reversed by steroid or other treatment, may represent exposure of the patient to greater risk than benefit.

A more reasonable approach may be the use of low doses of both cyclosporine and azathioprine for long-term maintenance. We use this approach whenever blood levels of cyclosporine that prove to be the minimal possible for adequate immunosuppression appear to be associated with significant nephrotoxicity. Such would be the case, for example, in a patient for whom gradual lowering of cyclosporine levels results in consistent improvement in renal graft function until he or she suddenly develops an episode of acute rejection 10 days after a new blood level is attained that would have been thought to be acceptable. The addition of azathioprine in doses of 0.5 to 1.0 mg·kg$^{-1}$ per day may prove adequate to prevent rejection in such patients.

In addition, this approach is appealing for dealing with another group of problematic patients. Several centers, including ours, have had particular difficulty with cyclosporine dosing in pediatric patients who have had liver transplants.[76] On many occasions the blood cyclosporine levels fall dramatically in these children during an episode of gastroenteritis. These patients appear to continue to be at risk for the development of acute rejection at almost any time, even several years after transplantation. Instances of severe rejection, eventually leading to the need for retransplantation, have been seen in several such children with intestinal malabsorption in whom blood levels of the drug, despite what would seem to be quite adequate dosing with cyclosporine, were virtually undetectable. The hope is that low doses of azathioprine may protect these individuals against the development of rejection during these intervals of poor drug absorption.

The reader is cautioned that convincing evidence to support the validity of either of these approaches is still lacking. Kahan points out that the idea that low doses of azathioprine are at all effective may be erroneous, since the drug acts as a competitive inhibitor of nucleotide incorporation into DNA, a phenomenon that would be expected to be dose dependent.[62] On the other hand, Kahan goes on to admit, studies by Squifflet et al. in animals do suggest a synergistic effect between low-dose azathioprine and cyclosporine.[100]

Thus far the use of the monoclonal antibody OKT 3 in the United States has been limited to the treatment of rejection episodes that are resistant to conventional treatment (steroids, cyclosporine, and ATG) or for cases in which these conventional measures are contraindicated. The promising results obtained in kidney recipients and in liver recipients suggest that use of this drug may become much more common. In addition, other monoclonal antibodies are likely to become available. The ultimate form that this kind of therapy will take may involve the use of a library of monoclonal antibodies directed against a variety of cell lines (e.g., helper T cells, natural killer or NK cells), or mixtures of monoclonal (or even polyclonal) antibodies to be used at different intervals during the host's response to the new graft.

Attempts to induce donor-specific, immunological unresponsiveness in a host (and by definition maintain normal immunity to other antigens, such as infectious agents) have been successful in certain laboratory models using adult animals. Billingham, Brent, and Medawar were able to show that immunological tolerance to histocompatibility antigens could be induced by exposing neonatal mice to alloantigens.[101] In more recent times the use of either small doses or massive doses of antigen has led to tolerance in certain animal models. The mechanism for this effect is unclear, but may involve deletion of specific clones of reacting lymphocytes. Another approach involves the modification of donor antigens. Attaching radioactive isotopes or cell toxins to the antigens so that the reactive lymphocytes are destroyed when they react with the antigen is one such approach, but no clinical success has been obtained as yet.

Transplantation literature in the mid 1980's is replete with articles describing the experimental success of various approaches designed to induce tolerance. Much of this work was reported at the Tenth International Congress of The Transplantation Society in 1984 and published in several places.[102,103]

The observation in both experimental and clinical transplant models of the beneficial effects of prior exposure to donor antigens by blood transfusion supports the notion that the formation of some sort of antidonor antibody in the host may be important in preventing the development of immunity. These kinds of antibodies have been referred to as blocking antibodies because they appear to act to prevent or ameliorate rejection rather than promote it. They may be part of the recognized feedback control mechanisms of the immune response. A great deal of experimental effort is being directed toward the identification and characterization of such antibodies. The ability to promote the formation of such antibodies endogenously, or even the exogenous administration of such antibodies, holds the potential for ameliorating or perhaps even eliminating the immune response to a graft. On another tack, employment of anti-idiotype antibodies (antibodies directed against the antigenic features of the donor-specific antigen receptors on B and T cells that are reacting to the graft) has proven useful in altering the host response to a graft. Still another approach attempts to increase populations of circulating suppressor cells by combining the administration of antigen along with cyclosporine.

As other means of preparation of the recipient, several groups have revived an interest in total lymphoid irradiation, with and without donor or autologous bone marrow reconstitution.[104-106] Similar to the intent behind whole-body irradiation, the theory in this kind of therapy is that the host is presented with the donor antigens at a time when various elements of the host immune system have been temporarily destroyed. By the time these elements begin to regenerate, they may react to the graft as though it were self, much as Billingham, Brent, and Medawar witnessed when the immune system of neonatal mice matured in the presence of alloantigen, thus promoting tolerance. Reconstituting these recipients with donor bone marrow offers the theoretical advantage of assuring that the new immune system will view the graft as self, but carries the risk of severe graft-versus-host disease. Use of autologous stem cell lines to reconstitute radiated hosts may provide marrow elements that are immature enough to accept as self

the donor tissue, even after they propagate into more mature cell lines. In this setting, the closer the histocompatibility between host and donor, the more likely the attempt to achieve tolerance will be successful.

All of these approaches offer potential improvements in graft survival. Which ones, if any, will lead to the reliable induction of tolerance remains to be seen. Any technique that seeks to abrogate the immunological response after it begins to be manifested by signs of organ destruction should be considered treatment rather than prophylaxis and, as such, probably does not represent the kind of immunological manipulation that will lead to tolerance. On the other hand, pretransplant conditioning of the recipient or modification of the immune response during the induction phase, although potentially more costly and complicated, may lead to the promotion of unresponsiveness that is permanent, lasting even after the cessation of all exogenous immunosuppression.

With state-of-the-art immunosuppression, surviving recipients of a variety of solid organ transplants can be expected to obtain near-normal quality of life, including normal growth and development in children,[106,107] normal activity levels, and normal career aspirations.[107-111] The exceptions, for the most part, continue to be those in whom rejection cannot be controlled by the usual measures and in whom the potential for overimmunosuppression, with all of its deleterious effects, is greatest. The last 20 years have provided advances in surgical technique, critical care, nutrition, and the treatment of infectious diseases that have greatly improved our overall care of these patients. As a result, rejection (or the effect of our attempts to control it) is more than ever the most important barrier to the ultimate success of transplantation as a therapy. Thus, not only has the final chapter on immunosuppression not been written, it is not even within the realm of our current understanding of the immunology of rejection. That its pages may lie as yet unturned within the imagination of one or more of our contemporaries is what makes the field ultimately so exciting.

## REFERENCES

1. Hume EH: The Chinese Way in Medicine. Baltimore, The Johns Hopkins Press, 1940, pp 77–78.

2. Ullmann E: Experimentelle nierentransplanta-tion. Wein Klin Wochenschr 15:281, 1902.

3. Carrel A: La technique operatoire des anasto-moses vasculaires et la transplantation des vis-ceres. Lyon Med 99:859, 1902.

4. Carrel A: Remote results of the replantation of the kidney and the spleen. J Exp Med 12:146, 1910.

5. Gibson T, Medawar PB: The fate of skin homo-grafts in man. J Anat 77:299, 1942–43.

6. Medawar PB: The behaviour and fate of skin au-tografts and skin homografts in rabbits. (A report to the War Wounds Committee of the Medical Research Council). J Anat 78:176, 1944.

7. Medawar PB: A second study of the behaviour and fate of skin homografts in rabbits. J Anat 79:157, 1945.

8. Holman E: Protein sensitization in isoskingraft-ing. Is the latter of practical value? Surg Gy-necol Obstet 38:100, 1924.

9. Billingham RE, Brent L, Medawar PB: Quanti-tative studies on tissue transplantation immun-ity. II. The origin, strength and duration of ac-tively and adoptively acquired immunity. Proc R Soc (Biol) 143:58, 1954.

10. Moore FD: Give and Take: The Development of Tissue Transplantation. Philadelphia, WB Saunders Company, 1964, pp 58–66.

11. Hume DM, Merrill JP, Miller BR, Thorn GW: Ex-perience with renal homotransplantation in the human: Report of nine cases. J Clin Invest 34:327, 1955.

12. Merrill JP, Murray JE, Harrison JH, Guild WR: Successful homotransplantation of the human kidney between identical twins. JAMA 160:277, 1956.

13. Murray JE, Merrill JP, Harrison JH: Kidney transplantation between seven pairs of identical twins. Ann Surg 148:343, 1958.

14. Wilson RE, Dealy JB Jr, Sadowsky NL, et al: Transplantation of homologous bone marrow and skin from common multiple donors follow-ing total body irradiation. Surgery 46:261, 1969.

15. Mannick JA, Lochte HL Jr, Ashley CA, et al: A functioning kidney homotransplant in the dog. Surgery 46:821, 1959.

16. Murray JE: Remembrances of the early days of renal transplantation. Transplant Proc 13(suppl 1):9, 1981.

17. Schwartz R, Damashek W: Drug induced immu-nological tolerance. Nature 183:1682, 1959.

18. Calne RY: The rejection of renal homografts. In-hibition in dogs by 6-mercaptopurine. Lancet 1:417, 1960.

19. Zukowski CF, Lee HM, Hume DH: The prolon-gation of functional survival of canine renal homograft by 6-mercaptopurine. Surg Form 11:470, 1960.

20. Calne RY: Inhibition of the rejection of renal hom-ografts in dogs with purine analogues. Trans-plant Bull 28:445, 1961.

21. Calne RY, Alexandre GPJ, Murray JE: A study of the effects of drugs in prolonging survival of homologous renal transplants in dogs. Ann NY Acad Sci 99:743, 1962.

22. Murray JE, Merrill JP, Dammin GJ, et al: Kidney transplantation in modified recipients. Ann Surg 156:337, 1962.

23. Goodwin WE, Kaufmann JJ, Mims MM, et al: Human renal transplantation: I. Clinical expe-riences with six cases of renal homotransplan-tation. J Urol 89:13, 1963.

24. Starzl TE, Marchioro TL, Waddell WR: The re-versal of rejection in human renal homografts with subsequent development of homograft tol-erance. Surg Gynecol Obstet 117:385, 1963.

25. Hume DM, Magee JH, Kauffman HM, et al: Renal transplantation in man in modified recipients. Ann Surg 158:608, 1963.

26. Marchioro TL, Axtell KH, LaVia MF, et al: The role of adrenocortical steroids in reversing es-tablished homograft rejection. Surgery 55:412, 1964.

27. Starzl TE, Marchioro TL, Porter KA, et al: The use of heterologous antilymphoid agents in ca-nine renal and liver homotransplantation and in human renal homotransplantation. Surg Gyne-col Obstet 124:301, 1967.

28. Woodruff MFA, Anderson NF: Effect of lympho-cyte depletion by thoracic duct fistula and ad-ministration of antilymphocyte serum on the survival of skin homografts in rats. Nature 200:702, 1963.

29. Borel JF: The history of cyclosporin A and its significance. In White DJG (ed): Cyclosporin A: Proceedings of an International Conference on Cyclosporin A. New York, Elsevier Biomedical Press, 1982, pp 7–8.

30. Borel JF: Comparative study of *in vitro* and *in vivo* drug effects on cell mediated cytotoxicity. Im-munology 31:631, 1976.

31. Calne RY: The development of immunosuppres-sion in organ transplantation. In Morris PJ, Til-ney NL (eds): Progress in Transplantation. London, Churchill Livingstone, 1984, Vol 1, p 5.

32. Kostakis AJ, White DJG, Calne RY: Prolongation of the rat heart allograft survival by cyclosporin A. IRCS Med Sci 5:280, 1977.

33. Green CJ, Allison AC, Precious S: Induction of specific tolerance in rabbits by kidney allograft-ing and short periods of cyclosporin treatment. Lancet 2:123, 1979.

34. Dunn DC, White DJG, Wade J: Survival of first and second kidney allografts after withdrawal of cyclosporin A therapy. IRCS Med Sci 6:464, 1978.

35. Calne RY, White DJG, Rolles K, et al: Prolonged survival of pig orthotopic heart grafts treated with cyclosporin A. Lancet 1:1183, 1978.

36. Calne RY, White DJG: Cyclosporin A—A pow-erful immunosuppressant in dogs with renal al-lografts. IRCS Med Sci 5:595, 1977.

37. Calne RY, White DJG, Thiru S, et al: Cyclosporin A in patients receiving renal allografts from ca-daver donors. Lancet 2:1323, 1978.

38. Calne RY, Rolles K, White DJG, et al: Cyclo-sporin A initially as the only immunosuppres-sant in 34 recipients of cadaveric organs: 32 kid-neys, 2 pancreases, and 2 livers. Lancet 2:1033, 1979.

39. Calne RY, Rolles K, White DJG, et al: Cyclo-sporin A in clinical organ grafting. Transplant Proc 13:349, 1981.

40. Sells RA: A prospective randomized substitutive trial of cyclosporine as a prophylactic agent in human renal transplant rejection. Transplant Proc 15:2495, 1983.

41. Starzl TE, Weil R, Iwatsuki S, et al: The use of cyclosporine A and prednisone in cadaver kid-

ney transplantation. Surg Gynecol Obstet 151:17, 1980.

42. Starzl TE, Hakala TR, Rosenthal JT, Iwatsuki S, Shaw BW Jr: The Colorado-Pittsburgh cadaveric renal transplantation study with cyclosporine. Transplant Proc 15:2862, 1983.

43. Calne RY, White DJG, Evans DB, et al: Cyclosporin A in cadaveric organ transplantation. Br Med J 282:934, 1981.

44. Kahan BD, Van Buren CT, Flechner SM, et al: Cyclosporine immunosuppression mitigates immunologic risk factors in renal allotransplantation. Transplant Proc 15:2469, 1983.

45. Canadian Multicentre Transplant Study Group: A randomized clinical trial of cyclosporine in cadaveric renal transplantation. N Engl J Med 309:809, 1983.

46. Carpenter BJ, Tilney NL, Strom TB, et al: Cyclosporin A in cadaver renal allografts. Kidney Int 19:265, 1981.

47. Najarian JS, Strand M, Fryd DS, et al: Comparison of cyclosporine versus azathioprine-antilymphocyte globulin in renal transplantation. Transplant Proc 15:2463, 1983.

48. Sheil AGR, Hall BM, Tiller DJ, et al: Australian trial of cyclosporine (CsA) in cadaveric donor renal transplantation. Transplant Proc 15:2485, 1983.

49. Starzl TE, Iwatsuki S, Van Thiel DH, et al: Evolution of liver transplantation. Hepatology 2:614, 1982.

50. Oyer PE, Stinson EB, Jamieson SW, et al: Cyclosporin A in cardiac allografting: A preliminary experience. Transplant Proc 15:1247, 1983.

51. Shumway NE: Recent advances in cardiac transplantation. Transplant Proc 15:1221, 1983.

52. Copeland JG, Griepp RB, Bieber CP, et al: Successful retransplantation of the human heart. J Thorac Cardiovasc Surg 73:242, 1977.

53. Shaw BW Jr, Gordon RD, Iwatsuki S, Starzl TE: Hepatic retransplantation. Transplant Proc 17:264, 1985.

54. Shaw BW Jr, Gordon RD, Iwatsuki S, Starzl TE: Retransplantation of the liver. Semin Liver Dis 5:394, 1985.

55. Kahan BC, Reid M, Newburger J: Pharmacokinetics of cyclosporine in human transplantation. Transplant Proc 15:446, 1983.

56. Venkataramanan R, Burckart GJ, Ptachcinski RJ: Pharmacokinetics and monitoring of cyclosporine following orthotopic liver transplantation. Semin Liver Dis 5:357, 1985.

57. Stiller CR, Keown PA: Cyclosporine therapy in perspective. In Morris PJ, Tilney NL (eds): Progress in Transplantation. London, Churchill Livingstone, 1984, Vol 1, pp 11–45.

58. Starzl TE, Hakala TR, Rosenthal JT, et al: Variable convalescence and therapy after cadaveric renal transplantation under cyclosporin A and steroids. Surg Gynecol Obstet 154:819, 1982.

59. Van Buren CT: Four strategies to initiate immunosuppressive therapy: Strategy II—double drug. Transplant Immunol Ltr 2:2, 1985.

60. Ferguson R: Four strategies to initiate immunosuppressive therapy: Strategy IV—quadruple drug. Transplant Immunol Ltr 2:3, 1985.

61. Sommer BG, Ferguson RM: Three immediate postrenal transplant adjunct protocols combined with cyclosporine. Transplant Proc 17:1235, 1985.

62. Kahan BA: Four strategies to initiate immunosuppressive therapy. Transplant Immunol Ltr 2:1, 1985.

63. Slapak M: Four strategies to initiate immunosuppressive therapy: Strategy III—triple drug. Transplant Immunol Ltr 2:3, 1985.

64. Slapak M, Geoghegan T, Digard NJ, et al: The use of low-dose cyclosporine in combination with azathioprine and steroids in renal transplantation. Transplant Proc 17:1222, 1985.

65. Starzl TE, Iwatsuki S, Shaw BW Jr: Liver homotransplantation. In Sabiston DC Jr (ed): Textbook of Surgery. Philadelphia, WB Saunders Company, 1986, pp 457–468.

66. Burckart GJ, Venkataramanan R, Ptachinski R, et al: Cyclosporine absorption following orthotopic liver transplantation. J Clin Pharmacol. In press.

67. Gridelli B, Scanlon L, Seltman H, et al: Cyclosporine metabolism and pharmacokinetics following intravenous and oral doses in the dog. Transplant Proc 17:107, 1985.

68. Burckart G, Starzl TE, Williams L, et al: Cyclosporine monitoring and pharmacokinetics in pediatric liver transplant recipients. Transplant Proc 17:1172, 1985.

69. Cosimi AB, Colvin R, Burton R, et al: Use of monoclonal antibodies to T cell subsets for immunologic monitoring and treatment in recipients of renal allografts. N Engl J Med 305:308, 1981.

70. Cosimi AB, Burton RC, Colvin RB, et al: Treatment of acute renal allograft rejection with OKT3 monoclonal antibody. Transplantation 32:535, 1981.

71. Burton RC, Cosimi AB, Colvin RB, et al: Monoclonal antibodies to human T-cell subsets: Use for immunological monitoring and immunosuppression in renal transplantation. J Clin Immunol 2(suppl):142, 1982.

72. Thistlethwaite JR, Cosimi AB, Delmonico FL, et al: Transplantation. To be published.

73. Goldstein G, Schindler J, Sheahan M, et al: Orthoclone OKT3 treatment of acute renal allograft rejection. Transplant Proc 17:129, 1985.

74. Norman DJ, Barry JM, Henell K, et al: Reversal of acute allograft rejection with monoclonal antibody. Transplant Proc 17:39, 1985.

75. Kreis H, Chkoff H, Vigeral P, et al: Prophylactic treatment of allograft recipients with a monoclonal anti-T3$^+$ cell antibody. Transplant Proc 17:1315, 1985.

76. Fung JJ, Demetris AJ, Porter KA, et al: Use of OKT3 with cyclosporine and steroids for reversal of acute kidney and liver allograft rejection. Unpublished data.

77. Cosimi AB, Cho SI, Delmonico FL, et al: A randomized trial of OKT3 monoclonal antibody for hepatic allograft rejection. Transplant Proc. Unpublished data.

78. Reitz BA, Wallwork JL, Hunt SA, et al: Heartlung transplantation: Successful therapy for patients with pulmonary vascular disease. N Engl J Med 306:557, 1982.

79. Starzl TE, Iwatsuki S, Shaw BW Jr, et al: Pancreaticoduodenal transplantation in humans. Surg Gynecol Obstet 159:265, 1984.

80. Macedo C, Greenleaf GE, Sayers HJ, Orloff MJ:

Effect of whole pancreas transplantation on long-established kidney lesions of diabetes. Surg Forum 36:346, 1985.

81. Gil-Vernet JM, Fernandez-Cruz L, Andreu J, et al: Clinical experience with pancreaticopyelostomy for exocrine pancreatic drainage and portal venous drainage in pancreas transplantation. Transplant Proc 17:342, 1985.

82. Solinger HW, Kalayoglu M, Hoffman RM, et al: Results of segmental and pancreaticosplenic transplantation with pancreaticocystostomy. Transplant Proc 17:360, 1985.

83. Lillihei R, Simmons R, Najarian J, et al: Pancreatico-duodenal allotransplantation: Experimental and clinical experience. Ann Surg 172:405, 1970.

84. Caves PK, Stinson EB, Graham AE, et al: Percutaneous transvenous endomyocardial biopsy. JAMA 225:289, 1973.

85. Opelz G, Sengar DPS, Mickey MR, Terasaki PI: Effect of blood transfusions on subsequent kidney transplants. Transplant Proc 5:253, 1973.

86. Salvatiera O Jr, Vincenti F, Amend W, et al: Deliberate donor-specific blood transfusions prior to living related renal transplantation. A new approach. Ann Surg 192:543, 1980.

87. Salvatiera O Jr, Vinceenti F, Amend W, et al: Update of the University of California at San Francisco experience with donor-specific blood transfusions. Transplant Proc 14:363, 1982.

88. Ting A, Morris PJ: Powerful effect of HLA-DR match on survival of cadaveric renal allografts. Lancet 2:282, 1980.

89. Svejgaard A: DR matching and cadaver kidney transplantation. Transplantation 33:1, 1982.

90. Wood RFM, Thompson JF, Allen NH, et al: The consequences of conversion from cyclosporine to azathioprine and prednisolone in renal allograft recipients. Transplant Proc 15(suppl 1):2862, 1983.

91. Canafax DM, Sutherland DER, Ascher NL, et al: Cyclosporine nephrotoxicity in renal allograft recipients: Conversion to azathioprine to improve renal function. Transplant Proc 15(suppl 1):2874, 1983.

92. Flechner SM, Van Buren CT, Kerman R, Kahan BD: The effect of conversion from cyclosporine to azathioprine immunosuppression for intractable nephrotoxicity. Transplant Proc 15(suppl 1):2869, 1983.

93. Wood RFM, Thompson JF, Ting A, et al: A randomized controlled trial of short-term cyclosporine therapy in renal transplantation (trial II). Transplant Proc 17:1164, 1985.

94. Canafax DM, Martel EJ, Ascher NL, et al: Two methods of managing cyclosporine nephrotoxicity: Conversion to azathioprine, prednisone, or cyclosporine, azathioprine, and prednisone. Transplant Proc 17:1176, 1985.

95. Rocher LL, Milford EL, Kirman RL, et al: Utility of azathioprine in management of renal allograft recipients initially treated with cyclosporine. Transplant Proc 17:1185, 1985.

96. Tegzess AM, Donker AJM, Meijer S: Improvement in renal function after conversion from cyclosporine to prednisolone/azathioprine in renal transplant patients. Transplant Proc 17:1191, 1985.

97. Land W, Castro LA, Hillebrand G, et al: Conversion rejection consequences by changing the immunosuppressive therapy from cyclosporine to azathioprine after kidney transplantation. Transplant Proc 15(suppl 1):2857, 1983.

98. Vanrenterghem Y, Waer M, Michielsen P: A controlled trial of one versus three months' cyclosporine and conversion to azathioprine in renal transplantation. Transplant Proc 17:1162, 1985.

99. Flechner SM, Van Buren CT, Jarowenko M, et al: The fate of patients converted from cyclosporine to azathioprine to improve renal function. Transplant Proc 17:1227, 1985.

100. Squifflet JP, Sutherland DER, Field J, et al: Synergistic immunosuppressive effect of cyclosporin A and azathioprine. Transplant Proc 15(suppl 1):520, 1983.

101. Billingham RE, Brent L, Medawar PB: Actively acquired tolerance of foreign cells. Nature 172:603, 1953.

102. Facilitation of allograft survival and immunological tolerance. Transplant Proc 17:1015, 1985.

103. Najarian JS, Bach FH, Sutherland DER, Rapaport FT (eds): Transplantation Today. Orlando, Grune & Stratton, 1985, pp 1015–1152.

104. Cortesini R, Renna Molajoni E, Monari C, et al: Total lymphoid irradiation in clinical transplantation: Experience in 30 high-risk patients. Transplant Proc 17:1291, 1985.

105. Haas G, Halperin E, Dorseretz D, et al: Prolonging the immunosuppressive effects of lymphoid irradiation by suppression of T cell recovery prior to organ transplantation. Transplant Proc 17:1294, 1985.

106. Sampson D, Levin BS, Hoppe RT, et al: Preliminary observations on the use of total lymphoid irradiation, rabbit antihymocyte globulin, and low-dose prednisone in human cadaver renal transplantation. Transplant Proc 17:1299, 1985.

107. Gartner JC Jr, Zitelli BJ, Malatack JJ, et al: Orthotopic liver transplantation in children: 2-year experience with 47 patients. Pediatrics 74:140, 1984.

108. Urbach AH, Gartner JC Jr, Malatack JJ, et al: Linear growth following pediatric liver transplantation. Unpublished data.

109. Shaw BW Jr, Starzl TE, Iwatsuki S, Gordon RD: An overview of orthotopic transplantation of the liver. In Flye W (ed): Principles of Organ Transplantation. Philadelphia, WB Saunders Company, 1986.

110. Friedman EA: Kidney transplantation is the preferred therapy for uremia. Transplant Proc 17:1500, 1985.

111. Simmons RG, Anderson CR, Kamstra LK, Ames NG: Quality of life and alternate end-stage renal disease therapies. Transplant Proc 17:1577, 1985.

# 5

# Infection and Organ Transplantation

MONTO HO

Infection is probably second only to organ rejection as a primary concern of surgeons and physicians taking care of patients after organ transplantation.

Table 5–1 summarizes risk factors for infection in transplant recipients. Over the years we have systematically determined the role of many of these factors, particularly in the case of virus infections, and we have studied those for which we had little information. In many cases, precise information is still absent.

**TABLE 5–1. Risk Factors for Infections in Transplant Recipients**

1. Underlying disease and type of organ failure
2. Type of organ transplanted and trauma of surgery
3. Source of microbial pathogen
   a. Endogenous flora and latent infection
   b. Transmission via donated organ or tissue
   c. Transfused blood and blood products
   d. Environment (persons and physical)
4. Depression of host resistance
   a. Surgical factors
   b. Immunosuppression (azathioprine, cyclosporine, antithymocyte globulin, steroids)
   c. Host-vs-graft reaction (rejection)
   d. Graft-vs-host reaction

The underlying disease and type of organ failure are important factors. We have determined, for example, that liver transplant recipients who were receiving steroids or antibiotics before transplantation were at greater risk for subsequent fungus infection.[1] Bone marrow transplantation is a unique case because this is the only type of transplant in which the organ or transplanted tissue is nonfunctional for a significant time after transplantation. While awaiting bone marrow engraftment, the patient is severely immunosuppressed in terms of phagocyte and lymphocyte function and therefore at high risk for infection. Later a unique immunological reaction peculiar to bone marrow transplantation, the graft-versus-host reaction, might ensue. This type of reaction is also immunosuppressive, as it has been associated with activation of cytomegalovirus (CMV) infection in animals[2] and with CMV pneumonia in human patients.[3] Pneumocystis pneumonia is also frequently seen in bone marrow transplant recipients, often in conjunction with graft-versus-host reaction and/or signs of CMV pneumonia.[4] In many ways bone marrow transplantation is an extreme example of the hazards for infection after transplantation.[3,4]

49

## SOURCE OF PATHOGENS

The source of the microbial pathogens in patients is related to the type of transplantation. For example, endogenous flora in the gastrointestinal tract may be released if the integrity of this system is violated. One of our most important early findings from studying renal transplant patients was that the donated organ was the main source of primary infection by CMV.[5] The role of transfused blood in producing viral infections, particularly CMV infections, is also well documented.[4] This risk is a function of the type and amount of blood transfused. It is reduced in the case of leukocyte-poor blood or blood that has been frozen and stored. The risk is negligible if the number of units transfused during the operation is less than four or five. But it may well be significant in liver or heart transplantation in which much more blood than this may be used, although this specific point has not been studied.

The biological as well as physical environment may be a source of organisms for the transplant recipient. If the susceptibility of the host is unusually high, ordinarily avirulent environmental organisms may become infective. This is true in bone marrow transplantation, in which prodigious efforts at environmental isolation of the patient have been made from time to time.[3] Certain fungi, such as *Aspergillus*, which arise from the physical environment, are particularly troublesome. *Nocardia* is another important opportunistic fungus that is also assumed to come from the environment. *Candida*, on the other hand, is almost always endogenous. The large numbers of bacteria, both gram-negative and gram-positive, that are causes of wound and systemic infection after transplantation may arise either from the patient *per se* or from the hospital environment. There is no doubt that the hospital may be the source of significant pathogens, even though no particular precautionary measures are taken for renal, liver, heart, and heart and lung transplant recipients. Highly resistant bacteria, such as methicillin-resistant *Staphylococcus*, and multiply resistant *Pseudomonas* and *Enterobacter* may also be peculiar to certain hospitals. One important environmental organism in our institution is *Legionella pneumophila*. Every year since 1981 we have had about four to six cases of pneumonia due to this organism despite hyperchlorination of our hot water system.[6]

Whether this represents an irreducible minimum or a preventable problem remains to be determined. We have also noted that significantly more serious infections are caused by *Staphylococcus epidermidis* and *Candida* species. However, this is probably more the result of selective forces engendered by heavy use of antibiotics than of environmental spread.

## APPROACH TO INFECTIONS IN TRANSPLANT RECIPIENTS

Transplant recipients are frequently very ill with multiple disorders. The diagnosis and treatment of infections in these patients are a major challenge. An expert or, better, a group interested in infectious disease is a necessity in any center dealing with a significant number of transplantations. This group must be able and willing to work with other colleagues and be part of a team. An important problem is that the team may work at cross-purposes unless it is properly coordinated by a primary physician. The diagnostic microbiology laboratory is an essential part of the infectious disease expertise. It should be able to handle large numbers of specimens with dispatch and be able to provide expert diagnosis in bacteriology, virology, mycology, and parasitology. Depending on the type of transplantation, there may be need for surveillance cultures and serological studies. We have found periodical cultures of throat, urine, and buffy coat for CMV and herpes simplex virus to be useful in managing patients with heart, heart and lung, and liver transplants. They might also be very useful in bone marrow transplant recipients. They are probably no longer indicated in renal transplant recipients because significant morbidity from viruses in these patients is relatively low. Routine serological determinations are not required, but we have found that saving serum from the donor and the recipient, before and at intervals after transplantation, is a useful procedure. Frequently serological diagnosis is possible only if prior samples are available for observation of diagnostic rise. Serodiagnosis has helped us in the diagnosis and management of CMV, herpes simplex virus (HSV), Epstein-Barr virus (EBV), hepatitis A and B, toxoplasmosis, legionellosis, and HTLV-III infections. Infections are more frequent and more severe and complicated within the immediate post-transplantation period. Surveillance cultures and protocol samples are most useful when collected during the initial hospitalization and for three to six months after transplantation.

Proper therapy of infectious disease in transplant recipients, as in other patients, depends on specific diagnosis. We cannot go into details here, and only a few principles will be mentioned. Administration of antibiotics without proper indication is to be avoided. Antibiotics used for prophylaxis during surgery should be stopped shortly after surgery and not be used for more than 72 hours. My experience has been that febrile episodes of presumed infectious etiology without demonstrable site or cause, so common in the leukopenic patient receiving chemotherapy for lymphoproliferative cancer, are unusual in the transplant patient. By and large they are less immunosuppressed and their infections are diagnosable. Hence there is less need to use antibiotics for undiagnosed febrile episodes. The danger of abuse of antibiotics may not be apparent in individual cases, but becomes obvious after study of patient groups. They include the development of highly resistant gram-negative organisms (particularly to third-generation cephalosporins) and emergence of organisms, such as coagulase-negative *Staphylococcus*, and yeasts for which antibiotic treatment is still unsatisfactory.

Apparently nontoxic antibiotics may produce unexpected problems in the transplant recipient. These relate to compromised organ function and drug interactions. For example, it is now known that ketoconazole,[7] erythromycin,[8] and probably rifampin increase the half-life and toxicity of cyclosporine, presumably through inhibition of the cytochrome P-450 system.

## NONVIRAL INFECTIONS IN TRANSPLANT RECIPIENTS

### Kidney Recipients

Most symptomatic infections after transplantation are caused by bacteria. Characteristics of such infections may be obtained from data collected by our team from renal transplant recipients from 1978 to 1980, all of whom received classic azathioprine and prednisone therapy.[9] Fifty-nine patients were followed-up for 12 months, and all types of infections were recorded. Three patients died in six months, and nine patients died

after one year (15 per cent). Most of the infections (78 per cent) occurred in the first three months, while an additional 10 per cent of all infections occurred later, between three and twelve months after transplantation.

The four most common types of nonviral infections were infections of the urinary tract, lung, skin and wound, and peritoneal and perinephric region. There were 38, 13, 10, and 6 patients respectively who had these types of infection. Each patient had a mean 1.44 episodes of infection.

The most frequent infection was of the urinary tract. There were 50 episodes in 38 (64 per cent) patients. The type of organisms does not differ from urinary pathogens in other patient groups. The most common isolates were *Escherichia coli* (5), *Klebsiella* (4), *Pseudomonas aeruginosa* (3), and enterococci (2).

Pulmonary infections are examples of more severe infections. They were defined by clinical diagnoses based on the presence of fever, pulmonary infiltrates seen on x-ray examination, and frequently leukocytosis. Table 5–2 lists the causes of 25 episodes of pulmonary infection in 19 patients. Of these, 19 were due to bacteria, 2 to fungi, 2 to a protozoan, and 1 to CMV; in 4 cases of clin-

**TABLE 5–2. Pathogens Causing Pulmonary Infections in Renal Transplant Recipients Treated with Azathioprine and Prednisone**

| Pathogen | Times Isolated |
|---|---|
| **Bacterium** | 19 |
| *Staphylococcus aureus* | 5 |
| *Legionella micdadei* | 3 |
| *Legionella pneumophila* | 2 |
| *Pseudomonas aeruginosa* | 3 |
| *Hemophilus influenza* | 1 |
| Streptococcus (group A) | 1 |
| *Escherichia coli* | 1 |
| *Streptococcus faecalis* | 1 |
| *Serratia marcescens* | 1 |
| *Acinetobacter* | 1 |
| **Fungus** | 2 |
| Aspergillus | 1 |
| Nocardia | 1 |
| **Virus** | |
| Cytomegalovirus | 1 |
| **Parasite** | |
| *Pneumocystis* | 2 |

* Isolated together with another bacterium.
From Poorsattar A, Dowling JN, Ho M: Unpublished data.

ical pulmonary infection, no significant pathogens were isolated.

The severity of bacterial infections may be gleaned from the description of bacteremias (Table 5–3). Ten patients (17 per cent) had 13 episodes of bacteremia. Five patients died within one year after transplantation, but in only two patients were the deaths associated with the bacteremia. *Staphylococcus aureus* caused the most episodes.[9] In most cases the source of bacteria and cause of the bacteremias were determined.

It is instructive to compare these data to the more recent data on infections in renal patients treated with cyclosporine and prednisone.[9] After an initial randomized trial of azathioprine and cyclosporine therapy,[10] all transplant recipients in Pittsburgh since 1982 have been treated with cyclosporine and prednisone. In 64 renal transplant recipients receiving cyclosporine and prednisone, there was no mortality after six months. The number of nonviral (mostly bacterial) infections was significantly decreased; 41 per cent of the patients had a total of 39 episodes. Thus the mean number of nonviral infections per patient was 0.61 (as opposed to the previous 1.44 episodes per patient treated with azathioprine and prednisone).

The range of infections in the cyclosporine group was similar to that of patients treated with azathioprine. Urinary tract infection was still the most frequent and caused 40 per cent of all the infections. Only 3 of 64 (5 per cent) cyclosporine renal patients developed pulmonary infections, which is significantly less than in patients treated with azathioprine. All three episodes were due to gramnegative bacteria; none was due to staphylococcus, previously the most important pathogen. We noted a marked reduction of staphylococcus infection at other sites as well. This marked reduction in bacterial infections in renal recipients was not paralleled by a reduction in virus infections; it was also in contrast to infections in other transplant groups treated with cyclosporine (see below).

## Heart and Liver Transplant Recipients

In terms of proportion of patients infected and number of episodes per patient, the liver and heart transplant recipients had more nonviral infections than the renal patients: 53 per cent of the cardiac and 67 per cent of the hepatic transplant recipients developed nonviral infections. The mean number of infections per patient was 0.88 and 1.42 respectively.[9]

Table 5–4 describes perhaps the more important differences among the three groups. The sites of infection and mortality due to infection varied according to type of transplant.[11] Liver transplant recipients had primarily abdominal biliary tract and intestinal infections; kidney transplant recipients had urinary tract infections; while heart recipients had pulmonary and intrathoracic infections. These sites are clearly related to the site of operation and type of organ transplanted. The severity of infections in these

### TABLE 5–3.    Bacteremia in Renal Transplant Recipients

| Patient No. | Organism | Days PT | Associated Infection | Outcome PT |
|---|---|---|---|---|
| 33 | *Staphylococcus aureus* | 19 | Urinary tract infection | Died 6–12 mo |
|  | *Streptococcus faecalis* | 19 | Urinary tract infection |  |
|  | *Serratia marcescens* | 19 | Urinary tract infection |  |
| 11 | *Staphylococcus aureus* | 73 | Perinephric abscess | Alive 12 mo |
|  | *Bacteroides fragilis* | 186 | Source unknown |  |
| 2 | *Staphylococcus aureus* | 18 | Lung infection | Alive 12 mo |
| 15 | *Staphylococcus aureus* | 122 | Urinary tract infection | Died 4 mo |
| 90 | *Staphylococcus aureus* | 79 | Intravenous line | Died 3 mo |
| 44 | *Staphylococcus aureus* | 28 | Perinephric abscess | Alive 1 yr |
| 6 | Streptococcus (group A) | 160 | Urinary tract infection | Alive 1 yr |
| 12 | *Escherichia coli* | 47 | Source unknown | Died 3–6 mo |
| 50 | *Escherichia coli* | 7 | Wound infection, peritonitis | Alive 1 yr |
| 59 | *Bifidobacterium* | 46 | Perinephric abscess | Alive 1 yr |

PT = post transplantation.
From Poorsattar A, Dowling JN, Ho M: Unpublished data.

**TABLE 5–4.** Site of Infections According to Type of Transplant in Recipients Treated with Cyclosporine

| Type of Transplant | Frequent Sites of Infection | | % Bacteremia | % Fungemia | % Infection-Associated Deaths |
| --- | --- | --- | --- | --- | --- |
| | Site | % of all infections | | | |
| Kidney | Urinary tract | 41 | 5 | 0 | 0 |
| Heart | Pulmonary and intrathoracic | 38 | 24 | 0 | 27 |
| Liver | Abdominal and gastrointestinal | 35 | 30 | 16 | 40 |

Data taken from Ho M, Wajszczuk CP, Hardy A, Dummer JS, Starzl TE, Hakala TR, Bahnson HT: Infections in kidney, heart and liver transplant recipients on cyclosporine. Transplant Proc 15:2768–2772, 1983.

three groups varied considerably as seen from the frequency of bacteremia. Its incidence was low in the case of kidney recipients (5 per cent), and relatively high in heart (24 per cent) and liver (30 per cent) transplant patients. More important is the fact that 40 per cent of deaths in patients with liver transplants were associated with severe infections. As opposed to this, no death in the renal transplant group could be attributed to infection.

The types of organisms that infected the three different transplant groups also differed. These differences are illustrated in Figure 5–1. The first two bars represent the proportion of infections in patients who were receiving a randomized trial of azathioprine and cyclosporine. As already pointed out, patients taking azathioprine had more bacterial (nonviral) infections and more gram-positive

and staphylococcal infections. The proportion of patients with gram-negative infections was not significantly different in renal patients treated with azathioprine or cyclosporine or in heart and liver recipients.

## FUNGUS INFECTIONS IN TRANSPLANT RECIPIENTS

It is well known that systemic fungal infections, particularly due to *Candida, Aspergillus, Cryptococcus,* and *Nocardia,* occur sporadically in many types of immunosuppressed patients, including transplant recipients. However, when we had the opportunity to compare infections in different types of transplantation, it became clear that severe and frequent fungus infections are a special problem of liver transplant recipients.[1,9,11] The predominant fungi were yeasts

**Figure 5–1.** Comparison of proportion of patients who develop bacterial, fungal, and viral infections among (1) renal patients treated with azathioprine and prednisone; (2) comparable renal patients treated with cyclosporine and prednisone; (3) cardiac patients treated with cyclosporine and prednisone; and (4) liver patients treated with cyclosporine and prednisone. (From Dummer JS, White LT, Ho M, Griffith GP, Hardesty RL, Bahnson HT: Morbidity of cytomegalovirus infection in recipients of heart or heart-lung transplants who received cyclosporine. J Infect Dis 152:1182–1191, 1985, with permission of authors and publisher.)

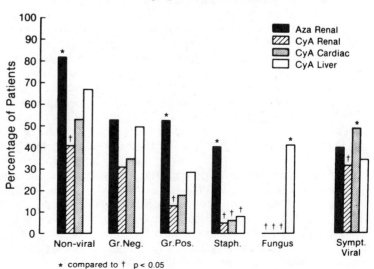

Proportion of Transplant Patients with Symptomatic Infections

* compared to † p < 0.05

of the *Candida* species. Leukopenia, immunosuppression, excess use of antibiotics, and abdominal surgery are known predisposing factors of this type of infection.[12] All transplant recipients receive many antibiotics and undergo immunosuppression, and liver transplant surgery uniquely involves entering the upper gastrointestinal tract, which has sites of normal candidal colonization.

We studied 62 liver transplant recipients and found that 26 (42 per cent) had 30 episodes of severe fungal infections. Superficial mucosal infections by *Candida* were excluded. Of 30 episodes of fungal infections, 22 were due to *Candida*, 6 to *Aspergillus*, and 1 each to *Cryptococcus* and *Mucor*. There were 10 episodes of disseminated candidal infection, and 13 candidal infections were associated with death.[1] Dissemination was defined as infection at two anatomically noncontiguous sites, at least one of which almost always involved the site of operation, such as the wound, biliary tree, peritoneal cavity, abdominal drainage sites, or chest. Only 41 per cent of the episodes of candidal infection resolved. The remainder of the patients died, although it is at times difficult to determine the importance of the fungus infection in such deaths. All 6 patients with *Aspergillus* infection had infections of the lung and died. The mortality after two months of follow-up after transplantation in the group without fungus infections was 8 per cent (3/36), while the mortality in 26 patients with fungus infections was 69 per cent (18/26). These infections occurred primarily in the immediate post-transplantation period. All except 3 of the 26 patients became infected within eight weeks after transplantation. The most frequent time of occurrence was within the first week.

The following factors were significantly associated with increased fungal infections: preoperative administration of steroids or antibiotics, longer transplant operation time, and reoperations after transplantation for corrective surgery or for retransplantation. Patients with fungal infections also had received more antibiotics and had more bacterial infections. The type of pathology underlying the transplantation was also an important factor. Patients with primary biliary cirrhosis had significantly fewer fungal infections as well as lower mortality than patients with other diseases, such as chronic active hepatitis, carcinoma, hepatoma, and primary sclerosing cholangitis. Fungal infection was associated with rejection episodes.

Whether there is a causal relationship and which is the cause and which is the effect is not known. It has not been determined whether better monitoring of immunosuppressants can help reduce fungus infections. Other measures that remain to be studied and might be preventive are reduction of candidal colonization prior to surgery and more directed and regulated use of antibiotics.

## VIRUS INFECTIONS IN TRANSPLANT RECIPIENTS

About 40 to 50 per cent of transplant patients develop some form of symptomatic virus infection (see Fig. 5–1). One of the most striking features about them is that only a few viruses are culpable.[13] These are viruses that remain latent in humans and hence become ready pathogens when antiviral resistance is compromised. They are also agents that by and large infect patients with congenital or acquired cellular immune deficiency, including acquired immune deficiency syndrome (AIDS).

The most important group of viruses that produce morbidity in transplant recipients is the herpesvirus group, DNA viruses that include CMV, HSV types I and II, varicella-zoster (VZ), and EBV. Adenoviruses have also been implicated, particularly in bone marrow transplant recipients. By routine virus cultures of 1051 recipients, Shields et al.[14] found that 51 (4.9 per cent) of the cultures were positive. Ten (one fifth) of these patients were symptomatic; four had pneumonia, two had nephritis, and two hepatitis. Occasionally adenovirus hepatitis has been seen in children after liver transplantation (E. Yunis, personal communication). This virus may be more pathogenic in marrow recipients, as it has been associated with a graft-versus-host reaction and may also represent reactivation of an endogenous, latent infection.

Papovaviruses represent another DNA virus that is prone to latent infection. Warts, caused by human papillomaviruses, are an important problem in renal transplant recipients, particularly long-term survivors.[13]

The incidence of herpes simplex infections varies in different series.[13] We found that in 94 renal, heart, and liver recipients treated with cyclosporine, 47 per cent had evidence of herpes simplex infection when mouthwashes and urine were routinely cultured; only about half (21/44) were symptomatic.[9]

In the same group of 94 patients, 4 developed herpes zoster.

Most of the herpes simplex infections in transplant recipients are self-limited episodes of oral-labial reactivation, indistinguishable from the course in normal subjects. At times, perhaps less commonly than in leukopenic patients with lymphoproliferative disorders, a progressive mucocutaneous lesion may develop.[15] We have also observed genital herpes, at times severe. Recently disseminated vesicular eruption due to HSV type II developed in two patients after receiving kidneys from one seropositive donor (JS Dummer et al., unpublished data).

Herpes simplex infections can now be treated with oral or intravenous acyclovir, while herpes zoster may be treated with acyclovir, 500 mg/m$^2$ IV three times a day.

**Cytomegalovirus Infection.** CMV infection and some other virus infections in transplant recipients may be documented by culturing mouthwashes, blood buffy coat, or urine, or by showing a rise in antibodies against CMV. Only a fraction of infected patients are symptomatic. The proportion of infected patients to diseased patients varies with the type of immunosuppression and the type of transplantation.

The distinction between primary and secondary or reactivated infections should be clearly understood. The first occurs in the seronegative "virgin," while the second represents activation of a latent infection of a seropositive "immune" person. This is not a problem with virus infections that do not become latent or when acquired immunity is almost absolute. But in the case of CMV, clinical disease may result from either type of infection. There may be a source of confusion in infections in a previously seropositive patient, as it may not be possible to distinguish reinfection from activation. Indeed, reinfection may occur, as shown by mapping of nucleic acid fragments, but it is not the rule.[16]

Typically the primary CMV infections are more symptomatic.[17] There are two situations in transplantation in which this may not be apparent. One is in bone marrow transplantation,[3,4] in which the morbidity due to CMV is generally high and resembles that of primary infection. The patient may have to re-establish his or her immune status after marrow engraftment irrespective of the prior serological status. The second situation is when morbidity due to reactivation infection is increased. The Minnesota group reported that the morbidity of primary and reactivation infection in renal transplant recipients was about the same.[18] Higher morbidity of their reactivated infections may have been due to a greater degree of immunosuppression as a result of the use of antithymocyte globulin in addition to azathioprine and prednisone (see below).

The most important source of primary CMV infection is probably the transplanted organ.[5,19] This hypothesis was proposed largely on the basis of clinical-epidemiological correlations. We found that seronegative recipients became infected only if their donors were seropositive. In the series of Betts et al. all the seronegative recipients who received kidneys from seropositive donors became infected.[19] These simple observations had an important corollary: Normal seropositive subjects almost always carry latent virus in their tissues that is potentially activatable. This also explains why reactivation infections in many series of seropositive transplant recipients approached 100 per cent.[4] As with other herpesvirus infections, CMV infections are basically incurable.

Attempts to isolate the latent virus or to demonstrate it by hybridization techniques in blood or other tissues from seropositive subjects have almost all been unsuccessful. However, in bone marrow recipients it has recently been found that the endonuclease restriction pattern of a fortuitous isolate from a donor and a later isolate from the recipient were identical.[16] In renal transplant recipients who received kidneys from the same donors, CMV isolates were shown to be identical, suggesting that they came from the same source.[18]

CMV infection is frequently asymptomatic, even in the immunosuppressed, but it may have protean clinical manifestations. A febrile episode, lasting from weeks to a month or two, is the most common presentation. Atypical lymphocytosis may be absent, but if seen, there may be less than 10 per cent lymphocytes. It is usually absent in more severe forms of CMV infection. One common feature is an increase in liver enzymes, but hyperbilirubinemia and jaundice are rare. Lymphadenopathy, splenomegaly, and pharyngitis, so common in EBV mononucleosis, are almost never seen in CMV infections. The next most common manifestation of CMV infection is interstitial pneumonitis. The pneumonitis is more likely to show an interstitial than an alveolar pattern, but nodules or cavities may be seen on x-ray films. The virus may be found in lung biopsies, or intranuclear inclusions may be seen in lung tissue. Association with *Pneumocystis* is particularly striking. CMV pneumonia may range from asymptomatic virus shedding to rapidly fatal pneumonia. Consistently, fever, nonproductive cough, and dyspnea associated with hypoxia are observed. Hypoxia is a poor prognostic sign. With reduction of immunosuppression, the course of CMV pneumonia may be benign, even though there is no satisfactory treatment. A new nucleoside antiviral, DHPG, is still under trial.

Other types of clinical manifestations include severe hepatitis, particularly in liver transplant recipients, retinitis, and CMV disease of the gastrointestinal tract. The last includes hemorrhage, colitis, and intestinal perforation. It is not unusual to find at postmortem examination, particularly in a liver, heart, or heart-lung recipient, widely disseminated evidence of CMV infection. Such widespread infection may be entirely unsuspected.

CMV INFECTION IN VARIOUS TRANSPLANT GROUPS. A comparison between CMV infection and morbidity from such infection in two different transplant groups is illustrated. The recent data on CMV infection in renal patients treated with cyclosporine in Pittsburgh are shown in Table 5–5. The rate of infection is 60 per cent, morbidity is low (8 per cent), and among patients with primary infection, significantly more are symptomatic. Even so, symptomatic disease was mild. Only three patients developed pneumonitis (2 per cent).

The infection rate and symptomatology of

CMV disease are different in heart and heart-lung recipients.[20] In 50 heart and 5 heart-lung recipients, 49 (89 per cent) become infected with CMV (Table 5–6); of those infected, 17 patients (35 per cent) became symptomatic. Among the symptomatic group there were 8 cases of CMV pneumonias, that is, 15 per cent of the entire group developed CMV pneumonia. There were 22 seronegative patients, 16 of whom developed primary infection. The remainder of the patients (33) were seropositive, and all (100 per cent) had reactivation infection.

More recent analysis of 18 heart-lung recipients suggests that they indeed not only have more CMV infection, but they also have more *Pneumocystis* and *Pseudomonas* pulmonary infections (JS Dummer et al., unpublished data). It appears that within this subgroup, heart-lung recipients are at greater risk than heart recipients for developing CMV and other infections.

The following differences among the renal, heart, and heart-lung groups are significant (compare Tables 5–5 and 5–6): The total number of CMV infections and primary and reactivation infections is higher in the heart and heart-lung groups. The proportion of patients in the heart and heart-lung groups developing symptomatic infections is significantly higher. The proportions of primary and reactivation infections in this symptomatic group may be individually higher than in the renal groups.

Liver recipients too have more significant CMV disease than renal transplant recipients. Since 1983 we evaluated the status of 65 adult liver transplant recipients; 40 (62 per cent) developed CMV infection. There were 16 symptomatic patients: Seven had CMV in the lung and evidence of pneumonitis or of dissemination with CMV found in various organs at postmortem examination. Four patients had CMV hepatitis as determined by histological evidence obtained from the biopsy. This is a very important finding, since such hepatitis may be confused with rejection.[21] Five patients had a viral febrile syndrome with a favorable outcome. The frequency of symptomatic infection and the type of morbidity resemble more the heart and heart-lung recipients than the renal group.

EFFECT OF IMMUNOSUPPRESSION ON CMV INFECTION AND MORBIDITY. The main effect of different immunosuppressive regimens is on the morbidity of CMV infection rather

**TABLE 5–5. Primary and Reactivated Cytomegalovirus Infections in Renal Transplant Recipients**

| Pretransplant Antibody State | Total No. Patients | No. Patients with Infections (% of Total) | No. Symptomatic Patients (% of infected) |
|---|---|---|---|
| Negative | 37 | 11/37 (30) | 5/11 (45) |
| Positive | 94 | 68/94 (72) | 5/68 (7) |
| | | | |
| Total | 131 | 79/131 (60) | 10/79 (13) |
| Morbidity | | | 10/131 (8) |

**TABLE 5–6.** **Primary and Reactivated Cytomegalovirus Infections in Heart and Heart-Lung Recipients**

| Pretransplant Antibody Status | Total No. Patients | No. Patients with Infections (% of Total) | No. Symptomatic Patients (% of infected) | No. Patients with CMV Pneumonia (% of infection) |
|---|---|---|---|---|
| Negative | 22 | 16/22 (73) | 11/16 (69)* | 5/16 (31) |
| Positive | 33 | 33/33 (100) | 6/33 (18)* | 3/33 (9) |
| Total | 55 | 49/55 (89) | 17/49 (35) | 8/49 (16) |
| Morbidity | | | 17/55 (31) | |

* P < 0.005, primary infections compared with reactivation infections.
Data from Dummer JS, White LT, Ho M, Griffith GP, Hardesty RL, Bahnson HT: Morbidity of cytomegalovirus infection in recipients of heart or heart-lung transplants who received cyclosporine. J Infect Dis 152:1182–1191, 1985.

than the rate of infection. The rate of infection is high in almost all types of major organ transplantation and has not been significantly reduced by any of the new immunosuppressive regimens.

In 1981 to 1983, we monitored the infections of renal transplant recipients randomly assigned to either cyclosporine or azathioprine immunotherapy[9] (see Fig. 5–1). The results on bacterial infection have already been presented. Viral infections, particularly asymptomatic and symptomatic CMV infections, occurred with about the same frequency in these two groups. On the other hand, we feel that another immunosuppressant, antithymocyte globulin, may be responsible for more **morbidity** due to CMV infection in kidney recipients than either cyclosporine or azathioprine.

This point is illustrated by comparison of data from Pittsburgh and Minnesota (Table 5–7). Renal transplant recipients received either azathioprine and prednisone or azathioprine, prednisone, and antithymocyte globulin. In Pittsburgh, 138 patients received the former form of immunosuppression, and there were only three incidents of CMV pneumonia (2.2 per cent). In Minnesota 349 patients received the latter form of immunosuppression, and 29 cases of CMV pneumonia (8.3 per cent) were reported.[22] The frequency of CMV pneumonia in renal transplant recipients treated with cyclosporine and prednisone immunosuppression (3/131, 2.3 per cent) was about the same as in patients treated with azathioprine and prednisone immunosuppression (2.2 per cent).

Morbidity due to CMV infection is differ-

**TABLE 5–7.** **Effect of Immunosuppression and Type of Transplant on Incidence of Cytomegalovirus Pneumonia**

| Type Transplant | Immuno-suppression | Total No. Patients | No. Patients with CMV Pneumonia (% of total) |
|---|---|---|---|
| **Pittsburgh Patients** | | | |
| Kidney | AZ-P | 138 | 3 (2.2) |
| Kidney | Cs-P | 131 | 3 (2.3) |
| Heart and Heart-Lung | Cs-P | 55 | 8 (15.0) |
| **Minnesota Patients** | | | |
| Kidney | AZ-P-ATG | 349 | 29 (8.3) |
| Kidney | Cs-P | 76 | 2 (2.6) |

AZ = azathioprine; P = prednisone; Cs = cyclosporine; ATG = antithymocyte globulin.
Data from Peterson PK, Balfour HH, Fryd DS, Ferguson R, Kronenberg R, Simmons RL: Risk factors in the development of cytomegalovirus-related pneumonia in renal transplant recipients. J Infect Dis 148:1121, 1983.

ent in different transplant groups. For example, in bone marrow transplant recipients, interstitial pneumonitis is a special problem. Nearly half of the recipients eventually develop interstitial pneumonitis, and 60 per cent of cases are associated with CMV. Mortality is 75 per cent.[3] This means that 45 per cent of transplant recipients may die of CMV pneumonia. So far, specific gamma globulin, interferon, and acyclovir have been tried for either prophylaxis or treatment without clear successes. The special problems in this group of patients are probably a result of extreme immunosuppression due to pretransplantation immunosuppressive conditioning, a period of absence of marrow function after transplantation, and severe host-versus-graft reaction.

**Epstein-Barr Virus Infection and Lymphomas in Transplant Recipients.** Both primary EBV and reactivation infections can occur after transplantation. Since seronegative adults are relatively rare, most authors have reported reactivation infections. We found previously that 32 per cent of renal transplant recipients had reactivation infection.[23] Conversion did not occur in three seronegative subjects. Cheeseman et al.[24] found that reactivation occurred only in patients who received antithymocyte globulin in addition to azathioprine and prednisone, and they suspected at times pneumonitis or pulmonary infiltrates due to EBV. The frequency of EBV infection in our present transplant population, detected by titering pretransplant and post-transplant sera for IgG antibody against virus capsid antigen (VCA), is presented in Table 5–8.[25] Of 134 renal, liver, heart, and heart-lung transplant recipients, 49 developed EBV infection (37 per cent).

**TABLE 5–8. Primary and Reactivated Epstein-Barr Virus Infections in Transplant Recipients 1981–1983**

| Pretransplant IgG anti-VCA | Renal | Liver | Heart and Heart-Lung | Total |
|---|---|---|---|---|
| Negative | 3/5* | 1/1 | 5/5 | 9/11 |
| Positive | 7/36† | 17/44 | 16/43 | 40/123 |
| Total Infections | 10/41 | 18/45 | 21/48 | 49/134 |
| % Infected | 24 | 40 | 44 | 37 |

\* Number with serological evidence of primary infection/total in category.
† Number with serological evidence of reactivation infection/total in category.

The clinical significance of these infections is difficult to evaluate. Patients with evidence of EBV infection may have different syndromes, with fever, leukopenia, transient pulmonary infiltrates, thrombocytopenia, and lymphadenopathy. The problem is that many or most of these patients also had evidence of CMV infection. We now also believe that the combination of CMV and reactivated EBV infections is more symptomatic then either alone. For example, of 15 heart and heart-lung transplant recipients with symptomatic CMV infection, 11 also had evidence of EBV infection. On the other hand, of 30 recipients with asymptomatic CMV infection, only three had evidence of EBV infection.[20]

**Primary EBV infection** is an important cause of morbidity, although it is relatively infrequent (Table 5–8). Of 11 susceptible, that is, pretransplant seronegative patients, nine developed primary infections. However, in terms of morbidity, these primary infections were disproportionately important; six of the nine patients with primary infections developed either lymphoma or lymphoproliferative syndrome. Seven patients developed this lymphoma syndrome after reactivation infection. One patient had evidence of chronic EBV infection and was not included in the table.[25] We therefore observed 14 instances of lymphomas in 498 transplant recipients from 1980 through June 1983. The relative frequency of this important complication in transplant groups was as follows: 2.5 per cent (8/315) in the renal group, 2.3 per cent (3/129) in the liver transplant recipients, and 9.3 per cent (5/54) in the heart and heart-lung transplant recipients. Clearly, the frequency of lymphomas in the heart and heart-lung transplant recipients was significantly higher than in the other groups. EBV lymphoproliferative syndromes have also recently been observed in pediatric liver recipients.

The significance of EBV infection in transplant recipients is being only gradually elucidated. At this time it appears particularly important to diagnose primary infections because these patients are prone to develop lymphomas. It is essential to have available a pretransplant serum. Primary infection may be diagnosed by observing a serological conversion from a negative pretransplant titer to a positive transplant titer. The type of antibodies to be determined is also an important factor. Heterophil agglutinins do not usually appear in these patients. The most reliable test is conversion of a serological rise of IgG antibodies against VCA. IgM antibodies against VCA are also helpful, but not sensitive. A rise in early antigen, particularly of the restricted type, is another means of detection. Such serological tests are unfortunately not rapid. In contrast to CMV, virus cultures are unfortunately not very helpful in the diagnosis of EBV infection because up to 25 per cent of normal individuals excrete the virus in their saliva.

Patients with lymphomas or lymphoproliferative syndrome in our series developed this complication within the first six months after transplantation. All of them had been receiving cyclosporine and prednisone. The lesion may manifest itself by a viral syndrome associated with cervical lymphadenopathy, gastrointestinal bleeding, intestinal obstruction, or other indications of a tumor, for example, a lung lesion or node in other parts of the body. Almost all such tumors have evidence of EBV activity demonstrated either by the presence of EBV nuclear antigen or by EBV DNA, as determined by hybridization techniques.[25] It is important to diagnose these tumors and the associated EBV infection quickly, because most are reversible if immunosuppression is stopped or reduced.[26] We do not find acyclovir useful. It is also possible that the frequency of these tumors has been reduced by better monitoring of immunosuppressants.

## SUMMARY AND CONCLUSIONS

Infections remain an important complication in transplant recipients. Almost all patients have bacterial infections of some sort. They may be life threatening in liver, heart, or heart-lung recipients. Infection should no longer be a significant cause of mortality in renal transplant recipients. More than half of all transplant recipients have evidence of viral infection, and a significant proportion of those will have evidence of morbidity due to cytomegalovirus (CMV) and Epstein-Barr virus (EBV). CMV infections are frequently asymptomatic, but patients with symptoms usually have viremia. They may develop a viral syndrome, pneumonitis, or dissemination. Fungus infections are a particular problem in liver transplant recipients. Forty-two per cent developed serious fungus infections, mostly due to *Candida*. Hepatitis due to CMV, which occasionally can end in destruction of the graft, is also a particular problem of this group. Clinically such infections are difficult to distinguish from rejection. Heart and particularly heart-lung recipients are prone to CMV infections and pneumonia. Interstitial pneumonitis, most often caused by CMV, is a special problem of bone marrow recipients. EBV infection, especially of the primary type, may be associated with the development of the lymphoma or lymphoproliferative syndrome. Better methods for prevention, early diagnosis, and treatment of all infections are needed.

ACKNOWLEDGMENTS: Studies from the author's laboratory were partially supported by NIH grant 1R01 AI 19377. Colleagues in our research were M. K. Breinig, J. S. Dummer, J. A. Armstong, A. Hardy, C. P. Wajszczuk, A. Poorsattar, and J. N. Dowling.

## REFERENCES

1. Wajszczuk CP, Dummer JS, Ho M, VanThiel DH, Starzl TE, Iwatsuki S, Shaw B Jr: Fungal infections in liver transplant recipients. Transplantation 40:347–353, 1985.
2. Dowling JN, Wu BC, Armstrong JA, Ho M: Enhancement of murine cytomegalovirus infection during graft versus host reaction. J Infect Dis 133:990–994, 1977.
3. Meyers JD, Thomas ED: Infection complicating bone marrow transplantation. In Rubin RH, Young LS (eds): Clinical Approach to Infection in the Compromised Hospital. New York, Plenum, 1981, pp 507–551.
4. Ho M: Cytomegalovirus: Biology and Infection. New York, Plenum, 1982.

5. Ho M, Suwansirikul S, Dowling JN, Youngblood LA, Armstrong JA: The transplanted kidney as a source of cytomegalovirus infection. N Engl J Med 293:1109–1112, 1975.
6. Shands KN, Ho JL, Meyer RD, Gorman GW, Edelstein PH, Mallison GF, Finegold SM, Fraser DW: Potable water as a source of legionnaires' disease. JAMA 253:1412–1416, 1985.
7. Ferguson RM, Fidelus-Gort R: The immunosuppressive action of cyclosporine in man. Transplant Proc 15:2350–2356, 1983.
8. Ptachinski RJ, Carpenter BJ, Burckart GJ, Venataramanan R, Rosenthal JT: Effect of erythromycin on cyclosporine levels. N Engl J Med 313:1416–1417, 1985.
9. Dummer JS, Hardy A, Poorsattar A, Ho M: Early infections in kidney, heart and liver transplant

recipients on cyclosporine. Transplantation 36:259–267, 1983.

10. Starzl TE, Hakala TR, Rosenthal JT, Iwatsuki S, Shaw BW Jr: The Colorado-Pittsburgh cadaveric renal transplantation study on cyclosporine. Transplant Proc 15:2459–2468, 1983.

11. Ho M, Wajszczuk CP, Hardy A, Dummer JS, Starzl TE, Hakala TR, Bahnson HT: Infections in kidney, heart and liver transplant recipients on cyclosporine. Transplant Proc 15:2768–2772, 1983.

12. Louria DB, Stiff DP, Bonnett B: Disseminated moniliasis in the adult. Medicine 41:307–337, 1967.

13. Ho M: Virus infections after transplantation in man. Arch Virol 36:259–267, 1977.

14. Shields AF, Hackman RC, Fif KH, Corey L, Meyers JD: Adenovirus infections in patients undergoing bone-marrow transplantations. N Engl J Med 312:529–533.

15. Ho M: Systemic viral infections and viral infections in immunosuppressed patients. In Galasso GL, Merigan TC, Buchanan RA (eds): Antiviral Agents and Viral Diseases of Man, 2nd ed. New York, Raven Press, 1984, pp 487–516.

16. Winston DJ, Huang ES, Miller MJ, Lin CH, Ho WG, Gale RP, Champlin RE: Molecular epidemiology of cytomegalovirus infections associated with bone marrow transplantation. Ann Intern Med 102:16–20, 1985.

17. Marker SC, Howard RJ, Simmons RL, Kalis JM, Connelly DP, Najarian JS, Balfour HH Jr: Cytomegalovirus infection: A quantitative prospective study of 320 consecutive renal transplants. Surgery 89:660–671, 1981.

18. Chou S: Acquisition of donor strains of cytomegalovirus by renal-transplant recipients. N Engl J Med 314:1418–1423, 1986.

19. Betts RF, Freeman RB, Douglas RG Jr, Talley TE, Rundell B: Transmission of cytomegalovirus infection with renal allograft. Kidney Int 8:387–394, 1975.

20. Dummer JS, White LT, Ho M, Griffith GP, Hardesty RL, Bahnson HT: Morbidity of cytomegalovirus infection in recipients of heart or heart-lung transplants who received cyclosporine. J Infect Dis 152:1182–1191, 1985.

21. Demetris AJ, Lasky S, Van Thiel DH, Starzl TE, Dekker A: Pathology of hepatic transplantation. A Review of 62 adult allograft recipients immunosuppressed with a cyclosporine/steroid regimen. Am J Pathol 118:151–161, 1985.

22. Peterson PK, Balfour HH, Fryd DS, Ferguson R, Kronenberg R, Simmons RL: Risk factors in the development of cytomegalovirus-related pneumonia in renal transplant recipients. J Infect Dis 148:1121, 1983.

23. Armstrong JA, Evans AS, Rao N, Ho M: Viral infections in renal transplant recipients. Infect Immun 14:970–975, 1976.

24. Cheeseman SH, Henle W, Rubin RH, Tolkoff-Rubin NE, Cosimi B, Cantell K, Winkle S, Herrin JT, Black PH, Russell PS, Hirsch MS: Epstein-Barr virus infection in renal transplant recipients. Ann Intern Med 93:39–42, 1980.

25. Ho M, Miller G, Atchison RW, Breinig MK, Dummer JS, Andiman W, Starzl TE, Eastman R, Griffith BP, Hardesty RL, Bahnson HT, Hakala TR, Rosenthal JT: Epstein-Barr virus infections and DNA hybridization studies in posttransplantation lymphoma and lymphoproliferative lesions: The role of primary infection. J Infect Dis 152:876–886, 1985.

26. Starzl TE, Nalesnik MA, Porter KA, Ho M, Iwatsuki S, Griffith BP, Rosenthal JT, Hakala TR, Shaw BW Jr, Hardesty RL, Atchison RW, Jaffe R, Bahnson HT: Reversibility of lymphomas and lymphoproliferative lesions developing under cyclosporine-therapy. Lancet 1:583–587, 1984.

# 6

# *Kidney Transplantation*

GWENDOLYN B. GRAYBAR
MARGARET TARPEY

## ANATOMY AND PHYSIOLOGY OF THE KIDNEYS

The kidneys serve the important function of maintaining balance of many substances essential to life, including water, electrolytes, and amino acids. In addition, they aid in the removal of endogenous and exogenous compounds and assist in the preservation of acid-base status. The mechanisms by which the kidneys maintain homeostasis are filtration, secretion, and reabsorption. These processes are controlled by a complex interplay of neural, hormonal, and intrinsic or autoregulatory factors, many of which are just now being described or understood.

### Anatomy

The kidney is composed of a cortex, medulla, renal pelvis, and ureter (Fig. 6–1). The medulla can be further divided into outer and inner layers, with the inner medullary layer having one or more papillary tips. The renal artery enters the kidney adjacent to the ureter and subdivides into interlobar, arcuate, and interlobular branches. An afferent arteriole then leads to the glomerular capillary network that re-forms into an efferent arteriole. A peritubular capillary network, which includes the vasa recta, is formed from the

efferent arterioles before becoming the renal venous system, with a configuration similar to the arterial system.[1]

The functional unit of the kidney, the nephron, is composed of a glomerular capillary network, surrounded by Bowman's space, leading into a tubular system made up of a proximal segment, a loop of Henle with descending and ascending limbs, a distal segment, and a collecting duct. The epithelial lining of this tubular system has distinctive conformations at various sites along its length, corresponding to the functions of the tubule at each point. Approximately two million nephrons within the human kidneys provide a reserve that allows an individual to maintain an active life with only one-quarter functional renal tissue.

Nephrons can be divided into two types: cortical and juxtamedullary. The cortical nephron arises from the superficial cortex, has a short loop of Henle and a simple peritubular capillary network. The juxtamedullary nephron arises from the deeper substance of the cortex, and its loop of Henle reaches varying depths into the medullary substance. Its efferent arteriole continues not only as a peritubular capillary network but forms a series of vascular loops known as the

61

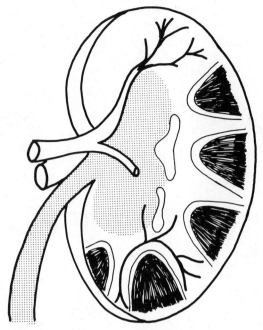

**Figure 6–1.** Renal anatomy.

vasa recta. The vasa recta also reach into the medulla, breaking into capillaries that surround the collecting ducts and loops of Henle, before re-forming into ascending bundles and joining the venous system.[2]

The juxtaglomerular apparatus is a combination of tubular and vascular cells found in the vicinity of the distal tubule and its corresponding glomerulus. It contains macula densa cells, specialized epithelial cells in the thick ascending limb, and early distal tubule, lacis cells, and granular cells found in the media of the afferent arterioles. The juxtaglomerular apparatus is involved in the secretion of renin and local production of angiotensin and appears to be involved in the autoregulation of glomerular filtration rate (GFR).[3,4]

### Innervation

There is sympathetic innervation to virtually all segments of the nephron, with input to all aspects of renal function, including water and electrolyte reabsorption. Alpha adrenergic receptors have been described in various tubular segments and play an important role in sodium, chloride, and water reabsorption and the regulation of sodium balance.[5] There are also alpha receptors in renal vascular tissue that mediate renin release.[6] Beta-adrenergic receptors have been found on juxtaglomerular apparatus granular cells

and stimulate renin release without causing renal vasoconstriction.[6] Dopaminergic receptors have also been located in the renal vasculature, and dopamine has been utilized clinically to increase renal blood flow and to enhance natriuresis.[7,8] However, the role of endogenous dopamine and the effects of renal nerve stimulation on renal vasodilation are unclear.

### Renal Hemodynamics

There are two sites of large pressure drops in the renal vasculature, the afferent and efferent arterioles, signifying these as the major sites of vascular resistance. A change in resistance at either site will alter renal blood flow; however, it is the differential resistance between the two arterioles that determines the glomerular capillary hydrostatic pressure and thus the GFR.

An increase in resistance at either afferent or efferent arterioles will result in a decline in renal blood flow. If the resistance of the afferent arteriole is elevated, glomerular filtration will also decrease. Alternately, if the resistance rises at the efferent arteriole, glomerular capillary hydrostatic pressure increases and GFR rises. Changes in glomerular filtration do not always mirror changes in renal blood flow, and it may be inaccurate to estimate alterations in GFR from changes in renal blood flow alone (Fig. 6–2).

### Autoregulation

As renal perfusion pressure (renal arterial–renal venous) increases from 80 to 180 mm Hg, renal blood flow remains constant. This indicates that renal vascular resistance rises along with elevations in perfusion pressure. As perfusion pressure increases, the GFR also remains constant, identifying the afferent arterioles as the site of the altered resistance. The constancy of renal blood flow and GFR, over a wide range of perfusion pressures, persists after adrenalectomy, renal denervation, and in the isolated perfused kidney, and has been termed autoregulation.

The mechanism of autoregulation has not been identified. Vascular smooth muscle contracts when it is stretched and relaxes when it is shortened.[9] This property in the afferent arteriole, described by Bayliss in 1902, may contribute to autoregulation as well as tubuloglomerular feedback. The flow rate of tubular fluid is sensed at the macula densa of the juxtaglomerular apparatus and

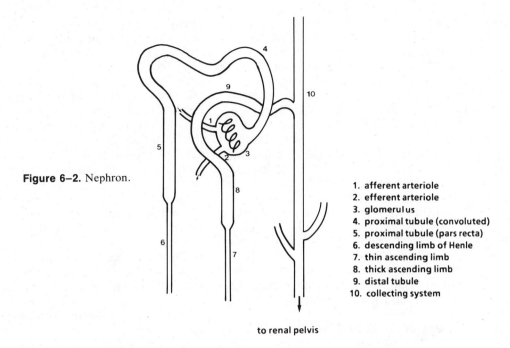

**Figure 6–2.** Nephron.

1. afferent arteriole
2. efferent arteriole
3. glomerulus
4. proximal tubule (convoluted)
5. proximal tubule (pars recta)
6. descending limb of Henle
7. thin ascending limb
8. thick ascending limb
9. distal tubule
10. collecting system

to renal pelvis

reflexly controls the filtration rate of the glomerulus to which that juxtaglomerular apparatus belongs. The variable that is sensed at the macula densa is not known precisely. Possibilities include the concentration of Na or Cl, the total amount of Na or Cl delivered to the macula densa, or tubular fluid osmolality. The effector mechanism is also unknown and may involve the renin-angiotensin system, renal sympathetic efferent nerves, or other vasoactive substances, possibly prostaglandins.[3]

## Renal Blood Flow and Oxygen Consumption

Renal blood flow is normally 3 to 5 $ml\cdot min^{-1}\cdot gm^{-1}$ tissue. This flow rate is several times greater than other "high-flow" organs such as the brain and heart. Renal oxygen consumption is directly related to renal blood flow, and the renal arteriovenous oxygen content difference (A-VDO$_2$) is approximately 2 ml $O_2\cdot dl^{-1}$. As renal blood flow falls to 1 $ml\cdot min^{-1}\cdot gm^{-1}$, oxygen consumption also declines with no change in A-VDO$_2$. When renal blood flow falls to 0.5 to 1 $ml\cdot min^{-1}\cdot gm^{-1}$, A-VDO$_2$ widens. At blood flow below 0.5 $ml\cdot min^{-1}\cdot gm^{-1}$ renal cells become ischemic and oxygen consumption again falls. These data have been interpreted as indicating that approximately 25 per cent of oxygen consumption is required for basal metabolism. The remainder is required to support active transport processes (especially for Na$^+$) within the tubular cells. With a stable sodium concentration, the amount of sodium filtered varies in direct proportion to the GFR; an increase in GFR requires more sodium reabsorption to maintain sodium balance. When GFR and thus sodium reabsorption cease, the remaining oxygen consumption reflects the basal metabolic requirements of renal tissue. In this range the kidneys extract more oxygen when the flow cannot increase to meet minimal needs.[10]

## Glomerular Filtration

Glomerular filtration occurs at the glomerular capillary between the afferent and efferent arterioles. The filtrate is formed according to the Starling equation:

$$Q = Kf((Pc - Pt) - (\pi c - \pi t))$$

where Q = volume of filtrate$\cdot min^{-1}$; Kf = filtration coefficient, which is dependent upon both capillary permeability and total surface area of capillaries; Pc = hydrostatic pressure within the capillary; Pt = hydrostatic pressure within Bowman's space; $\pi c$ = protein oncotic pressure within capillary; and $\pi t$ = protein oncotic pressure within Bowman's space.

Thus the same mechanisms that govern movement across systemic capillaries apply to the glomerular network. However, there are several properties that are unique to this system. Hydrostatic pressure tends to remain constant within the glomerular capillary, while it declines along the length of a systemic capillary. Glomerular capillaries are less permeable to protein; therefore, protein oncotic pressure in Bowman's space is less than interstitial oncotic pressure. Protein oncotic pressure rises along the length of the glomerular capillary, while hydrostatic pressure in Bowman's space is higher than tissue hydrostatic pressure. These factors result in a net ultrafiltration pressure that is slightly higher than in extrarenal capillaries. Kf is also greater for glomerular capillaries because of both increased total surface area and greater intrinsic permeability to small molecules. Thus, glomerular filtration is much greater than that found in systemic capillaries.

GFR can be measured with a substance that is only filtered, without further secretion or reabsorption. Creatinine is filtered but also is secreted in the renal tubules to some extent, and therefore creatinine clearance tends to overestimate GFR. However, creatinine clearance can be a useful guide to estimate GFR without having to resort to exogenous substances for a more accurate measure of GFR.

### Renin-Angiotensin-Aldosterone

Granular cells of the juxtaglomerular apparatus secrete renin, a proteolytic enzyme that converts renin substrate to angiotensin I. Angiotensin II is produced by the action of angiotensin-converting enzyme on angiotensin I. While there are high levels of angiotensin-converting enzyme in the lung, there is also high renal enzyme activity, suggesting not only systemic effects, but an important local role for angiotensin II. Angiotensin II is a potent vasoconstrictor, acting on vascular smooth muscle to raise vascular resistance. It also stimulates the secretion of aldosterone in the adrenal cortex, ultimately leading to increases in $Na^+$ reabsorption. Angiotensin II also has a direct effect on renal tubules to increase $Na^+$ reabsorption. Angiotensin II elicits, via a central mechanism, an increase in efferent nerve activity to the peripheral sympathetic nervous system, resulting in increases in cardiac output and total peripheral resistance.

The rate-limiting step in the production of angiotensin II is the release of renin from the juxtaglomerular apparatus granular cells. Renin release is controlled by a direct negative feedback effect of angiotensin II on the granular cells. In addition, independent of angiotensin II levels, a baroreceptor mechanism acts to decrease renin release when renal perfusion pressure rises. Alterations in the levels of NaCl at the macula densa also act independently to alter renin release. Finally, renal sympathetic activity can modulate renin release. Progressive activation of renal sympathetic nerves results in a series of additive effects on renin secretion. Juxtaglomerular granular cell beta receptors mediate the release of renin to levels of stimulation that do not cause renal vasoconstriction; at higher levels of renal sympathetic stimulation, at which renal vasoconstriction is present, a portion of renin release is mediated by renal vascular alpha receptors.[4]

Aldosterone acts to increase $Na^+$ reabsorption in the cortical and medullary collecting ducts by increasing $Na^+$ permeability of the luminal membrane, increasing $Na^+$, $K^+$-ATPase activity of the peritubular membrane and by increasing mitochondrial oxidative metabolism, thus providing more energy to the $Na^+$ pump.

### Sodium Balance

Approximately two thirds of filtered $Na^+$ is actively and passively reabsorbed in the proximal tubule, mainly as NaCl, $NaHCO_3$, and in co-transport with organic solutes. Water is then absorbed passively as a consequence of solute reabsorption, and tubular fluid is isosmotic at the end of the proximal tubule.[11] The thin descending limb of Henle is relatively impermeable to $Na^+$ and $Cl^-$, while water permeability is high. This results in the movement of water out of the thin descending limb, along an osmotic gradient, with tubular fluid being hyperosmotic at the beginning of the ascending limb. The thin ascending limb of Henle is permeable to $Na^+$ and $Cl^-$ and passive reabsorption occurs there, while $Na^+$ and $Cl^-$ reabsorption is active in the thick ascending limb and accounts for 25 per cent of reabsorption of filtered $Na^+$. Both thin and thick ascending limbs of Henle are impermeable to water, so that dilute tubular fluid is always present at the origin of the distal tubule. $Na^+$ reabsorption from the distal tubule and the collecting duct is active, with about 8 per cent of filtered $Na^+$ reabsorbed in the distal nephron.[11]

Control of $Na^+$ reabsorption is mediated by several factors, including glomerulotubular balance, alterations in GFR, the renin-angiotensin-aldosterone system, natriuretic hormone, and the renal sympathetic nerves. Generally a constant fraction of filtered $Na^+$ is reabsorbed in the proximal tubule, despite alterations in GFR, and thus in the filtered load of $Na^+$. This fraction is normally 0.67 of the filtered load. The balance between glomerulus and tubule allows for efficient recycling of $Na^+$ in the face of varying GFR. If GFR and the filtered $Na^+$ load increase, glomerulotubular balance provides for an increase in the total amount of $Na^+$ reabsorbed from the proximal tubule. Adjustments in reabsorption from more distal segments provide for further reclamation of $Na^+$ to maintain normal $Na^+$ levels. Spontaneous changes in GFR result in negative feedback mechanisms, which tend to return the GFR and filtered $Na^+$ load to normal.

GFR can also respond to changes in $Na^+$ intake to help preserve overall $Na^+$ and fluid balance. An increase in $Na^+$ intake often results in an increase in extracellular volume, blood pressure, and GFR. This secondary (as opposed to spontaneous) elevation in GFR raises the filtered $Na^+$ load and ultimately increases $Na^+$ excretion. An increase in $Na^+$ intake also results in depressed aldosterone levels, decreasing cortical and medullary collecting duct $Na^+$ reabsorption. This effect of $Na^+$ concentration on aldosterone levels is independent of any effect mediated by activation of the renin-angiotensin. The increase in $Na^+$ excretion seen following increased $Na^+$ intake cannot be fully explained by the alterations in GFR and aldosterone levels. A natriuretic factor appears to decrease $Na^+$ reabsorption in both the proximal and distal tubules.

Renal tubular adrenoreceptors play an important role in the regulation of $Na^+$ balance. Low-level renal sympathetic nerve activity results in increased tubular reabsorption of $Na^+$ in the absence of changes in mean arterial pressure, GFR, renal blood flow, or intrarenal blood flow. Affected segments include the proximal tubule, thick ascending limb of Henle, and the collecting duct. Neither inhibition of prostaglandin synthesis nor antagonism of angiotensin II altered the increase in $Na^+$ reabsorption.[6]

## Water Balance

The thirst mechanism and secretion of antidiuretic hormone (ADH) regulate water balance. When deprived of water, plasma becomes hyperosmolar, inducing thirst and increasing release of ADH from the posterior pituitary. ADH increases water permeability of the late distal tubule and the collecting ducts, generating hyperosmotic urine.

Concentrated urine is formed by the passive reabsorption of water along an osmotic gradient. The countercurrent multiplication of $Na^+$ and $Cl^-$ reabsorption without water in the ascending limb of Henle produces a progressive osmolar gradient from cortex to papilla. The countercurrent arrangement of the vasa recta prevents medullary blood flow from diluting the gradient. In the absence of ADH the dilute tubular fluid present at the beginning of the distal tubule is excreted without further water reabsorption despite the osmotic gradient.

The secretion of ADH is regulated by osmoreceptors in the anterior hypothalamus. These cells monitor extracellular fluid osmolality, possibly by alterations in their cell volume. In addition, extracellular fluid volume appears to modulate the effect of osmoreceptors so that ADH secretion is less for any given osmotic stimulus when extracellular fluid volume is expanded. A number of drugs, including morphine, barbiturates, and some oral hypoglycemic agents, demonstrate an antidiuretic effect. This effect may be due to enhanced secretion of ADH from the posterior pituitary or to potentiation of ADH effect at the tubular membrane.[12]

## Acid-Base Balance

The lungs excrete approximately 15,000 mM of $CO_2$ daily, as the by-product of oxidative metabolism, while the kidneys are responsible for the excretion of 60 mM of fixed acid, resulting from protein and phospholipid metabolism. In addition, they are responsible for the conservation of $HCO_3^-$, the major plasma buffer component. Normally, greater than 99 per cent of the filtered $HCO_3^-$ is predominantly reabsorbed in the proximal tubule by the action of carbonic anhydrase in the luminal membrane. Fixed acid is secreted as a combination of both titratable acid, mainly $NaH_2PO_4$, and neutral ammonium salts. $NH_3$ is derived from amino acid catabolism within renal tubular cells. Neutral $NH_3$

**TABLE 6–1.    Percentage Reabsorption of Filtered Substance**

|  | H$_2$O* | Na$^+$ | K$^+$ | HCO$_3$$^-$ |
|---|---|---|---|---|
| Proximal tubule | 66 | 66 | 70 | 90 |
| Loop of Henle | 25 | 25 | 25 | 2 |
| Distal tubule | 3 | 5 | −15† | 8 |
| Collecting duct | 4 | 3 | 10 |  |
| Total | 99+ | 99+ | 90 | 99.9+ |

\* Under conditions of maximal ADH.
† K$^+$ is secreted in the distal tubule.
Data from references 2, 13, and 14.

is lipid soluble and passes into the tubular lumen, where it can combine with secreted H$^+$. The charged NH$_4$$^+$ ions are then trapped within the tubular lumen and excreted as NH$_4$Cl or (NH$_4$)$_2$SO$_4$. About 75 per cent of fixed acid is excreted as an ammonium salt, with the remainer as titratable acid. There is a large reserve for acid excretion as ammonium ion, rising as much as fivefold in some states of chronic acidosis.[13]

## Potassium Balance

K$^+$ is both absorbed and secreted in various parts of the nephron. Eighty per cent of filtered K$^+$ is reabsorbed by both active and passive processes in the proximal tubule and ascending limb of Henle. Normally, K$^+$ is secreted in the distal tubule and cortical collecting duct. Outer medullary collecting ducts may either secrete or reabsorb K$^+$, while inner medullary collecting ducts only reabsorb K$^+$. Net urinary K$^+$ excretion is thus governed by alterations in net secretion in the late distal tubule and collecting duct and is influenced by the electrochemical gradient for K$^+$ between tubular cell and lumen, and the flow rate of Na$^+$ and water to the distal nephron.[14]

## Phosphate and Calcium Balance

Both phosphate and calcium excretion are under the control of parathyroid hormone (PTH). In the presence of PTH, phosphate excretion from the kidney is enhanced with diminished reabsorption from the proximal tubule. Phosphate reabsorption is dependent upon sodium reabsorption in the proximal tubule; however, the movement of phosphate does not appear to be one of simple co-transport with sodium. Approximately 70 per cent of filtered calcium is actively reabsorbed along the proximal tubule. In addition, there is reabsorption in the thick ascending limb

and in the distal tubule and cortical collecting duct. While the overall effect of PTH is to enhance calcium reabsorption, proximal reabsorption is inhibited by PTH. Active calcium reabsorption in the distal nephron is increased by PTH, which is without effect in the ascending limb of Henle. The effects of PTH on calcium movement in the distal nephron occur independently of any changes in sodium or potassium transport.[15]

## HISTORY OF RENAL TRANSPLANTATION

Ullmann[16] first transplanted a dog's kidney from its normal position to its neck in 1902. The graft produced urine flow. However, he did not continue his experiments; neither did Decastello, another Viennese physician who reported the first dog-to-dog transplantation in the same year.[17]

Alexis Carrel also began his work with kidney transplants in 1902, which he continued for nearly 40 years. Carrel was the outstanding surgeon in the field of transplantation.[18] His technique for vascular anastomoses is still utilized today. In addition, Carrel experimented with hypothermic preservation and the immune response. He insisted on strict asepsis, noting that most of his dogs died of infection. With his close friend Charles Lindbergh, he developed a perfusion pump in 1935. He was awarded the first Nobel prize for the United States in Physiology and Medicine in 1912 for his work on renal allografts in cats and dogs.[19] In 1914 Carrel wrote, "The surgical side of the transplantation of organs is now complete because we are now able to perform transplantation of organs with perfect ease and excellent results from an anatomical standpoint, but as yet these methods cannot be applied to human surgery for the reason that homoplastic transplantations are almost always unsuccessful from the standpoint of the functioning of the organs. All of our efforts must now be directed toward the biological methods which will prevent the reaction of the organisms against foreign tissue and allowing the adapting of homoplastic grafts to their hosts."[17]

Jaboulay, Carrel's teacher, transplanted the kidneys from a pig and a goat to the limbs of humans with chronic renal failure in 1906. Each functioned for only one hour. Jaboulay's experiments were the first recorded human transplants, although Ullmann reported in 1914 that he had done similar transplants in 1902.[17]

Ernst Unger, in 1909, after performing more than 100 kidney transplants in dogs, transplanted the kidney of a stillborn baby to a baboon. The graft never functioned. In the same month he transplanted an ape's kidney to a young girl dying of renal failure. Following this failure, Unger concluded that there was a biochemical barrier to transplantation. Voronoy performed the first human allograft in 1933 and carried out six renal transplants by 1949, none of which functioned.[17]

In 1946 the Peter Bent Brigham Hospital initiated its major interest in transplantation when Hufnagel, Hume, and Landsteiner transplanted a cadaver kidney to a young woman dying of acute renal failure. She was believed to be too sick to be moved to the operating room. The kidney was anastomosed to her brachial vessels on the ward. It immediately made urine and she improved. However, the graft had to be removed after 48 hours. Meanwhile, the patient entered the diuretic phase and did well.[20] The first living-related transplantation was performed in 1953 from a mother to son whose solitary kidney was damaged in a road accident. The kidney functioned for nearly a month before being rejected.[17]

Hume et al.[21] in 1955 reported the Brigham experience with nine renal transplants. Six were from donors who had died during cardiovascular surgery; two received their kidneys from patients with hydrocephalus undergoing ventriculoureteral shunts that necessitated removal of one of their kidneys, and the last was from a patient with cancer of the ureter. One patient's kidney functioned for $5\frac{1}{2}$ months, two for 2 months, one for one month, and five did not function at all. One kidney that regained function had been anoxic for $1\frac{1}{2}$ hours. Although somewhat encouraged, the authors concluded that renal homotransplantation had no place for humans at that time.

The first kidney transplantation between identical twins was done on December 23, 1954, again at the Peter Bent Brigham Hospital.[22] The graft functioned well, and the patient's condition improved. In contrast to the 13 previous human homotransplants in which the kidneys were anastomosed to the femoral vessels, Merrill's group elected to place the kidney in the pelvis. Previous transplants utilized a cutaneous ureterostomy, introducing infection, and uniformly resulted in hydro-

nephrosis. Based on their animal experiments, Merrill et al.[22] implanted the ureter directly into the bladder.

Total-body irradiation was employed for immunosuppression between 1959 and 1962. Results were poor and mortality high. Calne[23] found that 6-mercaptopurine (6-MP) successfully prolonged renal allograft survival in dogs. Kuss et al.[24] reported in 1962 the first successful chemical immunosuppression for renal transplantation with a nonrelated donor. They utilized 6-MP and prednisone in a patient who had previously been irradiated. Newer derivatives of 6-MP such as azathioprine (Imuran) yielded better immunosuppression with less toxicity. Subsequently Starzl et al.[25] and Murray et al.[26] combined azathioprine and prednisolone with remarkable results.

Najarian et al.[27] stressed the importance of "renal protective mechanisms," including hydration, diuresis, and maintenance of normal blood pressure to the living-related donor to decrease the high early failure rate. Great improvements in tissue typing and dialysis occurred during the remainder of the 1960's.[17,28] Further survival of the graft improved markedly with preoperative blood transfusions.[29,30]

Since its introduction by Calne et al.[31] in 1978, cyclosporine has increased graft survival, particularly for cadaveric transplants. Cyclosporine selectively inhibits T-lymphocyte blastogenesis. Current data reveal that with cadaveric renal transplantation 80 per cent of grafts survive for one year compared to 4 per cent reported in 1964.[32]

Kidney transplants were formerly done only in large academic institutions. Currently, with increased safety and efficacy, they are being performed in community hospitals throughout the world.

## DONOR NEPHRECTOMY

### The Living Related Donor

The living related donor (LRD) should be in good health with good renal function demonstrated in both kidneys. Particularly when the end-stage renal disease (ESRD) in the recipient is of hereditary nature, as in polycystic kidney disease, the not-to-be-donated kidney must be shown to be normal. A history of diabetes, neoplasia, significant hypertension, or other major disease generally precludes consideration as an LRD. Preoperative laboratory tests include complete blood count, biochemical profile including both fasting and two-hour postprandial blood sugar determinations, chest roentgenography, and ECG. Urine studies include urinalysis, culture and sensitivity, and creatinine clearance. If the findings in intravenous pyelography are normal, aortography is done to determine the presence of multiple renal arteries, but it may also reveal other pathology such as unilateral fibromuscular dysplasia.[33] If only one kidney has multiple arteries, the other one should be donated. If both have multiple arteries, the choice should be the one that has larger arteries or with the greatest distance between them.

Each child receives one antigen haplotype from each of his parents. Although ABO blood type identity is not essential, most ABO-incompatible transplants are followed by acute rejection. However, the donor should not have any major blood group antigens not present in the recipient.

Once the patient is well hydrated, general endotracheal anesthesia is induced. A Foley catheter is inserted and then the patient is placed in the lateral position. Generally the left kidney is removed, unless it is determined to be the better of the two kidneys. The left renal vein is larger, thus making the transplantation easier. Some surgeons prefer to take the right kidney in women, as it is more susceptible to problems during pregnancy.[34]

Figure 6–3 depicts the LRD nephrectomy, which requires considerably more time than routine nephrectomy, because of the need for meticulous dissection and resting. A reversed S-shaped incision is made over the lower rib cage, curving inferiorly along the lateral margin of the rectus. The subperiosteal resection of the 11th rib allows better exposure than that of the 12th. The pleural and peritoneal cavities are avoided if possible. The renal vein is dissected to the vena cava. Tension on the renal artery will induce spasm and cyanosis of the kidney. The ureter is dissected free and cut at the level of the

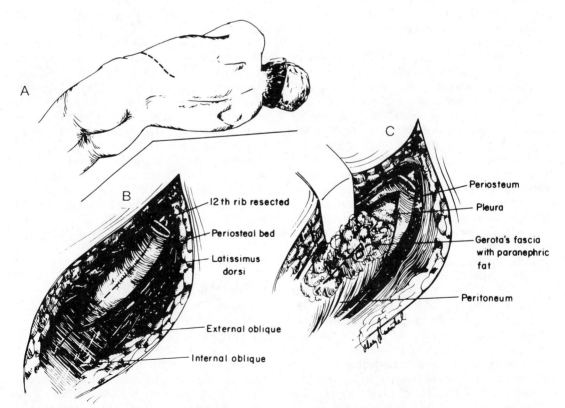

**Figure 6–3.** Living related donor nephrectomy. (From Cosimi AB: The donor and donor nephrectomy. In Morris PJ (ed): Kidney Transplantation. New York, Grune & Stratton, 1984, p 81, with permission of the author and publisher.)

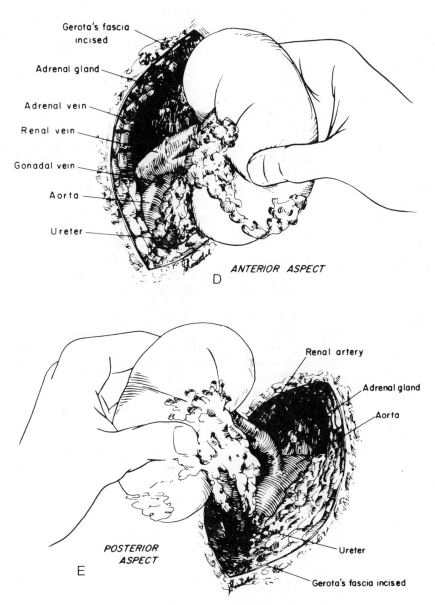

Gerota's fascia incised

Adrenal gland

Adrenal vein

Renal vein

Gonadal vein

Aorta

Ureter

ANTERIOR ASPECT

D

Renal artery

Adrenal gland

Aorta

Ureter

Gerota's fascia incised

POSTERIOR ASPECT

E

**Figure 6–3.** (*continued*)

pelvic brim. Good urine output should be observed. After dissection is complete the kidney is "rested" for 10 minutes to decrease arterial spasm. The renal artery is clamped and then the renal vein. After the renal vessels are clamped and ligated the kidney is given to the transplant surgeon. The renal artery is immediately flushed at a pressure of 100 mm Hg with 4°C solution until the venous effluent is clear. As the ischemic time is short, composition of the flush solution is not as critical as it is with cadaveric kidneys. While good results have been reported with chilled Ringer's solution, most transplant surgeons use their preferred flush solution for LRD's as for cadaveric kidneys. The kidney is then placed in ice slush in a sterile closed container and taken to the operating room of the recipient. The wound is closed, the surgeon checking once more to see if either the pleural or peritoneal cavity has been entered.

Postoperatively the LRD's may have prolonged ileus resulting from the periaortic dissection, possibly injuring the autonomic nerves. Most of the perioperative morbidity is caused by atelectasis (3 per cent), urinary tract infections (4 per cent), wound problems (2 per cent), and pneumothorax.[34] Occasionally, technical problems such as avulsion of the renal artery may occur. The perioperative mortality is 0.1 per cent and is usually the result of pulmonary embolism. Most LRD's are ready for discharge within a week and able to return to work in 3 or 4 weeks.[33] About 16 LRD's have died as a result of their donation. This and the marked improvement in survival of cadaveric grafts have led some to question whether LRD transplants should continue. Nevertheless, the majority feel that LRD's are far from obsolete and use of them will continue.

## The Cadaveric Renal Donor

Ideally the donor should be less than 35 years of age. However, with the current shortage of donors, 60 to 65 years is the accepted upper age limit for consideration as a cadaveric renal donor. Generally the creatinine clearance declines each year after the age of 50 so that the creatinine clearance of a normal 60-year-old is decreased by 35 per cent.[35] The potential donor must have good renal function, as evidenced by normal serum BUN and creatinine levels (a terminal increase in creatinine to 3 mg per dl is acceptable) and must be free of diabetes, significant hypertension, sepsis, drug abuse, and malignant disease (except primary CNS tumors and low-grade skin cancers).

An *en bloc* technique for bilateral neph-

rectomy is preferred for the following reasons: warm ischemia time is decreased, renal arterial spasm is decreased, kidneys may be initially washed out with the aorta used as a conduit, the chances of disrupting the intima of the renal artery are decreased, the technical problems associated with recognition and management of multiple renal arteries are minimized, and there is greater flexibility in the utilization of the kidneys.[36] When only the kidneys are to be harvested, a bilateral subcostal, long midline T incision is made from the symphysis pubis to the sternal notch (Fig. 6–4). The abdomen is explored thoroughly for unsuspected disease. The mesocolon is freed from the cecum to the diaphragm and medially to the midline. The entire bowel is freed and rotated to the upper left and retracted out of the abdomen. The entire dissection is done so that the kidneys may be removed easily and quickly. The distal aorta is ligated proximal to the bifurcation (Fig. 6–5). The ureters are freed, leaving the adventitia along their entire length. The kidneys are mobilized without dissection near the hila. Clamps are positioned around the aorta and vena cava proximal and distal to the renal vessels as seen in Fig. 6–6. The distal clamps are fastened and the vessels ligated. The ureters are severed deep in the pelvis and urine production noted. Five minutes later the proximal aortic clamp is closed

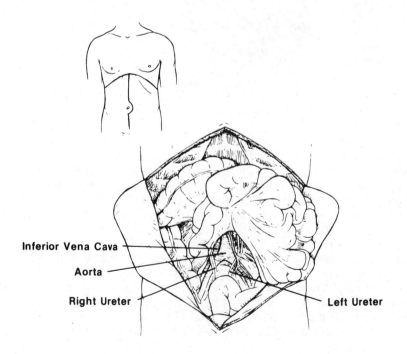

**Figure 6–4.** Incision for cadaveric nephrectomy. (From Phillips MG: Cadaver donor nephrectomy. In Glenn JF (ed): Urologic Surgery. Philadelphia, JB Lippincott Company, 1983, p 329, with permission of the author and publisher.)

Inferior Vena Cava

Aorta

Right Ureter

Left Ureter

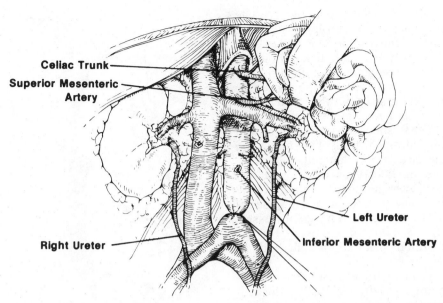

**Figure 6–5.** Cadaveric nephrectomy. Exposure of kidneys and ligation of distal aorta. Note larger left renal vein. (From Phillips MG: Cadaver donor nephrectomy. In Glenn JF (ed): Urologic Surgery. Philadelphia, JB Lippincott Company, 1983, p 329, with permission of the author and publisher.)

and the aorta ligated. The proximal clamp is then closed and the vena cava ligated. The specimen is removed *en bloc* and placed on another sterile table. Both kidneys are then immediately flushed with cold (0 to 4°C) solution via the aorta until completely blanched, usually about 10 minutes. The kidneys are then separated in a basin of ice flush.

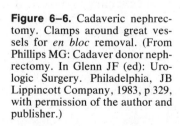

**Figure 6–6.** Cadaveric nephrectomy. Clamps around great vessels for *en bloc* removal. (From Phillips MG: Cadaver donor nephrectomy. In Glenn JF (ed): Urologic Surgery. Philadelphia, JB Lippincott Company, 1983, p 329, with permission of the author and publisher.)

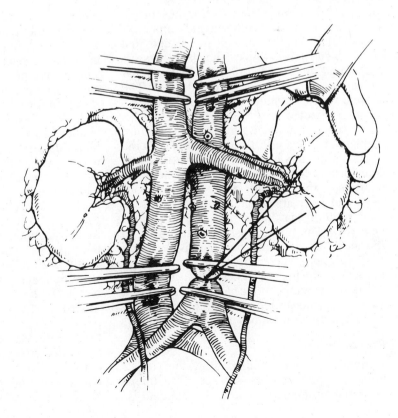

An aortic cuff is left with each kidney. The kidneys are placed in a sterile plastic bag. About 200 ml of flush solution is added, and the bag is securely tied and packed in ice.

The time of cross-clamping of the proximal aorta and any warm ischemia time need to be charted. Warm ischemia time is the time after the aorta has been clamped until the kidneys have been flushed with iced solution and also any time during the transplantation when the renal vessels are reclamped. Warm ischemia time should not exceed 60 minutes and generally averages about 3 minutes. The spleen and about 10 lymph nodes may be removed for tissue typing. The great vessels are ligated, the abdomen is closed, and the usual preparations made to take the body to the morgue.

Harvesting of multiple organs from a cadaver may improve the viability of the kidneys because of the extra care and special techniques used to protect the kidneys during the procedure. Rosenthal et al.[37] emphasized that when the heart, pancreas, liver, and kidneys are to be harvested, wide exposure is essential. A sternal notch to the pubic incision is made as in Figure 6–7. Segmental removal of the pancreas is done first, followed by mobilization of the liver. The kidneys are mobilized next as seen in Figure 6–8. A suture is placed around the superior mesenteric artery but not tied. The aorta and vena cava are isolated, and cannulas are placed just above their bifurcations. The great vessels are ligated and divided distally. After heparinization, the liver is perfused first. The splenic vein is cannulated and iced Ringer's solution injected into the portal system. As the heart is removed, the caval veins are clamped, leaving as little as possible with the heart and as much as possible for the liver. The aorta is cross-clamped, and cardioplegic solution is injected into the aorta. The kidneys and liver are flushed with an intracellular solution via the aorta to prevent warm ischemia. The portal flush is changed to an intracellular solution. The heart is removed first with no adverse affects on the liver and kidneys. The liver is taken next. Then the kidneys are removed *en bloc* with aorta and vena cava, separated, and prepared as described above for kidney procurement.

## Preservation

Simple surface cooling allows up to 12 hours of preservation storage. Treatment with mannitol extends the allowable cold is-

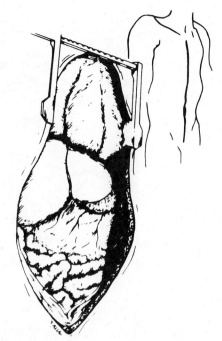

**Figure 6–7.** Incision for multiple organ harvesting. (From Rosenthal JT, Shaw BW Jr, Hardesty RL, et al: Principles of multiple organ procurement from cadaver donors. Ann Surg 198:617, 1983, with permission of the authors and publisher.)

chemia time to 16 hours. Transportation and tissue typing of patients and kidneys may necessitate longer periods of preservation. These have been made possible through pulsatile machine perfusion and use of flush solution followed by cold storage.

A flush solution with electrolyte content similar to intracellular rather than extracellular fluid used as cation exchange is believed to be detrimental.[38] Cold storage inhibits the active transport of sodium and potassium, which are then distributed via Donnan equilibrium. The cells gain water and swell because of the oncotic pressure generated by the intracellular proteins. The composition of the kidney flush solution (Euro-Collins) currently used at the University of Alabama at Birmingham consists of $KPO_4$ 115 mEq·L$^{-1}$, $NaHCO_3$ 20 mEq·L$^{-1}$, $KCl$ 15 mEq·L$^{-1}$, dextrose 31.6 gm·L$^{-1}$, and heparin 10,000 $\mu$·L$^{-1}$. $PO_4$ is the major anion in preservation solutions and is only semipermeable into cells, decreasing the likelihood of edema. In addition, it is a buffer within the physiological range and chelates calcium.[39] Hypertonic solutions should reduce cellular swell-

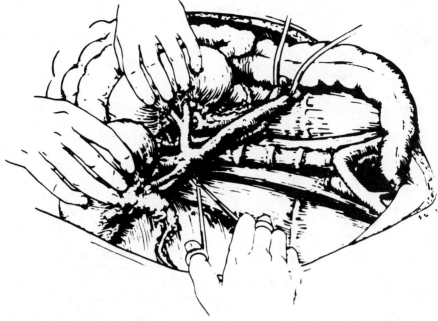

**Figure 6–8.** Mobilization of kidneys during multiple organ harvesting. (From Rosenthal JT, Shaw BW Jr, Hardesty RL, et al: Principles of multiple organ procurement from cadaver donors. Ann Surg 198:617, 1983, with permission of the authors and publisher.)

ing. Thus, dextrose and mannitol are used as impermeant agents. Compared to conventional Collins' or Sacks' solutions, a marked improvement in cellular ultrastructure was found when sucrose was used in an isotonic solution.[40] The addition of furosemide was not beneficial; in fact, large doses were nephrotoxic.[41] Excellent clinical response has resulted from cold storage up to 24 hours. Although some have advocated storage at 40°C for up to 48 hours, extending cold storage beyond 40 hours has resulted in a high incidence of acute tubular necrosis with less than optimal renal function.[42] However, patients can be supported by dialysis during acute tubular necrosis, which may last several weeks with subsequent adequate renal function.

Continuous hypothermic machine perfusion provides effective preservation for more than 48 hours.[41] Both continuous and pulsatile pumps have been used. Decreasing flow rates and rising perfusion pressures may indicate inadequate preservation. It was recommended that kidneys with flows of less than 80 to 100 ml/min be discarded. An estimated 25 per cent of kidneys would have to be discarded if these guidelines were followed. Therefore, Sampson et al.[43] transplanted 100 machine-preserved kidneys re-

gardless of their flow rates and found no correlation between flow rate and renal function at 1, 3, or 12 months. Current figures for wasted kidneys are 4 per cent with perfusion and 3 per cent with cold storage.[44] Loss is due to prolonged storage time and perfusion errors. No differences between perfusion and cold storage can be detected in optimally harvested kidneys with less than 24 hours' storage. However, pulsatile perfusion may be preferable when the donor status is less than optimal, e.g., upper age limit, hemodynamic instability, non-O type donors in whom tissue typing has not been started and up to 72 hours storage is anticipated. There has been a gradual decline in machine preservation over the past decade with a corresponding increase in cold storage (Fig. 6–9). In most cases, ice storage is simpler, safer, more economical, and as effective as machine storage.

A new perfusate including adenosine and $PO_4$ to replenish stores of adenosine triphosphate depleted during storage, resulted in immediate graft function of 87 per cent and one-month graft function of 97 per cent. Cyclosporine was used for immunosuppression. More recently Belzer's group[45] found that the addition of a 24-hour period of cold storage with the same adenosine phosphate solution resulted in no detrimental effect fol-

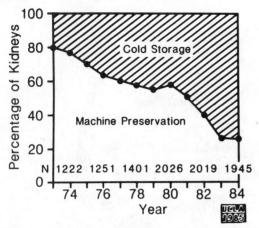

**Figure 6–9.** Percentage of kidneys preserved by cold storage and machine preservation. (From Terasaki PI, Toyotome A, Mickey MR, et al: Patient, graft and functional survival rates: An overview. In Terasaki PI (ed): Clinical Kidney Transplants 1985. Los Angeles, UCLA Tissue Typing Lab, 1985, p 1, with permission of the authors and publisher.)

lowing 48 hours of perfusion, thus facilitating national and international sharing of kidneys.

## SURGICAL TECHNIQUES OF KIDNEY TRANSPLANTATION

### Vascular Anastomoses

The right iliac fossa is preferred over the left, as the right iliac vein is more superficial. Also, the takeoff of the left hypogastric artery is much sharper, and the sigmoid colon may make exposure on the left more difficult. However, the left iliac fossa may be used whenever the right cannot, e.g., following prior transplantation. An oblique or curvilinear incision is made, beginning parallel to the inguinal ligament up to the iliac crest. The iliac vessels are carefully dissected. The lymphatic chain around the iliac vessels should be carefully ligated to prevent the formation of a lymphocele.

Although some surgeons prefer to do the arterial, many surgeons prefer to do the venous anastomosis first.[46] There is less movement of the kidney if the venous anastomosis is completed first. Maximum mobility of the iliac vein is needed to prevent renal vein thrombosis. The iliac vein is clamped near the vena cava and down near the inguinal ligament or with a partial occluding clamp such as a Satinsky clamp. An ellipse about the diameter of the renal vein is cut. Three or four stay sutures are placed as seen in Fig-

ure 6–10A. The renal vein anastomosis is done. The renal artery is anastomosed end to end with the internal iliac (hypogastric) artery in LRD transplants. In cadaveric transplants the renal artery is anastomosed end to side with the external iliac artery. Heparin saline flush is injected to prevent air emboli (Fig. 6–10B and C). If the internal iliac artery is either too arteriosclerotic or too small, the renal artery may be anastomosed end to side to the external iliac artery as it is in cadaveric transplants. Less dissection is necessary, and it takes less time when utilizing the external iliac. A patch of aorta is used with cadaveric transplants, decreasing the likelihood of development of renal artery stenosis. An aortic or Carrel patch may also be used with multiple renal arteries.

After adequate hydration and filling pressures have been achieved, the vascular clamps may be released. The proximal venous clamp is released first, then the distal venous, followed by the arterial. In cadaveric transplants the distal arterial clamp is released first, followed by the proximal. The color of the kidney should change from gray to pink, and the kidney should become firm and pulsating. Bluish mottling may result from vasospasm. Papavarine may be injected directly into the renal artery. Blood flow to the kidney may be temporarily increased by momentarily clamping the distal external iliac artery. A tight, too firm kidney may herald acute tubular necrosis. The bleeding is controlled with packing or additional sutures. Reclamping may be necessary, but introduces reperfusion injury when the kidney is warm and unprotected. Thus all efforts need to be made to ensure that the anastomoses will function prior to release of the clamps.

### Ureteral Anastomosis

The transplanted ureter may be anastomosed to the recipient's bladder or ureter. The advantage of ureteroneocystostomy is that it may be utilized when the recipient's ureter is unfit because of reflux, stenosis, or infection. The disadvantages are that it requires tunneling of the ureter through the bladder mucosa and a three-layer closure, the bladder may become infected, and there may be necrosis of either end of the ureter or stenosis at the tunnel in the bladder wall.[46] The ureteroneocystostomy is performed by tunneling the ureter from the midline to either lateral wall of the bladder, avoiding the recipient's native ureters. Laterally the bladder

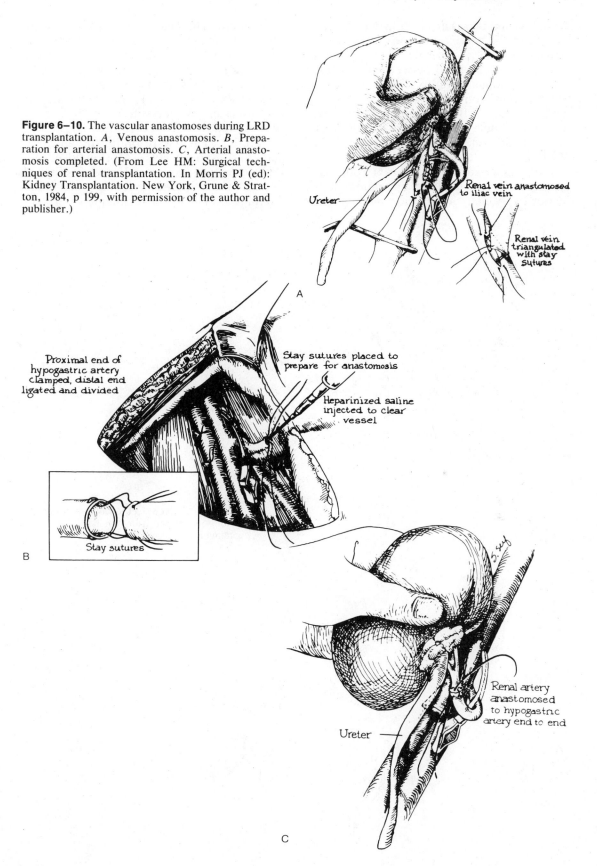

**Figure 6–10.** The vascular anastomoses during LRD transplantation. *A*, Venous anastomosis. *B*, Preparation for arterial anastomosis. *C*, Arterial anastomosis completed. (From Lee HM: Surgical techniques of renal transplantation. In Morris PJ (ed): Kidney Transplantation. New York, Grune & Stratton, 1984, p 199, with permission of the author and publisher.)

Ureter

Renal vein anastomosed to iliac vein

Renal vein triangulated with stay sutures

A

Proximal end of hypogastric artery clamped, distal end ligated and divided

Stay sutures placed to prepare for anastomosis

Heparinized saline injected to clear vessel

Stay sutures

B

Renal artery anastomosed to hypogastric artery end to end

Ureter

C

becomes thin, increasing the chances for leak formation. To decrease the possibility of necrosis, as little as possible of the ureter is used. The fascial band between the bladder and the abdominal wall is ligated to prevent ureteral adhesions and kinking. A recent modification of the ureteroneocystostomy uses a small hole in the anterior bladder without tunneling and a one-layer closure (Fig. 6–11).

The primary advantages of ureteroureteral anastomoses are simplicity and minimum infection, especially with prior bladder contamination. The main disadvantage is the relatively high incidence of fistula formation. This technique is unsuitable for patients in whom urine is made from their old kidneys.

If an ileal conduit is necessary it should be created six weeks prior to the transplant with the stoma on the opposite side. Glass et al. recently reported five cases and reviewed the literature.[47] They were optimistic about results and graft survival. McDonald et al.[48] reported good results with pre-existing cutaneous ureterostomy prior to renal transplantation. Whichever technique of ureteral

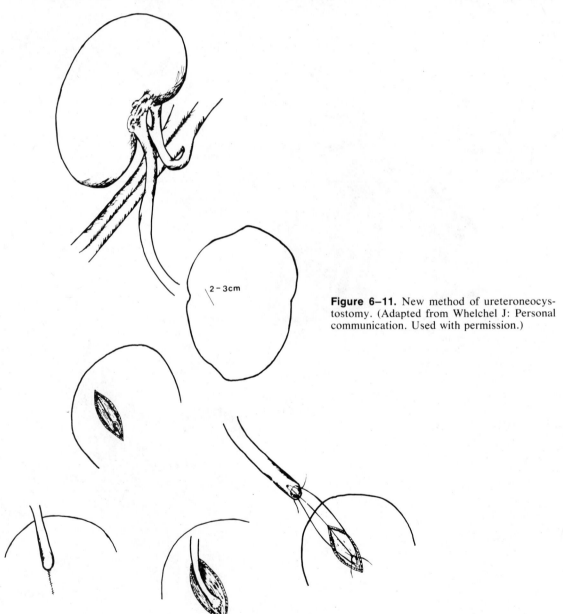

2 – 3 cm

**Figure 6–11.** New method of ureteroneocystostomy. (Adapted from Whelchel J: Personal communication. Used with permission.)

anastomosis is utilized, it should be the one best suited for the patient; meticulous attention should be given to every surgical detail and hemostasis in these immunosuppressed patients prone to infection and poor wound healing.

## Surgical Considerations for the Pediatric Patient

Although earlier results of transplantation in pediatric patients were dismal, recent data are encouraging.[49] In fact, some centers report, in comparison to adults, a higher percentage of uremic children living with a functioning transplant. The results of transplantation in children under the age of two years were particularly discouraging. So et al.[50] recently reported nine successful transplants in infants under the age of one year. Infants with end-stage renal disease have severe growth retardation as well as an encephalopathy that may not be reversed by dialysis. Dialysis in small children is difficult at best and poorly tolerated. Transplantation results not only in an improved psychosocial situation for the child, but better growth development.[50] Thus it is advised that transplantation be performed as soon as possible when the child develops ESRD. Although pediatric donors may be preferable in recipients under 10 kg, adult kidneys may be utilized with a transabdominal approach.[49] The renal artery and vein are anastomosed end to side with the common iliac vessels. In very small recipients it may be necessary to anastomose to the aorta and vena cava. When possible, the ureter should be anastomosed to the recipient's ureter. If not, the ureter should be implanted in the bladder using an antireflux technique.

## Transplant Nephrectomy

Rejection of a kidney that has been in place for months or years can make the transplant nephrectomy difficult. The usual approach is through the original incision, but an abdominal approach may be necessary if there is a mycotic aneurysm or an abscess. The pedicle may be mass ligated or the vessels separately dissected and ligated. Meticulous hemostasis is again essential.

## SURGICAL COMPLICATIONS

Although technical complications account for only about 5 per cent of graft failures, they do represent possible preventable losses of both graft and patient. Early recognition may save some grafts.

### Vascular

**Arterial.** Despite careful hemostasis at the time of surgery an occasional patient may require re-exploration for hemorrhage or hematoma. Renal artery thrombosis is quite rare, occurring in 1/800 in one series, and is said always to be due to a technical error at the time of surgery.[51] Precipitating causes include intimal flaps, arteriosclerosis, hypercoagulable states, and damage during harvesting or perfusion. The diagnosis is suspected by sudden anuria and confirmed when a renal scan shows no uptake.[52] Thrombosis of a lower pole artery affects the blood supply to the ureter. Warm ischemia time of greater than one and a half hours usually irreversibly damages the graft, and transplant nephrectomy is needed.

Persistent worsening diastolic hypertension without other signs of rejection is characteristic of renal artery stenosis. The incidence ranges from 3 to 10 per cent and is greater in LRD transplants in which an aortic cuff cannot be used. A bruit is present whenever the stenosis is greater than 65 to 80 per cent.[53] In most cases the stenosis is in the donor artery beyond the anastomosis. Causes include scar formation in the periadventitial tissue as an immunological response to the generalized homograft reaction, angulation or torsion of the renal artery, faulty surgical technique, trauma from the perfusion cannula, rejection, and arteriosclerosis. The diagnosis is made by arteriography. While the renal artery stenosis may occasionally resolve spontaneously, it generally does not. The renin level is increased. The hypertension may become unresponsive to medication. Captopril may result in acute but reversible deterioration of GFR and renal function.[54] Recently Trachtman et al. reported the successful use of captopril in the treatment of post-transplant renal artery stenosis in a child.[55] No decrease in renal function was detected. Initial trials of percutaneous transluminal angioplasty (PTA) revealed good but only temporary results.[53] Therefore PTA was recommended only when surgery was contraindicated or when its effectiveness was very doubtful, as in chronic rejection. However, some have reported better results, and PTA is now recommended as the first choice.[56] Surgical correction carries a high risk of graft loss. The patient's hypertension should subside within days following repair by PTA or surgical correction.

**Venous.** Primary venous thrombosis is rare. As with arterial thrombosis, it may be the end result of severe rejection. Precipitating causes include angulation of the iliac vein, pressure from hematoma or lymphocele, and thrombosis of the iliac vein. Symptoms of venous thrombosis include oliguria or anuria, proteinuria, and hematuria. While some surgeons have "always been able to reverse the process by systemic heparinization" and do not recommend venous thrombectomy,[51] others use heparinization only if re-exploration seems too risky. Venous hypertension may occur if a large accessory vein is not anastomosed or if a pediatric kidney is transplanted using a continuous suture for the venous anastomosis. Partial renal vein obstruction may occur secondary to iliac vein thrombosis. When first seen, patients have swelling of the leg and thigh on the same side as the graft. The kidney is swollen and has decreasing function.[51]

**Lymphocele.** A lymphocele is a collection of lymph that has leaked from the donor kidney lymphatics that were not ligated at the time of transplantation. The incidence ranges from 2 to 18 per cent and is now believed to be the most frequent surgical complication causing decreasing renal function during the post-transplantation period.[57] Lymphoceles usually occur following cadaveric transplantation and only rarely after LRD transplantation. Since transplantation is an extraperitoneal procedure, the accumulated lymph cannot be reabsorbed by the peritoneum. The first complaint is usually a feeling of fullness and discomfort. It is not particularly painful. Lymphedema causing swelling of the ipsilateral leg occurs in 10 per cent. Ultrasound reveals a collection of fluid between the kidney and the bladder; hydronephrosis may also be seen. The treatment is surgical drainage and creation of a large peritoneal window allowing lymph to be reabsorbed by the peritoneum.[51]

## Ureteral and Bladder Complications

Ureteral fistula or stenosis may occur. Vascular insufficiency is the primary cause of ureteral urinary extravasation and is more common after ureteral-ureteral anastomoses than after ureteroneocystostomy. Arterial branches to the ureter arise near the hilum traveling through the fatty tissue. Thus, excessive dissection must be avoided; the perihilar fat and sufficient areolar tissue are left around the ureter. The second most common cause of ureteral leak is too much tension on the anastomosis from the shaft of the ureter. Signs and symptoms of ureteral leak include decreasing urine output, pain, and decreasing renal function. The diagnosis and site may be determined by intravenous pyelography (IVP). Indigo carmine may be given intravenously during surgery to locate the leak precisely. Early diagnosis may prevent graft loss. If there is no renal function, sonography may confirm the diagnosis. Early ureteric stenosis is secondary to constriction of the ureter by the bladder and may result in necrosis. Late ureteric stenosis may be due to rejection, with marginal blood supply causing scarring.[51] The ureter may also be obstructed by abscess, lymphocele, or stones. Calculus formation is extremely rare following renal transplantation, with only about 80 reported cases. It may be mistaken for rejection. The calculi may be removed by percutaneous nephrolithotomy.

Bladder leaks are more common after repeat grafting. The incidence has significantly decreased since synthetic sutures such as polyglycolic acid (Dexon) and polyglactin (Vicryl) have been used instead of catgut. The diagnosis is suspected when there is clear fluid draining from the wound or a mass developing near the incision. Bladder leaks are relatively painless at first, as the pain fibers arise from the parietal peritoneum. The most common sign is hematuria. Leaks occurring several weeks after transplantation are usually only seen in diabetics. Bladder leaks need to be surgically corrected as soon as possible.

**Infection.** Deep wound infections around the kidney posterior to the external oblique fascia occur in less than 1 per cent of patients and require prompt surgical drainage. Graft removal may be necessary. Severe infection may disrupt the arterial anastomosis, causing massive hemorrhage. Superficial wound infections occur in about 1 per cent of patients and do not affect the prognosis of the patient or graft. The primary source of transplant infections is bladder contamination. Frank bladder infection is reason to postpone even cadaveric transplantation. Urinary tract infections decrease in frequency three months following transplantation. Most are asymptomatic and have a benign course. However, occasionally patients develop septicemia resulting in graft failure. Thus, routine urine cultures should be obtained. With the exception of diabetic nephropathy, neither the original renal disease nor the presence of vesicoureteral reflux were found to be predisposing factors. However, females were twice as likely to develop urinary tract infections as males.[58] Infectious complications are discussed in Chapter 5.

## Transplant Rupture

Transplant rupture most commonly occurs within the first two weeks following transplantation when the graft is the most swollen from severe acute rejection. The rupture occurs along the line of least resistance along the posterior convex border. It may also be associated with ischemia, biopsy, and other trauma. Typically the rupture begins while the patient is undergoing dialysis and is heparinized. It is quite painful and, as it expands, hematocrit decreases. Hyperkalemia unresponsive to dialysis may be present. Small, early ruptures may be diagnosed by ultrasound as hypoechoic masses associated with adjacent posterior perirenal fluid collection. These represent both intrarenal and extrarenal hematomas. Rarely, small ruptures are present and can be oversewn. If rupture is not detected early, circulatory collapse and loss of graft function occur. Usually irreversible rejection is present, necessitating graft removal. Transplant rupture may cause a severe consumptive coagulopathy.

## Femoral Neuropathy

Rarely reported, femoral neuropathy may result in weakness and numbness after renal transplantation. The causes may be either the self-retaining retractors or technical difficulties secondary to atheromatous plaques in the kidney.[59]

## ANESTHETIC MANAGEMENT OF THE LIVING RELATED DONOR

On the preoperative visit the anesthesiologist should expect to see a healthy patient. The upper age limit is usually set at 60 years for consideration as an LRD. If the anesthesiologist finds anything suspicious the transplant surgeon should be notified. In particular, mild hypertension, especially in male donors over the age of 50, may increase the incidence of late hypertension in the donor.[60] Other conditions that if undetected in their early stages might lead to renal problems sooner than if the patient had not donated include nephrosclerosis, diabetes, and mild pyelonephritic scars.

In 100 LRD's from the Mayo Clinic the mean creatinine was 0.98 (range 0.65 to 1.68) prior to donation and 1.2 10 to 20 years later (range 0.80 to 1.80).[60] The conclusion is that kidney donors did not suffer progressive loss of renal function. Long-term follow-up studies of LRD's have found that they continued to feel they had made the right choice and, given the same circumstances, would do it again.[61] After rejection of the kidney he donated to his sister, one patient of ours said to give it back to him and he would give her his other one! In addition, patients report heightened self-esteem and an increased positive outlook on life.

Competent adults may consent to surgery and anesthesia. The fact that the operation may not be beneficial does not affect the power to consent to it. In several early cases when transplants were done only between identical twins, the Supreme Judicial Court of Massachusetts found that the consent of the underage child and parents was valid. In each case the court determined that the child donor comprehended the need for surgery and would be psychologically harmed if he did not donate and his twin died.[62]

Hydration of the LRD must be optimal. In our institution, on the evening before surgery an intravenous infusion of 5 per cent dextrose in 0.45 per cent NaCl is begun at a rate of 125 ml·hr$^{-1}$ and increased to 250 ml·hr$^{-1}$ at 5 AM on the day of the operation.[63] Najarian et al. were the first to recognize what they called renal protective mechanisms in the LRD.[27] The protocol of Najarian et al. included giving 15 ml·kg$^{-1}$ of 5 per cent dextrose in 0.45 per cent NaCl intravenously at least one hour before induction of anesthesia, strictly maintaining normal blood pressure with fluid and plasma, and not giving any vasopressors. If urine output dropped below 1.5 ml·min$^{-1}$, 12.5 to 25 gm of mannitol were given. Mannitol was also given 30 minutes prior to removal of the kidney. They found a 40 per cent failure rate in the control group compared to 5 per cent in the "renal protective group."[27]

The following monitors are used routinely for LRD's: ECG, esophageal stethoscope, arterial blood pressure, urine output, temperature, oxygen analyzer, and end-tidal $CO_2$. Pulse oximetry is becoming routine. A second intravenous infusion is started upon arrival of the LRD in the operating room. Anesthesia induction is generally with thiopental, *d*-tubocurarine, and succinylcholine. Fentanyl, diazepam, and lidocaine are also frequently administered during induction, depending on the preferences of the anesthesiologist. Maintenance is generally with isoflurane. Fentanyl may supplement the inhalational anesthetic throughout the procedure. An argument against nitrous oxide can be made. One of the most frequent complications of donor nephrectomy is pneumothorax. This is particulary true for surgeons who deliberately enter the pleural cavity, resectioning the 10th rib for exposure of the kidney.

The majority of reported anesthetic complications were related to difficult intubation. Others included corneal abrasion and brachial plexus palsy. Following induction the patient is turned to the lateral position with care taken to protect the axilla and brachial plexus. As the kidney rest is raised, the blood pressure is closely monitored and maintained at normal levels with fluids and lightening of anesthesia. Vasopressors should be avoided. Ventilation is controlled to ensure eucarbia throughout the operation. This is particularly essential during the 10- to 15-minute "resting period" before closing of the vascular clamps. Hypercarbia and hypocarbia are potent inducers of renal artery spasm.[64,65] Thus end-tidal $CO_2$ monitoring is quite helpful.

Mannitol and furosemide are administered before the ureter is cut and during the resting period. Heparin is injected before clamping of the renal vessels at the end of the rest period. The cross-clamp time is noted in the anesthetic record as well as in the transplant records. After removal of the kidney, protamine is administered slowly. Before closing the wound, the surgeons explore for diaphragmatic and pleural leaks. Upon emergence from the anesthesia and extubation, the patient's breath sounds should be auscultated. Although chest roentgenograms are routine, a difference in breath sounds may confer a greater sense of urgency.

## ANESTHETIC MANAGEMENT OF THE CADAVERIC DONOR

The majority of potential cadaveric organ donors are in community hospitals where most traumatic injuries are treated. Regional organ banks aid in the retrieval and transport of organs. Members of the organ bank team endeavor to make the organ donation a positive and safely expedient experience for the family, referring physician, and hospital. Responsibilities of the transplant coordinators include public and professional education, donor surveillance and management, and assisting with organ procurement, preservation, and transportation.

Once the next of kin has given permission for organ donation, it is incumbent upon all to ensure the best chances for success of the transplant organs. Before surgery begins the anesthesiologist should check for properly prepared consents, a death note in the chart, specimens collected for tissue typing, drugs that may be asked for by the nephrectomy team, and any paperwork expected by the transplant team, i.e., cross-clamp time and so on. The anesthesia team supports the cadaveric donor until the aorta is cross-clamped. The "rule of 100's" states that systolic arterial pressure should be greater than 100 mm Hg, the urine output greater than 100 ml·hr$^{-1}$, and the arterial $P_{O_2}$ greater than 100 mm Hg. Blood pressure should first be supported by optimal hydration. Post-transplant renal failure is directly related to hypotension in the donor. Large volumes of balanced salt solutions (up to 1000 ml·hr$^{-1}$) may be required, particularly when diabetes insipidus is present. Diabetes insipidus is characterized by high output of urine (greater than 200 ml·hr$^{-1}$) of low specific gravity and osmolality with an associated rise in serum sodium. Other volume expanders such as hetastarch or albumin may be useful. Pitressin is utilized in diabetes insipidus to avoid dehydration by increasing reabsorption of water from the tubules. Its use should be discontinued, if possible, before removal of the cadaveric organs, as it increases the incidence of acute tubular necrosis and graft failure after transplantation. If crystalloid and colloid infusions are insufficient to maintain systolic pressure greater than 100 mm Hg, dopamine may be used. Although up to 10 μg·kg$^{-1}$·min$^{-1}$ is acceptable prior to organ removal, as low a dose of dopamine as possible should be used. Prenephrectomy use of dopamine to the cadaveric donor increases the incidence of acute tubular necrosis and graft failure. The combined use of dopamine and Pitressin results in 20 per cent of kidneys that never function in the recipient. Other vasopressors should not be used either. Mannitol and furosemide may be used to promote diuresis.

Generally, controlled ventilation is provided with 100 per cent oxygen. A pulse oximeter may be helpful to determine the patient's continued good oxygenation. An end-tidal $CO_2$ monitor should be used, as hypercarbia and hypocarbia decrease renal blood flow.[64,65] Other monitors used routinely include the electrocardiograph, sphygmomanometer, thermometer, and esophageal stethoscope.

Muscle relaxants are used to aid surgery and to blunt spinal reflexes. Wetzel et al.[66] recently reported that upon incision all cadaveric organ donors had significant increases in systolic and diastolic blood pressures as well as heart rate. The authors suggested that there might be some residual brain stem function even though irreversible brain stem damage has occurred from which brain death is inevitable.[66]

Multiple organ procurements involve considerably more care by the anesthesia team. In the event of sudden cardiovascular collapse during organ procurement, the aorta may be quickly cannulated and the kidneys perfused. However, removal of the pancreas, liver, heart, and lungs requires meticulous dissection, since these organs do not tolerate lengthy warm ischemia.[37] The anesthesia team must carefully monitor fluid and electrolyte balance as well as cardiovascular function. Blood replacement averages 4 units in adults and 2 units in children during multiple organ procurement.[37] Hypothermia may lead to cardiac arrest. Heated humidifiers, fluid warmers, and other measures to maintain normothermia should be employed. Warm fluids may be placed directly around the heart after the incision is made. Once the aorta has been cross-clamped, the ventilator is discontinued and monitoring devices removed. At this time, it is difficult not to contemplate what might have happened without the catastrophe that claimed the life of the donor. But it is better that his or her organs live on to help overcome another's misery than to be buried forever.

## MANAGEMENT OF THE KIDNEY TRANSPLANT RECIPIENT

### Preoperative Evaluation

Prior to 1971 when Congress provided funding for end-stage renal disease (ESRD),

the majority of persons with uremia "died unobtrusively without the benefit of surgical intervention." In 1968, 1500 patients were estimated to be receiving dialysis. In 1977, 80 per million population developed ESRD. By 1982, 91 per million, or 70,000 Americans, were undergoing dialysis at a cost of more than $1.6 billion.[67] Marked racial predispositions exist in development of ESRD: The annual figures are 108 per million blacks and 44 per million whites.[68] In Europe, the incidence is 22 per million per year. Hypertension accounts for ESRD in only 10 per cent of whites but in nearly 50 per cent of blacks. The incidence of essential hypertension in the general population is 10 per cent, while it exceeds 30 per cent in blacks.[69] Nephrosclerosis complicating essential hypertension occurs more frequently in blacks than whites.

The underlying renal diseases for the 1177 patients who underwent renal transplantation at the University of Alabama in Birmingham from 1968 to 1984 are summarized in Table 6–2. Certain renal diseases may recur in the transplanted kidney and may contraindicate transplantation, including rapidly progressing glomerulonephritis with high titers of antiglomerular basement membrane antibodies, active lupus erythematosus, and Wegener's granulomatosis.

There are several stages of chronic renal failure. Decreased renal reserve is first and is associated with a loss of up to 60 per cent of nephron mass. Clinically it is asymptomatic. The creatinine clearance gradually declines from 100 per cent to 20 per cent of

**TABLE 6–2. Underlying Renal Disease Before Transplantation**

| Disease | No. | % |
| --- | --- | --- |
| Glomerulonephritis | 479 | 41 |
| Hypertension | 198 | 17 |
| Diabetes | 108 | 9 |
| Unknown disease | 85 | 7 |
| Pyelonephritis | 66 | 6 |
| Other disease | 65 | 5 |
| Polycystic disease | 56 | 5 |
| Obstructive uropathy | 36 | 3 |
| Alport's syndrome | 30 | 3 |
| Hypoplasia-dysplasia | 20 | 2 |
| Lupus nephritis | 18 | 1 |
| Congenital nephrotic syndrome | 16 | 1 |

Data from 1177 patients who had renal transplantation at UAB from 1968 to 1984. (Courtesy of AG Diethelm. Used with permission.)

## TABLE 6–3. Signs and Symptoms of Uremia

**Behavioral, mental, or neurological**
  *Depressive:* fatigue, asthenia, malaise, mental dullness, shortening of concentration, memory defects, sluggishness or heaviness, anorexia, drowsiness by day, suicidal thoughts, thanatophobia, stupor, precoma, coma
  *Irritative:* anxiety, fasciculations, twitching, headache, cerebellar signs of ataxa, asterixis, abnormal gait, vertigo, compulsive actions, central nausea, convulsions
  *Psychiatric:* personality change, bizarre behavior (e.g., compulsive, paranoid) phobias, organic psychosis, selective amnesia, denial, food and drug kleptomania
  *Peripheral:* pruritus, paresthesias, burning foot, restless leg syndrome, foot flap and drop, monoplegia, paraplegia, sensory and motor defects, bladder atony and dysfunction
  *Ophthlamic:* nystagmus, miosis, asymmetric pupils (anisocoria), blurring, amaurosis, the red eye syndrome due to conjunctival irritation from calcium deposits, band keratopathy
**Gastrointestinal**
  *Membrane problems:* cheilitis, glossitis, stomatitis, parotitis, esophagitis, enteritis, pancreatitis, colitis, ileus
  *Functional problems:* anorexia, dysgeusia and ageusia, nausea, vomiting, hematemesis, constipation, diarrhea, abdominal distention
  *Structural problems:* peptic and colonic ulceration
**Cardiovascular-pulmonary**
  Pericarditis, acute and constrictive
  Cardiomegaly
  Pleuritis
  Congestive heart failure
  Change in blood pressure
  Arrhythmias
  Vascular calcification
  Accelerated atherosclerosis
  Cheyne-Stokes and/or Kussmaul breathing
**Hematological**
  Anemia (normochromic normocytic)
  Bleeding abnormality (prolonged bleeding time, abnormal platelet aggregation)
  Lymphopenia, mild thrombocytopenia
**Dermatological**
  Pallor
  Excoriations and pruritus
  Urea frost
  Purpura and ecchymosis
  Rash
    Pseudo-clubbed fingers of severe hyperparathyroid bone disease
    Brown nail of uremia
  Cutaneous and subcutaneous calcification
  Peripheral tissue necrosis and ulceration
**Metabolic**
  Musculoskeletal muscle pain and weakness, proximal myopathy, bone pain, bone fractures
  Aseptic necrosis of bone
  Disturbances in multiple endocrine systems
  Carbohydrate intolerance
  Hyperlipidemia
  Gout and pseudogout
  Washing and abnormalities in protein metabolism
**Sexual and reproductive**
  Impotence
  Decreased libido
  Reduced nocturnal penile tumescence
  Infertility
  Amenorrhea
  Frigidity
  Gynecomastia
  Galactorrhea

**TABLE 6–3. Signs and Symptoms of Uremia** (*Continued*)

**Immunological**
  Reduced T-cell-mediated immune function
  Impaired phagocytosis and chemotaxis
  Atrophy of the lymphoid system including thymus
  Reduced immune surveillance of neoplasia
**Miscellaneous**
  Reduced wound healing
  Hypothermia
  Impaired response to pyrogen

From Schreiner GE: Uremia. In Massry SG, Glassock RJ (eds): Textbook of Nephrology. Baltimore, Williams & Wilkins, 1983, p 452, with permission of author and publisher.

normal values. Although these patients should be carefully followed by their internists, they present little concern to the anesthesiologist. The second stage is renal insufficiency or the transitional stage. These patients have mild increases in BUN and creatinine. The creatinine clearance decreases from 20 per cent to 5 per cent of normal. Patients have limited ability to compensate for excess water and salt loads. Hypovolemia may be devastating, leading to overt renal failure. ESRD or uremia is symptomatic with anemia and other biochemical abnormalities occurring when creatinine clearance is reduced to below 5 per cent of normal. Uremia simply means urine in the blood. Unable to be excreted, the urinary solutes collect throughout the body, interfering with cellular metabolism in every organ system (Table 6–3).[70] The impact of uremia on every organ system in the body plays an important role in the anesthetic plan.

### Gastrointestinal Disorders

Anorexia, nausea, vomiting, hiccups, dysgeusia, and either diarrhea or constipation may be some of the earliest symptoms of ESRD. Of particular importance to the anesthesia team is the delayed gastric emptying time of 300 to 700 minutes.[71] Duodenitis occurs in 60 per cent, gastritis in 22 per cent, and esophagitis in 13 per cent of patients with ESRD. Gastrointestinal bleeding is common. Patients with peptic ulcer disease should be considered for ulcer surgery prior to renal transplantation. Many of the gastrointestinal problems can be relieved by dialysis and decreased dietary protein, or by transplantation. Phenothiazines and nasopharyngeal stimulation may help control hiccups.[69] Even without a history of hepatitis, many dialysis patients are chronic carriers of hepatitis

B surface antigen. Australia antigen–associated hepatitis, chronic hepatic venous congestion, and hemosiderosis occur frequently.

### Neurological and Psychiatric Disorders

Decreased attention span, memory, and concentrating ability are some of the earliest signs of uremia. General irritability, anxiety, depression, and psychosis occur. Suicide and suicidal tendencies are frequent. Institution of dialysis may initially cause exhilaration, but repeated episodes of depression follow. Uremic encephalopathy with more subtle nervous dysfunction, including impaired mentation and generalized weakness, may persist despite adequate dialysis. Dialysis is associated with two CNS disorders: dialysis dysequilibrium syndrome (DDS) and dialysis dementia (DD). DDS occurs with the initiation of dialysis resulting in headache, nausea and vomiting, blurred vision, muscle twitches, disorientation, hypertension, and seizures. Recent dialysis techniques have decreased the severity of these symptoms.[72]

Dialysis dementia occurs in patients who have been undergoing hemodialysis for more than two years. Speech disorders, including slurring, stuttering, and hesitancy, occur early and in 90 per cent of patients with DD. Affective disorders progressing to dementia occur in 80 per cent, motor disturbances in 75 per cent, and convulsions in 60 to 90 per cent. Symptoms initially occur during dialysis, but then become constant, progressing to death in six months. Alfrey et al.[73] found that compared to normal, the aluminum content of gray matter of patients with DD was increased elevenfold, and in other patients undergoing hemodialysis who did not have DD it was increased threefold. Deionization of the water used to prepare the dialysate has markedly decreased the incidence of DD. However, DD has been reported in patients receiving peritoneal dialysis and in children with renal failure who were not being dialyzed but were taking aluminum hydroxide antacids. Also, there are sporadic cases of DD unrelated to aluminum and of uncertain cause. The onset of DD in 70 per cent of cases is associated with hospitalization for another medical illness. Immobilization causes release of aluminum from bone.

During the preoperative visit, the anesthesiologist should question all renal failure patients for signs of neuropathy. Uremic peripheral neuropathy is characterized by sensations of pins and needles in the feet, the burning feet syndrome. The discomfort may be partially relieved with movement, in which case it is called the restless leg syndrome. The lower extremities are involved before the upper. Pathologically there is loss of the large myelinated fibers and secondary demyelination.[69] The presence of neuropathy is an indication to begin dialysis, as it should arrest the degenerative process. Transplantation almost invariably reverses the neuropathy.[69] The autonomic nervous system may also be involved. Abnormalities may include defective sweat gland function, abnormal response to Valsalva's maneuver, decreased baroreceptor sensitivity, decreased elevation of blood pressure with exercise, and hypotension unresponsive to volume loading during dialysis. Ventricular tachycardia and cardiac arrest have been reported following the administration of succinylcholine to patients with uremic neuropathy.[74,75]

### Cardiovascular Disorders

Most patients with ESRD are hypertensive. When a patient with renal failure is not hypertensive, one should suspect profound extracellular volume (ECF) depletion, excessive antihypertensive medication, previous bilateral nephrectomy, or a rare salt-losing renal disease. Uncontrolled hypertension will further damage the kidneys. Methyldopa tends to increase GFR while beta blockers decrease GFR. Propranolol may adversely affect patients with a BUN level greater than 25 mg per dl. Clonidine and prazosin can be useful in the treatment of hypertension. Minoxidil is also effective in ESRD, but may be associated with sodium retention, hypertrichosis, and pericardial effusions.[69]

Sodium nitroprusside and diazoxide are used in hypertensive crises. Intravenous labetalol is effective for acute hypertension. However, long-term administration of labetalol alone or with a thiazide may not be effective for severe hypertension. Captopril is the only orally effective angiotensin-converting enzyme inhibitor available in North America. It is effective in controlling hypertension mediated by the renin-angiotensin system. However, patients with renal failure have a high incidence of complications with captopril, including worsening of renal function.[54] Dialysis ameliorates hypertension in the majority of ESRD patients. About 10 to 15 per cent will have refractory hypertension with hyperreninemia. In the past, bilateral nephrectomy was the primary treatment, but is now performed for only a few specific indications. Renal transplantation usually cures hypertension associated with nephrosclerosis.

Left ventricular hypertrophy and congestive heart failure associated with the uremic state result from a number of factors, including hypertension, volume overload, anemia, atherosclerosis, pericarditis, and negative inotropism from acidosis, hyperkalemia, and hypermagnesemia. In addition, dialysis fistulas and grafts normally have flow rates of 250 to 750 ml·min$^{-1}$, but they may be as high as 2 L·min$^{-1}$, leading to high output heart failure.[76] Deaths from coronary artery disease in ESRD far exceed those in hypertensive or normal persons, approximating those in type II hyperlipidemia. Triglycerides are increased in ESRD. Renal transplantation may markedly improve cardiac function in patients with severe left ventricular dysfunction and ESRD. Cardiac conduction abnormalities may develop, particularly in the presence of hyperkalemia.

Two types of pericarditis occur in ESRD. Uremic pericarditis develops late in uremia or in poorly hemodialyzed patients. It responds to dialysis, is associated with few symptoms, has clear fluid, and rarely leads to tamponade. Dialysis-related pericarditis develops earlier, does not respond to dialysis, and is associated with pain, fever, and leukocytosis. The fluid is hemorrhagic, and tamponade occurs not infrequently.[69]

### Hematological Disorders

Anemia develops as the serum creatinine exceeds 3 mg/dl. Causes include decreased erythropoietin production with the loss of renal parenchyma, bone marrow suppression, hemolysis from oxidizing drugs with an abnormal pentose phosphate pathway, hemolysis from microangiopathic lesions, iron deficiency secondary to blood loss, decreased iron absorption due to phosphate-binding antacids, deficiency of folic acid and vitamins $B_{12}$ and $B_6$ and protein, and secondary hyperparathyroidism, which inhibits erythropoiesis, increases red cell turnover, and induces myelofibrosis.[77] Parathyroidectomy may improve the condition.

Although some accept a hematocrit of 20 per cent, most prefer a hematocrit of 24 per cent or higher for kidney transplantation. Patients with ESRD appear to do quite well with lower values of hematocrit for other surgical procedures. The levels of 2,3-diphosphoglycerate (2,3-DPG) increase in patients with ESRD, but not to the extent in nonrenal patients with the same degree of anemia. Thus, ESRD patients rely on increased cardiac output and a change in the oxygen-hemoglobin affinity for tissue oxygenation. Telangiectases and bleeding tendencies in uremia are related to platelet dysfunction, thrombocytopenia, abnormal platelet factor 3, excess heparin from dialysis, abnormal prothrombin consumption, and the like.

In the early 1970's it was believed that blood transfusion should be avoided in patients awaiting renal transplantation to prevent antibody formation from precluding a crossmatch. A decline in graft survival ensued. Opelz et al. reported that blood transfusion prior to renal transplantation increased graft survival.[29] The use of donor-specific transfusions has markedly improved graft survival in living related mismatched haplotypes[30,78] (Fig. 6–12). Ten to thirty per cent of recipients may develop antibodies that may delay transplantation while the titers decrease. The incidence of sensitization may be decreased by using stored rather than fresh blood or by giving azathioprine. The patients at greatest risk for becoming sensitized are women with multiple pregnancies and patients with a previous graft loss.[78] The issue of blood transfusion prior to transplantation is also discussed in Chapters 1 and 2.

### Musculoskeletal Disorders and Hyperparathyroidism

Bone diseases occurring with ESRD include osteomalacia, osteoporosis, osteosclerosis, and osteitis fibrosa cystica. They result from vitamin D deficiency, aluminum and magnesium toxicity, calcium and phosphate deficiency, and hyperparathyroidism. Vitamin D is needed for calcium absorption from the intestine and for bone mineralization. The hydroxylation of dietary 25-hydroxyvitamin $D_3$ to 1,25-dihydroxyvitamin $D_3$, the most active form of vitamin D, occurs in the kidney and thus is impaired in ESRD. Phosphate retention leads to hypocalcemia and in turn increases parathyroid hormone (PTH) secretion. Dietary phosphate, particularly dairy products, should be restricted. Aluminum hydroxide decreases phosphate absorption. Calcium supplements are pre-

**Figure 6–12.** Results of donor-specific blood transfusion in one-haplotype mismatched LRD transplants. (From Whelchel JD, Shaw JF, Curtis JJ, et al: Effect of pretransplant stored donor-specific blood transfusions on early renal allograft survival in one-haplotype living related transplants. Transplantation 34:326, 1982, with permission of the authors and publisher.)

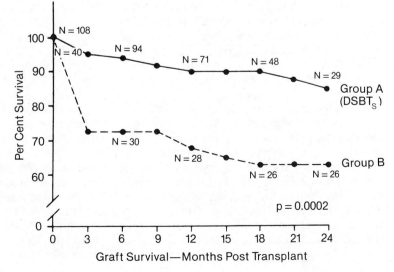

scribed as well as 1,25-dihydroxyvitamin $D_3$. Correction of metabolic acidosis is beneficial. Marked increases in serum and tissue aluminum are seen in patients with ESRD. PTH increases intestinal absorption of aluminum. Aluminum modulates bone acid and alkaline phosphatases and the response to PTH and 1,25-dihydroxycholecalciferol. The longer patients undergo dialysis the higher is the aluminum content in their bones. Deionized water for the dialysate can decrease the incidence of osteomalacia from 70 per cent to 15 per cent.[79] Metastatic calcifications may occur in the eyes, viscera, skin, arteries, and joints. Soft tissue calcifications are generally due to poor dietary control of phosphate. Arterial calcifications are some of the earliest radiographic complications of dialysis and are believed to be related to aluminum, which inhibits the enzymes involved with ATP, and magnesium, which mediates the toxic effects of aluminum and uremia on the heart. Once established, aluminum toxicity may be treated with desferrioxamine, which relieves symptoms of both dialysis osteomalacia and encephalopathy.[79]

One of the major hormonal imbalances in ESRD is increased PTH. PTH increases calcium in cells of the heart, brain, peripheral nerves, blood vessels, red blood cells, skin, muscle, and cornea. Intracellular calcium is critical to nearly all metabolic and enzymatic cellular functions. Changes in the intracellular-extracellular fluid $Ca^{++}$ ratio alter membrane permeability. PTH changes membrane phospholipids, in turn, altering agonist-receptor interactions. PTH is catabolic, resulting in accumulation of nitrogenous compounds in ESRD. Parathyroidectomy prior to ESRD has been shown to prevent the increase in calcium in nervous tissue. Goldstein et al.[80] have shown a direct correlation between PTH levels and EEG alterations in ESRD (Fig. 6–13). Serum parathyroid hormone is consistently elevated in osteitis fibrosa.

PTH inhibits erythropoiesis. This effect is masked in patients with primary hyperparathyroidism with normal kidneys producing erythropoietin. Only 5 to 21 per cent of patients with primary hyperparathyroidism are anemic.[81] In ESRD, the erythropoietin production is inadequate and the full inhibitory effects of PTH may be seen. PTH also decreases red cell survival, induces bone marrow fibrosis, and has pronounced cardiovascular effects. The heart cells may have

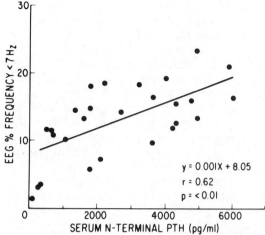

**Figure 6–13.** Effects of parathyroid hormone on EEG below 7 Hz in dialysis patients. (From Goldstein DA, Feinstein EI, Chui LA, Pattahiraman R, Massry SG: The relationship between the abnormalities in electroencephalogram and blood levels of PTH in dialysis patients. J Clin Endocrinol Metab 51:130, 1980, with permission of the authors and publisher.)

specific receptors for PTH activation, which causes tachycardia. Early cell death may occur. Left ventricular function improves after parathyroidectomy in ESRD.[81] PTH plays an important role in the regulation of organ blood flow by relaxing vascular smooth muscle and decreasing vascular resistance, including the coronary arteries.[82] PTH may affect carbohydrate metabolism, causing glucose intolerance, elevated insulin levels, insulin resistance, glycogenolysis, and gluconeogenesis. These effects are not seen in ESRD in the absence of PTH. Medical management may control most cases of secondary hyperparathyroidism, but fails in about 30 per cent. Suppression of PTH requires high-normal to slightly hypercalcemic levels in ESRD. The accumulation of PTH may be prevented by dietary phosphate restriction and/or 1,25-dihydroxyvitamin $D_3$. Thus, PTH may be one of the most important toxins of uremia. "The concept that PTH is a uremic toxin is unique, since it is the first time in the history of the search for uremic toxins that one may identify a toxin whose source could be controlled, allowing us to prevent its accumulation and to reduce its levels if they are already elevated."[81]

Although the incidence of secondary hyperparathyroidism appears to be decreasing,[83] the longer patients receive dialysis the more likely it is to develop. Chronic pyelonephritis is associated with a greater incidence of both secondary hyperparathyroidism and vitamin D osteomalacia. ESRD from analgesic abuse nephropathy results in particularly severe secondary hyperparathyroidism.[84] Diabetics have a significantly decreased incidence of severe secondary hyperparathyroidism. Whether the patient is undergoing hemodialysis or continuous ambulatory peritoneal dialysis does not affect the incidence of secondary hyperparathyroidism.

In 1960 Stanbury, Lumb, and Nicholson reported the first subtotal parathyroidectomy for renal osteodystrophy.[85] Total parathyroidectomy with an autograft of a small portion of one of the glands either to a pocket in the sternocleidomastoid[83] or to the forearm may be preferable to subtotal parathyroidectomy. The incidence of recurrence appears to be the same. Redo surgery may be easier when an autograft has been implanted and may be done under local anesthesia. Transient hypocalcemia should be expected between the third and fourth postoperative day as the bones begin to remineralize; it is treated with intravenous calcium.[83] Parathyroidectomy decreases the hyperlipidemia associated with ESRD.[83] Muscle weakness and atrophy, particularly of the lower extremities, occur with secondary hyperparathyroidism. Improvement in muscle strength is so rapid after parathyroidectomy that a reduction in PTH is a far more likely explanation than is resolution of atrophy. Osteitis fibrosa healed in 23 of 24 patients.[83]

Hypercalcemia in most patients resolves after transplantation.[86] Only 12 of nearly 1200 renal transplant patients required parathyroidectomy. Mild hypercalcemia—about 11 mg per dl—does not seem detrimental to the renal graft or to cause bone disease in the recipient.[83] There are no predictive factors to anticipate which patients will develop tertiary hyperparathyroidism. Exact indications for parathyroidectomy in tertiary disease remain unclear except for rapid decline in renal function and skeletal fractures. The primary goal of reduction of hyperfunctioning parathyroid tissue should be preservation of skeletal mineralization. Calcium levels above 16 mg per dl are considered a medical emergency, yet some patients with levels over 14 mg per dl will be quite symptomatic, particularly the elderly.[87] Thus, it is recommended that the calcium level be lower than 14 mg per dl prior to surgery.[87,88] The medical management of hypercalcemia includes optimal hydration with saline and monitoring of the central venous pressure. Furosemide is given every six to eight hours. Both saline and furosemide cause calciuria. The potassium level should be monitored and potassium replaced as needed.

### Diabetes

Diabetic nephropathy accounts for 25 per cent of new ESRD patients referred for dialysis.[89] The mean duration of diabetes mellitus prior to the onset of ESRD is 17.5 years. Twenty per cent of patients with type 1 or insulin-dependent diabetes mellitus (IDDM) develop ESRD before they are 30 years of age. Diabetic nephrosclerosis is the primary cause of death in 50 per cent of patients with IDDM. Survival rates have improved for IDDM patients who receive dialysis. In the early 1970's only 25 per cent survived 2 years. Currently 70 per cent of patients survive.[89] Older IDDM patients tend to do better with dialysis than with transplantation, while younger patients fare better following transplantation. Graft and patient survival do not differ between diabetic and nondiabetic recipients. Almost all IDDM patients who are candidates for renal transplantation have evidence of neuropathy, and all show improvement in the neuropathy following transplantation. Early transplantation may prevent blindness. Diabetic retinopathy progresses with use of hemodialysis. Psychological, social, and vocational rehabilitation are far more likely following renal transplantation than with hemodialysis. Insulin resistance is common in ESRD. Both continuous ambulatory peritoneal dialysis and hemodialysis improve the defect but do not restore insulin activity to normal. Impaired intracellular glucose metabolism or an abnormal transport system probably accounts for the insulin resistance of uremia.

### Drugs in End-Stage Renal Disease

ESRD is associated with a variety of derangements that predispose to adverse drug reactions. The pharmacokinetic and pharmacodynamic alterations include decreased renal excretion of drugs and their metabolites, decreased renal metabolism, altered bioavailability, hepatic metabolism and elimination, volume of distribution ($V_D$) from changes in protein binding, lipid solubility, and total body weight, and possible changes in end-organ response. Bennett et al. gathered an extensive list of guidelines for prescribing drugs in renal failure. Dosage adjustments for renal failure and the effects of dialysis for each drug are listed, as well as toxicity and adverse systemic side effects.[90]

In general, the loading dose of a drug in renal failure is similar to that for a patient without ESRD. One exception is digitalis. The binding of digoxin to myocardial receptors is decreased with uremia. The recommended loading dose is two thirds of a normal dose. Verapamil potentiates the effect of cyclosporine.[91] Post-transplant patients receiving both drugs may be prone to the nephrotoxic effects of cyclosporine.

Protein binding changes in ESRD become important when binding is greater than 90 per cent in patients with normal renal function.[90] Drug affinity for binding to albumin is decreased in renal failure. In addition, the plasma concentration of albumin is decreased in the nephrotic syndrome. Liver failure also decreases both drug affinity for albumin and its concentration. Acidic drugs bind primarily to albumin. Alpha$_1$ acid glycoprotein (alpha$_1$ AGP, or orosomucoid), lipoproteins, and albumin bind many cationic drugs such as those listed in Table 6–4.[92] The binding of these basic drugs is increased with those conditions listed in Table 6–5. Edwards et al.[93] showed that alpha$_1$ AGP was increased in all trauma patients within 24 hours of admission to the ICU, plateaued at five to seven days, and remained elevated for two to three weeks. The average free fraction of

### TABLE 6–4.  Basic Drugs That Bind to Alpha$_1$ Acid Glycoprotein

Propranolol
Lidocaine
Bupivacaine
Methadone
Quinidine
Dipyridamole
Imipramine
Prazosin
Perazine
Verapamil
Meperidine
Alfentanil

Modified from DeLeve LD, Piafsky KM: Clinical significance of plasma binding of basic drugs. Trends Pharmacol Sci 2:283, 1981, with permission of authors and publisher.

### TABLE 6–5.  Conditions That Increase Binding to Alpha$_1$ Acid Glycoprotein

Renal transplantation
Major surgery and trauma
Myocardial infarction
Malignant disease
Ulcerative colitis and Cushing's syndrome
Rheumatoid arthritis

Modified from DeLeve LD, Piafsky KM: Clinical significance of plasma binding of basic drugs. Trends Pharmacol Sci 2:283, 1981, with permission of authors and publisher.

lidocaine decreased from 0.28 to 0.15 in these trauma patients. Thus these patients required and tolerated otherwise toxic doses of lidocaine because of increased binding to alpha$_1$ AGP. Similar changes in protein binding of drugs have been noted for patients undergoing renal transplantation as well as during graft rejection.

### Patient Age

Life expectancy is increasing nearly every year. The incidence of ESRD increases with age. Although patients over the age of 45 to 50 years are no longer considered too great a risk for transplantation,[94] high-dose steroids are associated with excessive complications in older patients. Therefore, combinations of antilymphoblast globulin and low-dose prednisone or cyclosporine and low-dose steroids are used. Significant cardiac disease is more prevalent in the older population. Thus, Jordan et al.[94] performed coronary arteriography on all their patients prior to transplantation. Four patients underwent operation for coronary artery bypass grafts prior to transplantation.

Most pharmacological studies were done in young healthy volunteers. The effects of age on pharmacokinetics and pharmacodynamics are still being discovered. Both renal and hepatic clearances of drugs decrease with age. Lean body mass decreases and fatty tissue mass increases relative to total body weight with age. Lipid-soluble drugs such as diazepam and lidocaine are distributed more extensively in the elderly. The adverse effects from many of the benzodiazepines increase with age. Excessive bleeding from heparin also occurs with age. However, age does not appear to increase the risk of anesthesia or anesthetic complications.

## Preparation of the Recipient for Renal Transplantation

### Dialysis

Peritoneal dialysis was first employed in 1923 for renal failure. Intermittent peritoneal dialysis subsequently became utilized for patients with acute and some with chronic renal failure over the next several decades. Hemodialysis machines were introduced in Europe in 1948 and came into extensive use in the United States after 1950. The Tenckhoff catheter made continuous ambulatory peritoneal dialysis an effective alternative to both intermittent peritoneal dialysis and hemodialysis. Usually the catheters are inserted in the operating room with the patient under local anesthesia and sedated. Recently a new technique using a small instrument looking something like a rhinoscope permits placement of the catheters at the patient's bedside.[95] Continuous ambulatory peritoneal dialysis can allow the ESRD patient to live a reasonably normal life. Dialysis occurs while the patient is at work or play. Exchanges are repeated three to five times per day seven days a week. It requires a cooperative and capable patient and/or family member to perform the exchanges. Diabetics may benefit particularly from continuous ambulatory peritoneal dialysis because their vascular problems make long-term hemodialysis difficult. Congestive heart failure, hypertension, and anemia appear to respond best to continuous ambulatory peritoneal dialysis. Pericarditis, osteodystrophy, and neuropathy persist as problems.[96] Patients are allowed liberal fluid and protein intake to compensate for losses in the peritoneal dialysate. Blood chemistry values after a few weeks of continuous ambulatory peritoneal dialysis remain stable. Patients undergoing continuous ambulatory peritoneal dialysis show more favorable adjustments than hemodialysis patients in terms of self-esteem, general well-being, and vocational rehabilitation. Therefore, continuous ambulatory peritoneal dialysis is said to be the most physiological.

Dialysis is done 12 to 36 hours before transplantation to control blood pressure and potassium. The chart should state the patient's weight before and after dialysis as well as the patient's estimated dry weight. The dry weight is the minimum weight that has been achieved with dialysis without vascular collapse. Clear lung fields on roentgenography and ausculation and no ankle edema or congestive heart failure are present at dry weight. The patient's estimated dry weight compared to present weight helps estimate fluid status before surgery.

### Bilateral Nephrectomy

Before 1975 bilateral nephrectomy was routine prior to kidney transplantation, but resulted in significant morbidity (88 per cent) and mortality (11 per cent). Current indications for bilateral nephrectomy prior to renal transplantation include persistent pyelonephritis with bacteriuria, structural abnormalities of the urinary tract predisposing to infection, Goodpasture's syndrome, renin-dependent hypertension, certain rapidly progressing cases of glomerulonephritis, and polycystic kidneys with significant pain, persistent infection, bleeding, or excessive size.[97] When necessary, bilateral nephrectomy should be done six to eight weeks prior to transplantation. Bilateral posterior incisions are associated with lower morbidity and death rates than the anterior approach. Sheinfeld et al.[97] believe the initial excessive morbidity and mortality was a direct result of inadequate blood and fluid replacement. In their recent series there was no mortality and minimal morbidity. Average blood loss was 700 ml; mean fluid replacement was 6000 ml to maintain the central venous pressure at 5 to 10 cm $H_2O$ and hematocrit values at 25 per cent. The systemic vascular resistance falls following bilateral nephrectomy, and large amounts of fluids may be required to prevent hypotension and its sequelae of myocardial infarction, cerebral vascular accident, and thrombosed fistulas.

Patients who have undergone bilateral nephrectomy are more prone to hyperkalemia, anemia, vitamin D deficiency, and congestive heart failure from fluid overload. In the anephric state there is a direct relationship between the patient's plasma volume and blood pressure.

### Premedication

ESRD patients will have four times more unbound diazepam than patients with normal renal function. The half-life of diazepam is increased and the clearance for a single dose of diazepam decreased in ESRD.[98] The half-life of oxazepam is 25 hours in ESRD compared to 10 hours in normal subjects. Oxazepam is not dialyzable. It has been suggested that

ESRD increases the biliary excretion of oxazepam glucuronide. However, hydrolysis in the intestine results in reabsorption of oxazepam. Values of half-life of lorazepam for ESRD and normal subjects are similar to those of oxazepam. Repeated doses of lorazepam are associated with marked accumulation and greatly prolonged half-life in patients with ESRD in contrast to healthy subjects. Midazolam is a water-soluble, short-acting benzodiazepine. It is hydroxylated in the liver to inactive metabolites and has minimal renal excretion. Vinik et al. reported no differences in values of clearance or elimination half-life from a single dose of midazolam in renal failure patients compared to healthy volunteers.[99] Triazolam is a short-acting benzodiazepine with an elimination half-life of one and a half to five hours, resulting in less daytime sleepiness and better performance compared to both flurazepam and lorazepam. This drug is currently our benzodiazepine of choice.

The addition of a narcotic such as morphine may aid anxious patients. However, patients with ESRD are especially sensitive to morphine. As morphine, an organic base, is normally bound to plasma proteins, more active unbound fraction of morphine exists in patients with ESRD. Binding of morphine decreases with a decreasing pH. Protein-binding sites may bind with the increased organic acids associated with ESRD, again increasing the amount of free morphine. The pKa for morphine is 8.05. Therefore the amount of ionized morphine increases with acidosis. More morphine enters the CNS, as the blood-brain barrier is more permeable in uremia. Morphine is not dialyzable because of the relatively large size of the molecule. Patients with ESRD have been reported to have respiratory depression as long as six days after morphine which was reversible with naloxone administration.[100]

Meperidine is metabolized to normeperidine, which possesses half the analgesic potency of meperidine but twice the convulsant properties. Normeperidine is excreted in urine, and serum levels are undetectable in patients with normal renal function. A marked cumulative effect occurs in patients with renal failure. Seizures, which are reversible with naloxone, have been reported in patients with renal insufficiency who received meperidine for more than a week.[101] Meperidine 50 mg has been shown to result in greater respiratory depression than 10 mg of morphine or 75 μg of fentanyl in patients with ESRD.[102] Meperidine significantly decreases cardiac output and blood pressure while increasing systemic vascular resistance.

Metochlorpropamide and cimetidine or ranitidine may be given as part of the premedication. Ranitidine, unlike cimetidine, does not interfere with the hepatic cytochrome P450 metabolism of theophylline, diazepam, propranolol, lidocaine, or phenytoin.

### Perioperative Management of Diabetes

Hyperglycemic diabetics have an increased risk of renal transplant rejection, poorer wound healing, and higher rates of wound infection.[88] Steroids may significantly alter serum glucose levels. Therefore, whichever regimen is chosen for control of diabetes in the perioperative period, blood sugar should be measured frequently, and at least once intraoperatively along with electrolytes. For patients receiving steroids, the rate of insulin infusion[88] should be set at:

$$\text{insulin (units·hr}^{-1}） = \frac{\text{plasma glucose}}{100}$$

### Monitoring

The motto of the American Society of Anesthesiologists is *Vigilance*. There can be no doubt that the best monitor is a highly skilled, knowledgeable, vigilant anesthetist. However, there is an ever growing array of monitors to assist in maintaining vigilance over patients. At least half of all anesthetic deaths are believed to be preventable. Hypoxemia is the most common factor leading to anesthetic morbidity and mortality. Thus, detection of hypoxemia needs high priority, presumably while it is still reversible, prior to causing permanent damage. Oxygen saturation by pulse oximetry is recommended for all patients undergoing general anesthesia. Inadequate ventilation is the major cause of hypoxemia. Thus end-tidal $CO_2$ or $CO_2$ wave-forms, tidal and/or minute volume, and breath sounds should be monitored. Both hypercarbia and hypocarbia decrease renal perfusion.[64,65] Hypercarbia leads to hyperkalemia, possibly accounting for unexplained deaths reported in early series of renal transplants. Delivery of a low oxygen concentration is a much less frequent cause of hypoxemia. An oxygen analyzer placed on the expiratory limb is helpful.

Cardiovascular status is monitored by ECG, heart sounds, intermittent arterial blood pressure measurements, and patient temperature. Continuous ECG monitoring facilitates detection of hyperkalemia, which occasionally occurs during renal transplantation. Most patients who develop hyperkalemia greater than 6 mEq·L$^{-1}$, during renal transplantation come to surgery with normal blood concentrations of potassium.[103] Patients whose potassium before preoperative dialysis exceeded 6 mEq·L$^{-1}$ tend to have greater intraoperative increases. Laboratory facilities for rapid determination of electrolytes, blood gases, hematocrit, and glucose are essential for renal transplantation.

A noninvasive technique to monitor blood pressure is nearly always preferred. Any damage to a peripheral artery may preclude its later use for dialysis access. The one-minute monitoring of blood pressure afforded by the noninvasive machines is generally sufficient for monitoring the pressor response to intubation and optimal pressures at the time of clamp release. Monitoring of central venous pressure has become routine. Patients receiving immunosuppressive therapy are prone to infection. Pulmonary artery catheters result in higher infection rates.[104] Therefore, although pulmonary artery catheters may be more accurate monitors for volume expansion, their routine use is not warranted for kidney transplantation. In the future, noninvasive measurement of left ventricular function by transesophageal echocardiography or microprocessor scintillation detectors may provide safer and more accurate data.

Body temperature is routinely monitored during renal transplantation. Some sort of humidification of the anesthetic gases is utilized to decrease the fall in temperature. An increase in intraoperative temperature may be seen if patients are treated with antilymphocyte globulin before surgery.[105]

## Choice of Anesthesia

The same priorities regarding the choice of anesthesia for renal transplantation exist today as they did over 20 years ago when Robert Virtue referred to "the safety of the patient, the needs of the surgeon, and the comfort of the patient, in that order."[106] Previously, patients frequently came to surgery with congestive heart failure with electrolyte imbalance and malignant hypertension. Twenty-three per cent came to renal transplantation with serum potassium levels

greater than 6 mEq·L$^{-1}$. Five per cent developed life-threatening arrhythmias usually associated with intubation.[107] Preoperative preparations have markedly decreased the risk of anesthesia in renal transplantation. Routine hemodialysis within 24 hours of transplantation was not instituted until the late 1960's.

Either inadequate regional or general anesthesia may result in the kidney's being coughed out of the abdomen. Should the vessels have to be reclamped and repaired, the warm ischemic time may result in loss of the graft. Most transplant surgeons are acutely aware of the potential complications of a patient bucking or coughing during and after the vascular anastomoses.

### Spinal and Epidural Anesthesia

The first patient to receive an LRD kidney transplant had a spinal anesthetic.[108] Spinal anesthesia was believed to be particularly advantageous, as the patients usually had congestive heart failure. Spinal anesthesia offered a "bloodless phlebotomy."[106] It also avoided the problems of uptake and distribution of the inhalation anesthetics in congestive heart failure.

Linke and Merin[109] advocated spinal anesthesia for the following reasons: ideal surgical field without worry about untoward effects of muscle relaxants; avoidance of tracheal intubation; relative safety with a full stomach; no concern about hyperkalemia and acidosis and anesthetic agents; and an awake, reactive, comfortable patient in the immediate postoperative period. One major advantage of epidural anesthesia is the addition of morphine to the local anesthetic. All patients are monitored in the surgical intensive care unit after renal transplantation. Rostral spread is decreased by orders for the head of the bed to be elevated 30 degrees except when central venous pressure is being measured. The ICU nurses are instructed to observe for gradual respiratory depression. Naloxone is available in the ICU. Continuous epidural anesthesia can be used equally successfully.

### General Anesthesia

As patients were better prepared and halothane replaced cyclopropane and ether, general anesthesia was recommended more frequently. A variety of reasons were given, including fear of an epidural hematoma from heparin (for dialysis, and previously many patients were heparinized for renal transplantation), psychological status of the patient, possible marked falls in blood pressures, uremic neuropathy, and dangers of infection.[110,111]

Regardless of the choice of anesthetic, a large-bore intravenous infusion apparatus is required. A vein on the dorsum of the hand is preferred to prevent damaging forearm veins that might be needed for vascular access in the future. However, peripheral venous access may be a problem in patients who have been receiving hemodialysis for several years. Triple-lumen central venous pressure catheters decrease the need for additional venous access. The intravenous infusion and blood pressure cuff should not be placed on the extremity that has a functioning dialysis access. The graft or fistula should be protected intraoperatively by covering with foam rubber. The presence of a bruit should be noted before and after the operation. Surgery results in a hypercoagulable state that may, in part, be responsible for clotting of dialysis accesses.

Prophylactic antibiotics are given before surgery starts. A single dose before surgery is as effective as multiple doses. Chloramphenicol and nafcillin (unless the patient is allergic to penicillin) are used because they are not excreted by the kidneys and have low toxicity. Aminoglycosides may potentiate neuromuscular blockade in addition to being nephrotoxic.

Anesthesia induction has been associated with the greatest number of complications in transplant patients, including cardiac arrest. Most of the earlier deaths were related to hyperkalemia. Acidosis may lower the level of potassium needed to cause arrest. Large polycystic kidneys may cause supine hypotensive syndrome. A balance needs to be attained between the delayed gastric emptying time and the complications associated with the pressor response to intubation. Preoxygenation followed by cricoid pressure should protect the airway from regurgitation even in the presence of a nasogastric tube. Adjuvants to blunt the cardiovascular response to intubation include propranolol, fentanyl, and lidocaine.

Thiopental remains the induction agent of choice for most patients undergoing renal transplantation.[112] No differences between induction dose and arterial or venous sleep concentrations were found in patients undergoing renal transplantation as compared to patients with normal renal function undergoing abdominal surgery.[113] In uremic patients, 56 per cent of thiopental is unbound compared to 28 per cent normally. Although the unbound portion of thiopental is increased in ESRD, volume of distribution and clearance are increased, and the half-life is unchanged. The higher brain concentrations are transient, as distribution and elimination are unchanged. As thiopental causes a significant fall in stroke volume, etomidate may be preferable for patients with known cardiac disease, since it has minimal cardiovascular effects and does not release histamine.

Intravenous narcotics may be utilized throughout the surgical procedure as part of the anesthetic technique. Meperidine, in addition to having a toxic metabolite,[101] depresses cardiac output more so than the other narcotics.[102] Fentanyl seems to be the narcotic of choice for anesthesia for renal transplantation. In patients with insulin-dependent diabetes mellitus the half-life of fentanyl has been shown to be prolonged and the clearance rate lower, as compared to non-IDDM patients undergoing renal transplantation. Diabetic microangiopathy probably decreases uptake from tissue stores, prolonging the elimination phase.[114] Alfentanil can be used as an alternative, since it has a short elimination half-life of 90 minutes and a more rapid blood-brain equilibrium of one to two minutes as compared to five to seven minutes for fentanyl.

Chronic anemia changes uptake and distribution of inhalation anesthetics by altering their blood-gas partition coefficients. In addition, in most patients with renal failure cardiac output is high and tissue oxygen extraction increased. All general anesthetics decrease GFR and water and electrolyte excretion in a dose-related manner. Recent studies using flow probes and microspheres have revealed that renal blood flow may not change even though GFR and urine output decrease.

Halothane was introduced with clinical anesthesia around the same time that kidney transplantations began to be successful. Shortly thereafter it was recommended for use during renal transplantation in low concentrations to avoid hypotension.

One per cent of enflurane is metabolized producing fluoride. Enflurane-induced nephrotoxicity has been reported in patients with pre-existing renal insufficiency. Although hundreds of patients have done well with enflurane anesthesia for renal transplantation,[115] flouride levels approximate 75 per cent of those reported to cause nephrotoxicity.[116]

Only 0.1 per cent of isoflurane is metabolized, and it does not result in significant levels of fluoride. The anesthetic is relatively insoluble. Thus, uptake and emergence are enhanced, particularly in the presence of anemia. Isoflurane causes less myocardial depression than either halothane or enflurane. Isoflurane anesthesia may result in tachycardia, particularly when the agent is used in combination with anticholinergic drugs, pancuronium, or meperidine. Fentanyl may be used to decrease the heart rate, the concentration of isoflurane, and postoperative pain. Isoflurane is often used for kidney transplantation.

Nitrous oxide is utilized less frequently for anesthesia for a variety of reasons, including a high incidence of nausea and vomiting, and the possibility of an enlarged pneumothorax if it should occur after recent insertion of a subclavian venous catheter. Ventilation is controlled to maintain eucarbia. Both hypercarbia[64] and hypocarbia[65] decrease renal perfusion and GFR.

## Muscle Relaxants

The rapid onset of action for **succinylcholine**, allowing optimal conditions for intubation shortly after injection, remains unequaled by any other available muscle relaxant. In patients with renal failure pseudocholinesterase levels are about 45 per cent of normal.[117] This, in part, is due to increased plasma volumes, but primarily results from impaired hepatic synthesis of serum cholinesterase by the uremic state. However, this decrease in pseudocholinesterase activity is not associated with clinically significant prolongation of action of succinylcholine.

Serum potassium increases by 0.2 to 0.5 $mEq \cdot L^{-1}$ following administration of 1 $mg \cdot kg^{-1}$ of succinylcholine in patients with or without renal failure;[118,119] d-tubocurarine failed to prevent the increase in either group. Patients with severe burns, massive trauma, neurological lesions, or severe abdominal infections may respond to succinylcholine with hyperkalemia sufficient to cause ventricular fibrillation. Study of a large series of patients with renal failure who were given succinylcholine failed to reveal the problem.[120,121] However, anecdotal reports of cardiac arrest[74] and ventricular tachycardia,[75] oc-curring after administration of succinylcholine to patients with ESRD prompted the authors to state that succinylcholine was contraindicated in renal failure. The presence of uremic or diabetic neuropathy may contraindicate the use of succinylcholine in patients with renal failure as it does for other polyneuropathies. Walton and Farman[121] reported a patient with uremic neuropathy in whom $K^+$ rose from 4.5 to 7.3 $mEq \cdot L^{-1}$ following the second dose of succinylcholine for bronchoscopy when there was no change in serum potassium with the first dose. Powell's patient developed ventricular tachycardia following a third dose of succinylcholine.[75] Koide and Waud[119] found a second dose of succinylcholine would raise serum potassium concentration more substantially than the first dose.

Succinylcholine may precipitate a variety of cardiac arrhythmias. Succinylcholine stimulates all cholinergic autonomic receptors, including the nicotinic receptors of both the sympathetic and parasympathetic ganglion and the muscarinic receptors in the sinus node. Sinus bradycardia occurs as a result of stimulation of cardiac muscarinic receptors in the sinus node. Second doses of succinylcholine are more likely to cause bradycardia. The bradycardia may be prevented by thiopental, atropine, or nondepolarizing relaxants. Nodal rhythms are also more common after a second dose of succinylcholine and may again be prevented by pretreatment with curare. Succinylcholine lowers the threshold of the ventricle to catecholamine-induced ventricular arrhythmias. Additive factors include intubation, hypoxia, hypercalcemia, surgical stress, and drugs such as tricyclics, monamine oxidase inhibitors, exogenous catecholamines, and halogenated anesthetics. Ventricular escape beats may also occur as a result of severe sinus and atrioventricular nodal slowing. Nigrovic[122] proposed that the first dose of succinylcholine releases norepinephrine from the presynaptic cholinergic receptors. The receptors remain insensitive for awhile. If during this period a second dose of succinylcholine is given, the full muscarinic effects may be seen. The initial catecholamine release may account for many of the adverse effects of succinylcholine attributed to hyperkalemia. The ECG effects of hyperkalemia and catecholamines are similar. The various drugs given to blunt the hemodynamic effects of succinylcholine may decrease norepinephrine release as well as $K^+$. The effects of catecholamines on denervated muscle are similar to those seen with succinylcholine.

Succinylcholine is hydrolyzed to succinylmonocholine and choline with less than 5 per cent appearing unchanged in the urine. Cholinesterase acts considerably slower in hydrolyzing succinylmonocholine to succinic acid and choline. Succinylmonocholine is more dependent on renal excretion and therefore accumulates in patients with renal failure receiving succinylcholine. It has one-twentieth the neuromuscular blocking properties of the dicholine. Hypocalcemia, hyponatremia, hypermagnesemia, and acidosis have been shown to prolong the action of both depolarizing and nondepolarizing muscle relaxants. Nonetheless, the duration of action of succinylcholine is not usually unduly prolonged in uremic patients. Bishop and Hornbein[123] reported two patients who were returned to surgery within hours of renal transplantation that had been performed with curare and reversed with neostigmine and pyridostigmine. Succinylcholine was given to each of the patients for the emergency procedures. In both patients there was complete neuromuscular blockade lasting one to two hours.

Both **d-tubocurarine** and **pancuronium** have been recommended for use during renal transplantation. However, there have been numerous reports of prolonged neuromuscular blockade following the use of these relaxants. The elimination half-life for d-tubocurarine is 231 minutes with good renal function and 330 without. ESRD patients are not more sensitive to the effects of d-tubocurarine, since the plasma concentration to produce a given twitch depression is similar, regardless whether the patient has renal failure or not.[124] The duration of action of repetitive doses of d-tubocurarine is progressively prolonged. ESRD patients who received multiple doses of d-tubocurarine developed prolongation of the effect, while in those who received a single dose there was no difficulty in reversal. Similarly, high or repeated doses of pancuronium in patients with renal failure resulted in marked prolonged duration.[125] There was considerable interpatient variability that was not related to either the patient's serum creatinine level or serum potassium level. The side effects of both drugs may be disturbing. d-Tubocurarine produces histamine release and gangli-

onic blockade, which may result in undesirable hypotension. The vagolytic and sympathomimetic properties of pancuronium may result in significant catecholamine release and ST depression.[126] Propranolol may blunt some of these effects if given before pancuronium.[127] The use of both pancuronium and d-tubocurarine may be discontinued in renal failure, like that of gallamine.

Pancuronium has two acetylcholine (ACh) moieties, one on the A ring and the other on the D ring of the steroid nucleus. The D-ring ACh is required for neuromuscular blockade, while the ACh on the A ring is responsible for the vagolytic and sympathomimetic effects. **Vecuronium** has only the D-ring ACh. While the duration of action of vecuronium is shorter than that for pancuronium, the onset of action is the same. In contrast to the other nondepolarizing relaxants, 0.08 $mg \cdot kg^{-1}$ vecuronium results in ideal intubating conditions, while the adductor pollicis muscle is depressed by only 40 to 60 per cent.[128]

The inhalational anesthetics enhance a vecuronium block. However, the halogenated anesthetics have less effect on vecuronium than they do on pancuronium or d-tubocurarine. Thus, vecuronium has a more predictable blockade, but it cannot be easily enhanced by increasing the concentration of the inhalation anesthetic.[129] Ketamine, fentanyl, gammahydroxybutyrate, and etomidate potentiate a vecuronium block. Only ketamine significantly prolongs the duration.[130]

Normally only 10 to 25 per cent of vecuronium is excreted in the urine. The primary means of elimination is the bile. Rapid hepatic uptake and biliary excretion account for the more rapid clearance and shorter elimination half-life seen with vecuronium than pancuronium in normal patients and patients with ESRD. Fahey et al.[131] found no significant differences in onset, duration, or recovery when a single bolus of vecuronium was given to patients undergoing renal transplantation. Meistelman et al.[132] did find a 32 per cent increase in the elimination half-life of vecuronium as compared to a 500 per cent increase with pancuronium in patients with ESRD. The dose of vecuronium that causes 50, 90, or 95 per cent block is not changed in patients with ESRD as compared with the control.[133] However, as seen in Figure 6–14, there were cumulative effects from repeated small doses of vecuronium. With the intraoperative monitoring of neuromuscular func-

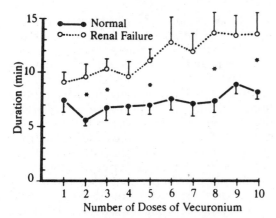

**Figure 6–14.** Cumulative effects of vecuronium in renal disease. (From Bevan DR, Donati F, Gyasi H, Williams A: Vecuronium in renal failure. Can Anaesth Soc J 31:491, 1984, with permission of the authors and publisher.)

tion, vecuronium blockade should be easily reversible. Hemodynamic changes induced by vecuronium are minimal.

**Atracurium** is another example of modern pharmacological engineering in pursuit of the ideal muscle relaxant. A curare-like molecule called petaline underwent spontaneous degradation in mild alkali. The reaction was described by Hofmann[134] in 1851, the same year Claude Bernard discovered the neuromuscular action of curare. Stenlake and colleagues synthesized a neuromuscular blocker that undergoes spontaneous degradation "by the well-known Hofmann elimination reaction."[135] While it was previously believed that Hofmann elimination was the major route of excretion, Nigrovic et al. have recently shown that ester hydrolysis may be the primary mode.[136]

The onset, duration of action, or recovery time for atracurium is prolonged by renal failure[137] (Table 6–6). de Bros et al.[138] found no significant differences in the pharmacokinetics and pharmacodynamics of atracurium in patients with renal failure under isoflurane anesthesia. Neither does hepatorenal failure prolong the plasma elimination half-life of atracurium. Thus, atracurium is the only available neuromuscular blocker that is unaffected by hepatorenal failure.

There is no apparent cumulative effect after multiple doses of atracurium in patients in whom renal function is absent.[139] At 90 seconds vecuronium results in poorer intubating conditions than atracurium. However, atracurium causes significant decreases in blood pressure while vecuronium does not.[140] High doses of atracurium result in significant histamine release, a 20 per cent decrease in arterial pressure, and an 8 per cent increase in heart rate. Patients with coronary artery disease may be particularly susceptible to doses of atracurium above 0.3 mg·kg$^{-1}$, which result in hypotension, possibly related to prior diuretic therapy.[141] Atracurium blockade is enhanced by both metabolic and respiratory alkalosis. Accordingly, spontaneous degradation of atracurium occurs more rapidly in lactated Ringer's solution (pH 6.5) than it does in normal saline (pH 5.85). Thus, atracurium infusions should be mixed with normal saline.[142]

Although high doses of laudanosine, the breakdown product of atracurium by Hofmann elimination, were found in 1899 to cause seizures in animals, no seizures have been reported in patients who have received atracurium.[143] Laudanosine crosses the blood-brain barrier, and its elimination half-life is considerably longer than that of atracurium, raising concern regarding repeated

**TABLE 6–6. Pharmacodynamics of Atracurium in Patients with Normal Renal Function and in Patients with Renal Failure**

| Patient Group | N | Onset (min) | Duration (min) | Recovery Time (min) |
|---|---|---|---|---|
| Normal | 10 | 1.8 ± 0.1 | 69.5† ± 5.2 | 10.5‡ ± 1.1 |
| Renal failure | 10 | 2.0 ± 0.4 | 77.4 ± 3.2 | 13.1 ± 3.2 |

Values represent mean ± SEM. †n = 7. ‡n = 8.
From Fahey MR, Rupp SM, Fisher DM, et al: The pharmacokinetics and pharmacodynamics of atracurium in patients with and without renal failure. Anesthesiology 61:699, 1984, with permission of authors and publisher.

doses or prolonged infusion of atracurium. Fahey et al.[137] found peak laudanosine levels of 327 ng·ml$^{-1}$ following a single dose of atracurium of 0.5 mg·kg$^{-1}$. Recently they reported an increase in the minimum alveolar concentration for halothane by as much as 30 per cent with similar levels of laudanosine in rabbits.[144] Laudanosine, a monoquaternary amine, is excreted renally. However, it seems unlikely that dangerous laudanosine concentrations will be achieved, even in anephric patients.[145]

**Priming Principle.** Many patients for renal transplantation require rapid sequence intubation, and yet succinylcholine may be contraindicated. None of the nondepolarizing muscle relaxants causes full paralysis as fast as succinylcholine. The use of small "priming" doses of the nondepolarizing muscle relaxants may be beneficial in these patients. Up to 75 per cent of neuromuscular receptors may be blocked without clinical effects. With 75 per cent of the receptors already blocked by the priming dose, the time required to achieve 90 per cent blockade is significantly reduced. The priming dose for atracurium is 75 to 80 μg·kg$^{-1}$[146] and for vecuronium 0.01 to 0.015 mg·kg$^{-1}$.[147] Small doses of pancuronium and d-tubocurarine (0.015 and 0.04 mg/kg respectively) may also be used as priming doses. The duration of action of the intubating dose will be decreased, necessitating earlier redosing.[147]

**Restoration of Neuromuscular Conduction.** In early reports of renal transplantation, several instances of cardiac arrest were described during attempts to restore neuromuscular conduction. These were most likely the result of concomitant electrolyte imbalance and acidosis.

Recently, latent myasthenia gravis was described when the action of the newer nondepolarizing muscle relaxants failed to be reversed following renal transplantation.[148] In the majority of patients with ESRD, neuromuscular blockade may be successfully antagonized with edrophonium, neostigmine, or pyridostigmine.

## Management During Surgery Prior to Revascularization

Just as it had been for bilateral nephrectomy in the early days of renal transplantation, fluid restriction was the rule for patients receiving a renal graft. As the result of routine use of preoperative dialysis, the anesthetist was confronted with dehydration and low blood volumes. Transplanted kidneys function far better when the patients are optimally hydrated. Diethelm et al.[63] emphasized that high-normal central venous pressure and diastolic pressure of 85 to 110 mm Hg helped ensure early maximal renal function. Patients with a mean pulmonary artery pressure greater than 20 mm Hg and a pulmonary artery diastolic pressure greater than 15 had a 6 per cent incidence of acute tubular necrosis following cadaveric transplantation as compared to 36 per cent when pulmonary artery pressures were lower.[149,150] Grundman et al.[151] recommended increasing the systolic pressure to 140 mm Hg at the time of clamp release, using dopamine if necessary. Maximal hydration at the time of releasing the clamps should also decrease the possibility of hyperkalemia from the flush solution in the transplanted kidney.

Therefore, it is the responsibility of the anesthesiologist to ensure that the patient is in optimal hemodynamic status before the vascular clamps are released. Each anastomosis takes 7 to 12 minutes unless there are technical problems such as double renal vessels. The central venous pressure is raised to 15 to 17 cm $H_2O$. Half-strength saline is our crystalloid of choice. The average blood loss is 200 ml. Packed cells are administered if necessary to increase the hematocrit to 24 to 25 per cent. Two units are kept ready in case of excessive bleeding following release of the vascular clamps. If it is not possible to attain a systolic pressure of 130 mm Hg by volume loading and lightening of the general anesthesia, up to 7 μg·kg$^{-1}$·min$^{-1}$ dopamine may be used. Other vasopressors should be avoided just as for the donors. During spinal or epidural anesthesia it may be difficult to increase the systolic pressure above 130 mm Hg, particularly if the patient's normal blood pressure is below 130 mm Hg.

Hypertension is rarely a problem in a well-dialyzed patient under anesthesia. If necessary, a variety of antihypertensive drugs may be utilized. Sodium nitroprusside is transformed in the liver to thiocyanate, which is excreted by the kidneys. However, anuric dogs have been shown to tolerate more sodium nitroprusside than normal dogs prior to appearance of toxic symptoms.[152] Sodium nitroprusside is dialyzable should it become necessary.[90]

In addition to methods of optimizing hemodynamic status and fluid balance, various pharmacological renal protectants are employed. The concept of oxygen supply-demand ratio is just as important for the kidney as it is for the heart. The susceptibility of the kidneys to failure during hypotension may seem strange, since there is a disproportionately high overall blood flow to the kidneys compared to oxygen consumption (Table 6–7). However, intrarenal blood flow is not homogeneous. The $Po_2$ falls drastically from the outer cortex to the inner medulla. The medulla normally has a $Po_2$ of 10 mm Hg, as seen in Figure 6–15A. The oxygen consumption–delivery ratio of the renal medulla is the highest of any organ (Table 6–7). Anemia does not cause anoxic damage to the medulla until the oxygen-carrying capacity is decreased substantially because of reactive renal vasodilation. Varying the arterial $Po_2$ over a wide range does not change the medullary $Po_2$. Other local factors such as pH and $Pco_2$ may affect the oxygen hemoglobin dissociation curve and critically change cellular oxygenation. Cytochrome $aa_3$, the terminal electron carrier of the mitochondrial chain, has a high affinity for oxygen. Only 2 per cent of the cytochrome is in reduced form in the liver or muscle. In contrast, 20 to 40 per cent is in reduced form in the kidney. The medullary thick ascending limb (mTAL) has relatively high oxygen demand to actively reabsorb sodium chloride and low oxygen supply from the medullary countercurrent exchange system.[153] The mTAL is thus particularly vulnerable to relatively mild insults. One of the earliest and most consistent defects in acute tubular necrosis is decreased solute reabsorption by the mTAL (Fig. 6–15B). If glomerular filtration continues while medullary hypoperfusion is present, mTAL injury may occur. Complete ischemia abolishes glomerular filtration and in turn protects the mTAL. Therefore, either decreasing the mTAL oxygen demand by inhibiting cellular transport or decreasing glomerular filtration will protect the mTAL. Furosemide produces oxidation of cytochrome $aa_3$, improving the oxygen balance in the mTAL. In addition, furosemide inhibits cell transport activity, protecting the mTAL and attenuating ischemic injury. Furosemide is given routinely prior to the release of the vascular clamps. Furosemide has been shown to be effective in many animal models and clinical studies of acute renal failure. However, there have been a number of studies showing negative results of furosemide in acute renal failure. The timing of furosemide administration appears to be important. In the studies with positive results it was given around the time of the injury. In another it was given 12 to 24 hours after the injury, making the acute tubular necrosis worse. In some studies in which negative results were obtained with furosemide, fluids had not been replaced. Intravascular depletion appears to negate the effects of furosemide. It may be nephrotoxic during hypotension.[153] Baek et al.[154] found the responses to furosemide to be predictive

**TABLE 6–7. Comparison of Balance of Oxygen Delivery and Oxygen Consumption in Several Organs***

| Region or Organ | $O_2$ Delivery | Blood Flow Rate (ml/min/100 gm) | $O_2$ Consumption | $O_2$ Consumption/ $O_2$ Delivery (%) |
|---|---|---|---|---|
| Hepatoportal | 11.6 | 58 | 2.2 | 18 |
| Kidney | 84.0 | 420 | 6.8 | 8 |
| Outer medulla | 7.6† | 190† | 6.0‡ | 79§ |
| Brain | 10.9 | 54 | 3.7 | 34 |
| Skin | 2.6 | 13 | 0.38 | 15 |
| Skeletal muscle | 0.5 | 2.7 | 0.18 | 34 |
| Heart | 16.8 | 84 | 11.0 | 65 |

* Measurements are in humans except for those from the outer medulla, in which case the estimates are from rats.
† The blood flow is estimated at 1.9 ml/min/gm. The oxygen content is estimated at 4 vol% (from standard dissociation curves for hemoglobin) assuming the arterial $Po_2$ at 15 to 20 mm Hg, highest recordings of tissue $Po_2$ in this region. The value is probably an overestimate of the actual oxygen delivery, since part of it is lost to the ascending vasa recta by countercurrent diffusion.
‡ This value is probably an underestimate because it is taken from slices including those from the inner medulla.
§ This is a minimum estimate (see † and ‡).
From Brezis M, Rosen S, Silva P, et al: Renal ischemia: A new perspective. Kidney Int 26:375, 1984, with permission of authors and publisher.

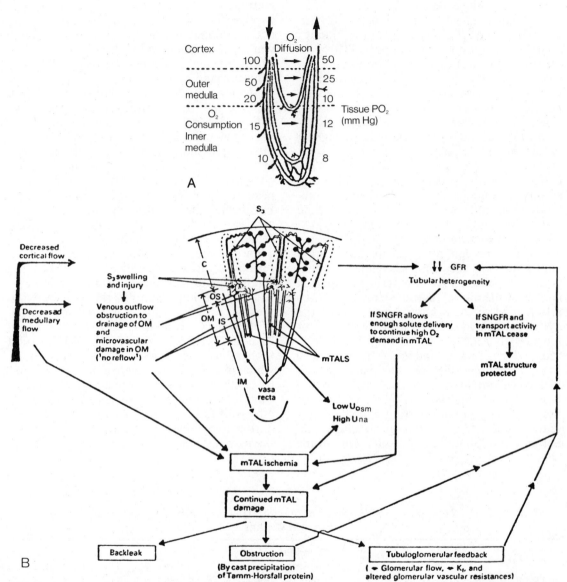

**Figure 6–15.** *A*, Countercurrent exchange of oxygen in the vas recta: Diffusion of oxygen between arterial and venous limbs minimizes the dissipation of the corticomedullary gradient of tissue oxygen tension. *B*, The hypothetical role of the medullary thick ascending limb in the pathophysiology of ischemic ARF. Medullary hypoperfusion is further aggravated by cell swelling and microvascular damage. mTAL ischemia may produce backleak, obstruction, and activation of tubuloglomerular feedback. If active transport ceases, the conditions are proper for return to normal structure in mTAL's with nonlethal injury. Thus, activation of tubuloglomerular feedback or obstruction may reverse or prevent morphologically demonstrable mTAL damage at the expense of a low GFR. Abbreviations: $S_2$ = pars recta of proximal tubule; mTAL = medullary thick ascending limb of Henle's loop; C = cortex; OM = outer medulla; OS = outer stripe; IS = inner stripe; IM = inner medulla; $U_{Osm}$ = urine osmolality; $U_{Na}$ = urinary sodium concentration; SNGFR = single nephron GFR; $K_1$ = glomerular capillary ultrafiltration coefficient. (From Brezis M, Rosen S, Silva P, et al: Renal ischemia: A new perspective. Kidney Int 26:375, 1984, with permission of the authors and publisher.)

of the severity of acute renal failure. No response meant that severe renal failure would follow. Furosemide may help convert oliguric renal failure to nonoliguric renal failure with its better prognosis.

Fifty grams of mannitol given just before revascularization of the graft resulted in development of acute tubular necrosis in only 3 of 22 patients, 1 of whom required dialysis. In contrast, acute tubular necrosis developed in 12 of 22 patients who received a placebo, all of whom required dialysis.[155] Mannitol increases plasma volume, filling pressures, and cardiac output, while decreasing systemic vascular resistance. Renal blood flow is increased to a greater extent than plasma volume is expanded. In addition to its osmotic action on the tubules, mannitol is a renal vasodilator. Mannitol increases the serum potassium by 0.4 to 0.7 $mEq \cdot L^{-1}$.[156] Thus the ECG should be observed following administration of mannitol.

Dopamine has been used successfully to treat oliguria resulting from a variety of conditions. Since dopamine affects $alpha_1$ and $alpha_2$ as well as $beta_1$ and $beta_2$ receptors in addition to dopaminergic $_1$ and $_2$ receptors, there are a number of possible mechanisms for the diuresis associated with dopamine. Dopaminergic $_1$ receptors are responsible for increases in renal blood flow and electrolyte excretion.[7] Dopamine reportedly improved post-transplantation renal function in dogs even when the kidneys were optimally harvested.[157] These findings were not collaborated by others.[151] Administration of dopamine to the recipient did improve function when the kidneys were harvested while the donor was hypotensive. In a prospective randomized trial of human cadaver kidney recipients in whom the kidneys had been harvested under optimal conditions, no benefit was found from dopamine given for the first four days post-transplantation.[158] Serum creatinine and the incidence of dialysis were the same in both groups. Although rejection occurred sooner in the dopamine group, the incidence was the same after three months. Kidneys that function immediately are rejected sooner than those that do not function immediately. Although a dose of only 2 $\mu g \cdot kg^{-1} \cdot min^{-1}$ was used, 3 of 25 patients developed heart rates of 120 to 170, necessitating withdrawal of dopamine. Thus, mannitol and furosemide are routinely given, but dopamine is reserved either for recipients who are hypotensive or for donors who are hypotensive or relatively elderly.

In conclusion, the anesthesiologist helps ensure optimal renal function by optimizing cardiac output and fluid balance, providing a good oxygen-carrying capacity, decreasing oxygen demands of kidneys with furosemide and mannitol, and improving the oxygenation status of mTAL with furosemide and renal vasodilation with dopamine, if necessary.

## Releasing the Clamps

The surgeons and the anesthesia team must all have completed their respective tasks of forming the anastomoses and optimizing the hemodynamic and pharmacological status of the patient prior to release of the vascular clamps. Upon release of the clamps the kidney should turn from gray to pink. Dopamine may be administered if the kidney appears mottled.

Hypertension sometimes developing upon release of the clamps may be attributed to renin release from the ischemic kidney upon reperfusion. Sometimes blood pressure decreases. Release of the vascular clamps releases fentanyl from the ipsilateral leg, resulting in a transient increase of plasma fentanyl concentration.[114] The blood pressure should be monitored every minute for several minutes following release of the clamps.

The central venous pressure commonly falls to 0 within a few hours after renal transplantation as the kidney begins to function. The patient may require 2 to 4 L of fluid to restore it to 5 or more. The fall appears to be out of proportion to the urine output, suggesting a decrease in vascular resistance, as following bilateral nephrectomy.[159] Urine output should be replaced milliliter for milliliter with half-normal saline in the immediate revascularization period. If the urine output is greater than 300 ml per half-hour after a few hours, some surgeons will limit the fluid intake to 300 ml per hour. Others continue to replace milliliter for milliliter to help ensure renal perfusion, but hyponatremia and hypokalemia may result.

Usually the endotracheal tube is left in place because high central venous pressure and anuria may lead to pulmonary edema, persistent oozing, or bleeding, which may require repeated surgery, and residual muscle relaxants and respiratory depression may necessitate ventilatory support. Naloxone may cause severe hypertension and should be used sparingly. As the vast majority of kidney transplants function in the immediate postoperative period, concerns regarding prolonged duration of the effects of morphine and normeperidine are not as much of a problem postoperatively as preoperatively.

Although some transplant surgeons let their patients return to the transplant ward, most surgeons prefer an intensive care environment.

### Early Complications

Cardiac complications remain the most serious cause of postoperative morbidity and mortality. Cardiac death occurs in about 1 per cent of patients, myocardial infarction in about 0.5 per cent, and serious arrhythmias in about 5 to 10 per cent of patients.[160] Hypertension should be vigorously controlled, as it threatens both patient and graft survival, especially in diabetics.[160,161]

Other nonsurgical complications occurring in the early post-transplantation period include acute and hyperacute rejection, acute tubular necrosis, cyclosporine nephrotoxicity, and sudden onset of diabetes. Hyperacute rejection begins within hours after transplantation and is the result of preformed cytotoxic antibodies. It is irreversible and requires transplant nephrectomy. The incidence has markedly decreased with serological crossmatching.

Cyclosporine has reduced the incidence of acute rejection. Acute rejection is characterized by increasing BUN and creatinine (without any other apparent cause) occurring within the first few months of transplantation. Patient noncompliance with medication should be considered if acute rejection occurs in the late post-transplantation period. A renal scan helps differentiate acute rejection from acute tubular necrosis or renal artery stenosis. A renal scan shows gradual improvement in estimated renal plasma flow with acute tubular necrosis and decreasing flow with acute rejection.[52,56] The treatment of acute rejection includes increased steroids and/or antithymocyte globulin. Early treatment of acute rejection decreases the likelihood of permanent damage from platelet aggregates and fibrin thrombi in the capillaries. Chronic rejection is progressive, irreversible, and untreatable, even with increased immunosuppression. It is the most common cause of a gradual increase in serum creatinine in the late post-transplantation period. The process may take two to ten years before complete graft failure occurs.

Acute tubular necrosis occurs in less than 3 per cent of LRD, but is present in nearly all cadaveric transplants to some degree; 20 to 30 per cent of cadaveric graft recipients require dialysis after transplantation. Unfortunately there is great interpatient variability with lack of correlation between cyclosporine levels and the degree of nephrotoxicity. Reduction in cyclosporine improves renal function.

Gastrointestinal complications occur, especially in the first three months after transplantation when high-dose steroids are used. Ulceration of the gastric or duodenal mucosa develops in 11 to 22 per cent. When hemorrhage occurs, the mortality exceeds 50 per cent. Cimetidine does not decrease the rate of this complication when given prophylactically or affect rejection episodes or graft survival.[162] Hemorrhagic pancreatitis can be lethal during the post-transplantation period.[163] Liver disease complicating renal transplantation is associated with 40 per cent mortality. Different kinds of infection can develop after kidney transplantation. The issue is addressed in Chapter 5.

### Long-Term Complications

Ten- and twenty-year survival of kidney grafts from parental donors is 46 and 29 per cent respectively; from sibling donors it is 43 and 35 percent; and from cadaveric donors it is 24 and 19 per cent, respectively. After transplantation from parents, patient survival rates at 10 and 20 years are 63 and 45 per cent respectively; from siblings, 51 and 38 per cent; and from cadavers, 40 and 30 per cent.[164] Mortality is higher after cadaveric transplantation because the greater immunosuppression needed leads to infection. In the first two years of the post-transplantation period, sepsis is the leading cause of death, followed by gastrointestinal, cardiac, and hepatic complications. After five years there was a decrease in septic deaths and an increase in the number of deaths from neoplasia. There is a sixfold increase in malignant disease in renal transplant patients compared to the general population. The risk increases with the longevity of the transplant. Excessive use of azathioprine appears particularly hazardous. High-dose steroids are associated with the greatest number of deaths due to infection. The use of lower doses of steroids supplemented with antithymocyte globulin and cyclosporine has helped decrease infectious complications. Cushing's syndrome develops in all patients after kidney transplantation. Patients who require more than 20 mg of prednisone per day to prevent rejection may eventually need transplant nephrectomy to prevent serious steroid complications.

Suicide accounts for 15 per cent of all deaths following renal transplantation.[165] The suicide rate is highest among younger recipients following graft loss.

Hypertension during the post-transplantation period is often caused by chronic rejection. However, a significant number of patients have hypertension associated with normal graft function. In such cases, bilateral nephrectomy should be considered. The native kidneys appear capable of inducing functional renal hemodynamic effects in the graft similar to those associated with chronic rejection and renal artery stenosis.[166] The renal nerves regenerate within about a year after transplantation and may mediate the hypertension. Hypertension in diabetics markedly decreases both patient and graft survival; 81 per cent of diabetics remain hypertensive after transplantation. In the 13 per cent who become normotensive, mortality is only 12 per cent; all have good graft function.[161] Thus, every effort should be made to control blood pressure during the post-transplantation period in diabetics. Methyldopa inhibits suppressor cells and could theoretically affect graft outcome. However, no adverse effects have been found with its long-term use after kidney transplantation.[167] Captopril may decrease renal graft function.[54]

About 10 to 20 per cent of renal transplant recipients develop avascular necrosis from tertiary hyperparathyroidism and steroid therapy. It occurs between the third post-transplantation month and the fifth post-transplantation year. Pain is the most common complaint, and the need for total hip replacement is determined by the severity of the pain. The femoral head is affected most frequently, followed by the femoral condyles, tali, and humeral head. Often more than one joint is involved. No HLA-identical recipient has developed osteonecrosis, indicating that the higher doses of immunosuppressives were responsible for the complication.

Histological changes of diabetic nephropathy, including hyalinization of the afferent and efferent arterioles, develop in the transplanted kidney. However, nearly all grafts continue to function well.[168]

Unusual complications following renal transplantation include clot anuria following renal biopsy obstructing the upper urinary tract, ligation of the ureter during herniorrhaphy, recurrence of Wegener's granulomatosis in the grafts, and recurrence of IgA nephropathy in the graft.

## RESULTS OF KIDNEY TRANSPLANTATION

The 1985 report of the UCLA Kidney Transplant Registry contains data from 133 centers throughout the world on 46,536 patients who had kidney transplantation since 1962.[169] The most important factor influencing graft survival is the transplant center itself, more so than any other variable (Fig. 6–16). Excellent centers have 24 per cent better

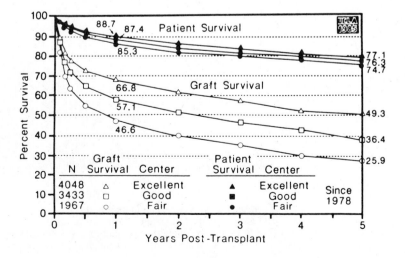

**Figure 6–16.** Influence of transplant center on patient and graft survival. (From Terasaki PI, Toyotome A, Mickey MR, et al: Patient, graft and functional survival rates: An overview. In Terasaki PI (ed): Clinical Kidney Transplants 1985. Los Angeles, UCLA Tissue Typing Lab, 1985, p 1, with permission of the authors and publisher.)

graft survival than fair centers. In part this may be because centers with excellent graft survival rates more often use blood transfusions and cyclosporine and type and match for HLA-A, -B, and antigens-DR than centers with only fair graft survival. Race, ischemia times, cytotoxic antibodies, original disease, and age of the recipient were not found to account for differences in the centers' results. The one-year graft survival rates in transplantations done since 1982 were 92 per cent when donors were HLA-identical siblings, 84 per cent when parents, and 65 per cent when cadavers. Five-year graft survival rates were 78, 60, and 40 per cent, respectively.

Cadavers account for the majority of the increasing number of kidney transplantations that are being performed each year (Fig. 6–17). Only 2 per cent of ESRD patients have suitable available LRD's.[170] The increasing efficacy and safety of renal transplantation, as well as public information, predict that a greater proportion of patients with ESRD will come to transplantation. Of the 70,000 Americans with ESRD in 1982, only 7 per cent received kidney transplants.

Figure 6–18 depicts graft survival in cadaveric transplants reported to the UCLA Registry since 1982 related to HLA matching. Survival was 79 per cent for zero mismatches and 59 per cent when all six were mismatched.[169] Matching for HLA-DR sig-

nificantly increases graft survival while HLA-A matching appears to be less important. Cyclosporine has increased graft survival to nearly 90 per cent when there are zero mismatches.[171] Cyclosporine and antithymocyte globulin for rejection have apparently increased graft survival at smaller transplantation centers that do less than 20 transplants per year, resulting in outcomes comparable to larger centers.[172] Since the mortality for the first year of dialysis is 10 per cent, transplantation does not increase risk to the patient. Renal transplantation offers the best source of complete rehabilitation to patients with ESRD and is less expensive than dialysis.[173] At the University of Alabama at Birmingham our current data for HLA haploidentical grafts show 90 per cent one-year and 88 per cent five-year survival. Ten percent of HLA-identical LRD grafts are rejected, indicating that there are other histocompatibility antigens (Fig. 6–19). Patient survival has increased to 95 per cent for the first post-transplant year as a result of earlier transplant nephrectomy; the return to dialysis does not increase patient mortality.[169]

The etiology of the ESRD accounts for some of the differences in outcome. Diabetics have a lower survival rate, which in turn affects graft survival (Fig. 6–20). Five-year survival rates are 63 per cent for diabetics compared to 83 per cent for patients with glomerulonephritis.[169] Cyclosporine has

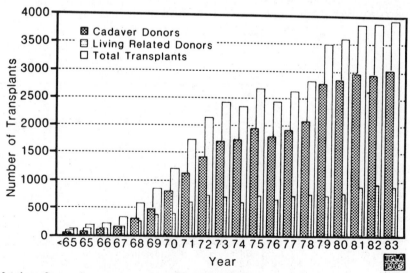

**Figure 6–17.** Number of transplants per year accumulated by the UCLA Transplant Registry. Cadaveric transplants have increased while LRD have remained constant. (From Terasaki PI, Toyotome A, Mickey AR, et al: Patient, graft and functional survival rates: An overview. In Terasaki PI (ed): Clinical Kidney Transplants 1985. Los Angeles, UCLA Tissue Typing Lab, 1985, p 1, with permission of the authors and publisher.)

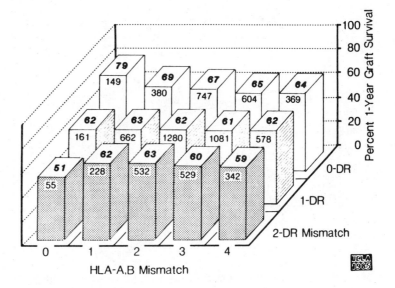

**Figure 6–18.** Effect of HLA-A, B and DR matching a one-year cadaveric graft survival. (From Terasaki PI, Toyotome A, Mickey MR, et al: Patient, graft and functional survival rates: An overview. In Terasaki PI (ed): Clinical Kidney Transplants 1985. Los Angeles, UCLA Tissue Typing Lab, 1985, p 1, with permission of the authors and publisher.)

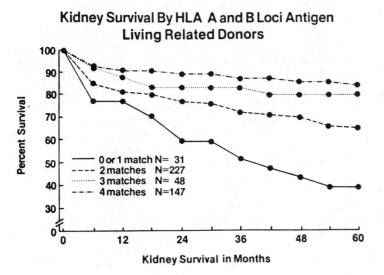

**Figure 6–19.** Results of LRD transplantation and HLA-A and B matching at UAB. Identical haplotype transplants result in 90 per cent one-year and 88 per cent five-year graft survival. (Courtesy of AG Diethelm.)

**Figure 6–20.** Patient and graft survival rates for recipients with various original diseases. Most notable is the lower patient survival rate among diabetics (DM) (62.9 per cent at five years) as compared with those with other diseases: nephrosclerosis (NS), 78.3 per cent; systemic lupus erythematosus (SLE), 79.6 per cent; polycystic kidney disease (PC), 80.4 per cent; pyelonephritis (PN), 82.1 per cent; glomerulonephritis (GN), 82.2 per cent). Graft survival varied more widely over a five-year period than did patient survival. The five-year graft survival rates were as follows: SLE, 28.1 per cent; NS, 34.5 per cent; DM, 34.7 per cent; PC, 39.9 per cent; PN, 40.1 per cent; and GN, 42.0 per cent. (From Terasaki PI, Toyotome A, Mickey MR, et al: Patient, graft and functional survival rates: An overview. In Terasaki PI (ed): Clinical Kidney Transplants 1985. Los Angeles, UCLA Tissue Typing Lab, 1985, p 1, with permissionof the authors and publisher.)

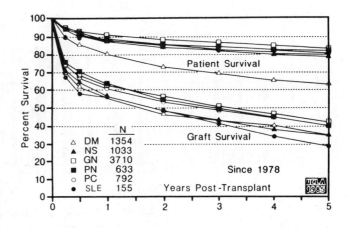

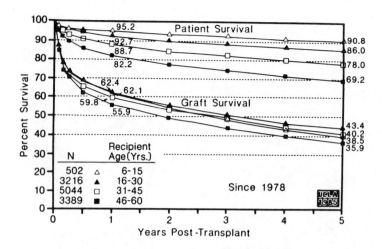

**Figure 6–21.** Effect of recipient age at time of transplant and survival rate. (From Terasaki PI, Toyotome A, Mickey MR, et al: Patient, graft and functional survival rates: An overview. In Terasaki PI (ed): Clinical Kidney Transplants 1985. Los Angeles, UCLA Tissue Typing Lab, 1985, p 1, with permission of the authors and publisher.)

been found particularly efficacious in ESRD secondary to chronic glomerulonephritis. When patient deaths are excluded, graft survival does not vary between diabetics and nondiabetics.[89,169] Although currently pancreatic transplant graft survival is only half that for renal, the combined procedure does not compromise the renal graft; the functioning pancreatic graft prevents recurrence of diabetic nephropathy and allows the patient to be insulin free.[174]

Patient age at the time of transplant may adversely affect both patient and graft survival (Fig. 6–21). Five years after transplantation, survival for patients 6 to 15 years of age was 91 per cent compared to 69 per cent for recipients age 46 to 60. However, there was only a 7 per cent difference in graft sur-

vival after five years between the age groups, indicating that older patients have a less severe rejection process.[169]

Survival of cadaveric first grafts is increased 15 per cent by a single pretransplant transfusion and 20 per cent by five transfusions over control recipients. Fewer transfusions are required to achieve maximum graft survival from LRD's, nulliparous women, and cadaveric recipients under 35 years. The effect of blood transfusions was independent and synergistic with HLA matching. The effect of blood transfusions is negligible in children, whereas it is rather remarkable in patients over the age of 35[175] (Fig. 6–22).

In most series of black recipients the graft survival rate is about 10 per cent lower, even

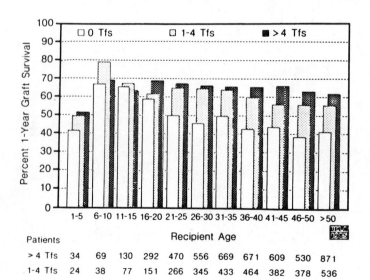

**Figure 6–22.** Transfusion effect and recipient age on one-year graft survival rate. (From Cecka M, Cicciarell J: The transfusion effect. In Terasaki PI (ed): Clinical Kidney Transplants 1985. Los Angeles, UCLA Tissue Typing Lab, 1985, p 73, with permission of the authors and publisher.)

| Patients | 1-5 | 6-10 | 11-15 | 16-20 | 21-25 | 26-30 | 31-35 | 36-40 | 41-45 | 46-50 | >50 |
|---|---|---|---|---|---|---|---|---|---|---|---|
| > 4 Tfs | 34 | 69 | 130 | 292 | 470 | 556 | 669 | 671 | 609 | 530 | 871 |
| 1-4 Tfs | 24 | 38 | 77 | 151 | 266 | 345 | 433 | 464 | 382 | 378 | 536 |
| 0 Tfs | 12 | 35 | 35 | 51 | 128 | 133 | 163 | 181 | 190 | 164 | 217 |

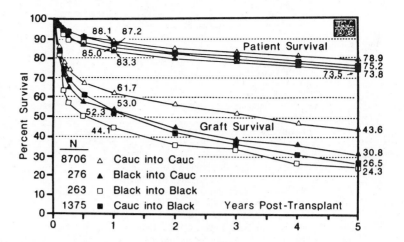

**Figure 6–23.** Racial effect and survival for cadaveric transplant since 1978. (From Terasaki PI, Toyotome A, Mickey MR, et al: Patient, graft and functional survival rates: An overview. In Terasaki PI (ed): Clinical Kidney Transplants 1985. Los Angeles, UCLA Tissue Typing Lab, 1985, p 1, with permission of the authors and publisher.)

for LRD and black-to-black transplants.[169] The best results are from Caucasian-to-Caucasian (Fig. 6–23). Socioeconomic factors are not believed to play a role, as patient survival is the same regardless of race. Poorer HLA matching may be a factor, since more than 98 per cent of the HLA-A and -B loci polymophisms have been identified for whites but far fewer have been identified for blacks.

The results of second and third kidney transplantations are markedly influenced by the first. If the first transplant was rejected for immunological reasons, graft survival was less in the second. If the first graft failed for technical reasons, the second had high survival rates. Cytotoxic antibodies do not influence second graft survival, particularly in HLA identical transplants. Early loss of the first transplant from acute rejection decreases the chances for survival of the second, while slow, chronic rejection of the first increases the chances for success. The success rate of retransplants has been slowly improving so that five-year survival rates for second transplants are now about 37 per cent. Diabetics appear to fare very poorly after second transplantation with graft survivals of only 24 per cent.

Thus, the first decades of renal transplantation have shown remarkable advances. Patients are now surviving ten or more years. They have a relatively normal life with productive vocations and active hobbies, including sports.[176] Pregnancy rates as well as live births are markedly higher following renal transplantation than they are in patients having dialysis.[177] Male fertility is also increased.[176]

Just as Carrel noted in 1914, the future of

successful transplantation must await the full elucidation of the immunological response. For, although enormous strides have been made, the full story behind the paradox of the body destroying a nonpathogenic, life-sustaining organ is still not known. The future of transplantation remains closely interwoven with that of immunology.

## REFERENCES

1. Beeuwkes R: The vascular organization of the kidney. Annu Rev Physiol 42:531, 1980.
2. Valtin H: Renal Function, Mechanisms Preserving Fluid and Solute Balance in Health. Boston, Little, Brown and Company, 1983.
3. Wright FS, Briggs JP: Feedback control of glomerular blood flow, pressure, and filtration rate. Physiol Rev 59:958, 1979.
4. Keeton TK, Campbell WB: The pharmacologic alteration of renin release. Pharmacol Rev 32:81, 1980.
5. Koepke JP: Renal responses to stressful environmental stimuli. Fed Proc 44:2823, 1985.
6. DiBona GF: Neural regulation of renal tubular sodium reabsorption and renin secretion. Fed Proc 44:2816, 1985.
7. Frederickson ED, Bradley T, Goldbert LI: Blockade of renal effects of dopamine in the dog by the DA₁ antagonist SCH 23390. Am J Physiol 249 (Renal Fluid Electrolyte Physiol 18) F236, 1985.
8. Hilberman M, Maseda J, Stinson EB, et al: The diuretic properties of dopamine in patients after open heart operation. Anesthesiology 61:489, 1984.
9. Bayliss WM: On the local reactions of the arterial wall to changes of internal pressure. J Physiol 28:220, 1902.
10. Cohen JJ, Kamm DE: Renal metabolism relation to renal function. In Brenner BM, Rector FC (eds): The Kidney. Philadelphia, WB Saunders Company, 1981.
11. Berry CA: Heterogeneity of tubular transport pro-

cess in the nephron. Annu Rev Physiol 44:181, 1982.

12. Schrier RW, Berl T: Disorders of water metabolism. In Schrier RW (ed): Renal and Electrolyte Disorders. Boston, Little, Brown and Company, 1980.

13. Tannen RL: Control of acid excretion by the kidney. Annu Rev Med 31:35, 1980.

14. Giebisch G, Stanton B: Potassium transport in the nephron. Annu Rev Physiol 41:241, 1979.

15. Dennis VM, et al: Renal handling of phosphate and calcium. Annu Rev Physiol 41:257, 1979.

16. Ullmann E: Experimentelle Nierentransplantation. Wien Klin Wochenschr 15:281, 707, 1902.

17. Hamilton D: Kidney transplantation: A history. In Morris PJ (ed): Kidney Transplantation. New York, Grune & Stratton, 1984, p 1.

18. Shaw R, Stubenbord WT: Alexis Carrel: Contributions to kidney transplantation and preservation. NY State J Med 80:1438, 1980.

19. Moseley J: Alexis Carrel, the man unknown. Journey of an idea. JAMA 244:1119, 1980.

20. Moore FD: Give and Take: The Development of Tissue Transplantation. Philadelphia, WB Saunders Company, 1964, p 14.

21. Hume DM, Merrill JP, Miller BF, et al: Experiences with renal homotransplantation in the human: Report of nine cases. J Clin Invest 34:327, 1955.

22. Merrill JP, Murray JE, Harrison JH, et al: Successful homotransplantation of the human kidney between identical twins. JAMA 160:277, 1956.

23. Calne RY: The inhibition of renal homograft rejection in dogs by 6-mercaptopurine. Lancet 1:417, 1960.

24. Kuss R, Legrain M, Mathe G, et al: Homologous human kidney transplantation. Postgrad Med J 38:528, 1962.

25. Starzl TE, Marchioro TL, Waddell WR: The reversal of rejection in human renal homografts with subsequent development of homograft tolerance. Surg Gynecol Obstet 117:385, 1963.

26. Murray JE, Merrill JP, Harrison JH, et al: Prolonged survival of human-kidney homografts by immunosuppressive drug therapy. N Engl J Med 268:1315, 1963.

27. Najarian JS, Gulyossy PP, Stoney RJ, et al.: Protection of the donor kidney during homotransplantation. Ann Surg 164:398, 1966.

28. Terasaki PI, Marchioro TL, Starzl TE: In Histocompatibility Testing. Washington, National Academy of Sciences, 1965, p 83.

29. Opelz G, Sengar DPS, Mickey MR, Terasaki PI: Effect of blood transfusions on subsequent kidney transplants. Transplant Proc 5:253, 1973.

30. Salvatierra O, Vincenti F, Amend W, et al: Deliberate donor-specific blood transfusions prior to living related renal transplantation. A new approach. Ann Surg 192:543, 1980.

31. Calne RY, White DJG, Thiru S, et al.: Cyclosporin A in patients receiving renal allografts from cadaver donors. Lancet 2:1323, 1978.

32. Woodruff MFA: Ethical problems in organ transplantation. Br Med J 1:1457, 1964.

33. Cosimi AB: The donor and donor nephrectomy. In Morris PJ (ed): Kidney Transplantation. New York, Grune & Stratton, 1984, p 81.

34. John P, Kumar MSA, Samhan M, et al: The living donor for kidney transplantation: A review of 100 consecutive donors. In Abouna GM (ed): Current Status of Clinical Organ Transplantation. Boston, Martinus Nijhoff, 1984, p 163.

35. Rowe JW, Andres R, Tobin JD, et al: The effects of age on creatinine clearance in man: A cross-sectional and longitudinal study. J Gerontol 31:155, 1976.

36. Phillips MG: Cadaver donor nephrectomy. In Glenn JF (ed): Urologic Surgery. Philadelphia, JB Lippincott Company, 1983, p 329.

37. Rosenthal JT, Shaw BW Jr, Hardesty RL, et al: Principles of multiple organ procurement from cadaver donors. Ann Surg 198:617, 1983.

38. Collins GM, Halasy NA: Forty-eight hour ice storage of kidneys: Importance of cation content. Surgery 79:432, 1976.

39. Marshall VC: Renal preservation. In Morris PJ (ed): Kidney Transplantation. New York, Grune & Stratton, 1984, p 138.

40. Coffey AK, Andrews PM: Ultrastructure of kidney preservation: Varying the amount of an effective osmotic agent in isotonic and hypertonic preservation solutions. Transplantation 35:136, 1983.

41. Grundman R, Strumper R, Eichmann J: The immediate function of the kidney after 24 to 72 hour preservation. Transplantation 23:437, 1977.

42. Barry JM, Fischer S, Lieberman C, et al: Successful human kidney preservation by intracellular electrolyte flush followed by cold storage for more than 48 hours. J Urol 129:473, 1983.

43. Sampson D, Kaufman JM, Walzak P: Flow and function in machine-preserved kidneys. Br J Surg 65:37, 1978.

44. Mittal VK, Kaplan MP, Rosenberg JC, et al: Pulsatile perfusion: Better than hypothermic storage with cyclosporine as an immunosuppressant. Dial Transplant 14:136, 1985.

45. Belzer FO, Hoffman RM, Rice MJ, et al: Combination perfusion-cold storage for optimum cadaver kidney function and storage. Transplantation 39:118, 1985.

46. Lee HM: Surgical techniques of renal transplantation. In Morris PJ (ed): Kidney Transplantation. New York, Grune & Stratton, 1984, p 199.

47. Glass NR, Uehling D, Sollinger H, et al: Renal transplantation using ileal conduit in 5 cases. J Urol 133:666, 1985.

48. McDonald MW, Zincke H, Engen DE, et al: Adaptation of existing cutaneous ureterostomy for urinary drainage after renal transplantation. J Urol 133:1026, 1985.

49. Fine RN: Renal transplantation in children. In Morris PJ (ed): Kidney Transplantation. New York, Grune & Stratton, 1984, p 546.

50. So SKS, Nevins RE, Chang P-N, Mauer SM, et al: Preliminary results of renal transplantation in children under 1 year of age. Transplant Proc 17:182, 1985.

51. Belzer FO, Glass N, Sollinger H: Technical complications after renal transplantation. In Morris PJ (ed): Kidney Transplantation. New York, Grune & Stratton, 1984, p 404.

52. Diethelm AG, Dubovsky EV, Whelchel JD: Diagnosis of impaired renal function after kidney transplantation using renal scintigraphy, renal

plasma flow and urinary excretion of hippurate. Ann Surg 191:604, 1980.

53. Belorusov OS: Modern trends in surgical correction of arterial stenosis of transplanted kidney. Int Angiol 4:193, 1985.

54. Curtis JJ, Luke RJ, Whelchel D, et al: Inhibition of angiotensin—Converting enzyme in renal transplant patients with hypertension. N Engl J Med 308:377, 1983.

55. Trachtman H, Butt KMH, Gordon D, et al: The use of captopril to control hypertension in post transplant renal artery stenosis. Clin Nephrol 23:203, 1985.

56. Thomsen HS, Dorph S, Mygind T, et al: The transplanted kidney. Diagnostic and interventional radiology. Acta Radiol 26:353, 1985.

57. Nakstad P, Kolmannskog F, Kolbenstvedt A, et al: Computed tomography in surgical complications following renal transplantation. J Comput Assist Tomogr 6:286, 1982.

58. Cuvelier R, Pirson Y, Alexander GPJ, et al: Late urinary tract infection after transplantation: Prevalence, predisposition and morbidity. Nephron 40:76, 1985.

59. Yazbeck S, Larbrisseau A, O'Regan S: Femoral neuropathy after renal transplantation. J Urol 134:720, 1985.

60. Velosa JA, Anderson CF, Torres VE, et al: Long-term renal status of kidney donors: Calculated small risk of kidney donation. Transplant Proc 17:100, 1985.

61. Marshall JR, Fellner CH: Kidney donors revisited. Am J Psychiatry 134:575, 1977.

62. Dornette WHL: Consent and living donors of organs. Anesth Analg 52:311, 1973.

63. Diethelm AG, Aldrete JS, Sterling WA, et al: Large volume diuresis as a mechanism for immediate maximum renal function after transplantation. Surg Gynecol Obstet 138:869, 1974.

64. Dhabuwala CB, Bird M, Salamon JR: Relative importance of warm ischemia, hypotension and hypercarbia in producing renal vasospasm. Transplantation 27:238, 1979.

65. Hunter JM, Jones RS, Utting JE: Effect of acute hypocapnoea on renal function in the dog artificially ventilated with nitrous oxide, oxygen and halothane. Br J Anaesth 52:197, 1980.

66. Wetzel RC, Setzer N, Stiff JL, et al: Hemodynamic responses in brain dead organ donor patients. Anesth Analg 64:125, 1985.

67. Gentile DE: Proposed regulations governing reimbursement under the Medicare end stage renal disease program. Testimony before Subcommittee on Oversight of the Committee on Ways and Means, Serial 97-57:322, April 22, 1982.

68. Rostand SG, Kirk KA, Rutsky EA, et al: Racial differences in the incidence of end stage renal disease. N Engl J Med 306:1276, 1982.

69. Kuruvila KC, Schrier RW: Chronic renal failure. Int Anesthiol Clin 22:101, 1984.

70. Schreiner GE: Uremia. In Massry SG, Glassock RJ (eds): Textbook of Nephrology. Baltimore, Williams & Wilkins Company, 1983, p 452.

71. Grodstein G, Harrison A, Roberts C, et al: Impaired gastric emptying times in hemodialysis patients. Am Soc Nephrol 1979, p 182A.

72. Arieff AI: Neurological complications of uremia. In Brenner BM, Rector FC Jr (eds): The Kidney. Philadelphia, WB Saunders Company, 1981, p 2306.

73. Alfrey AC, LeGendre GR, Kaehney WD: The dialysis encephalopathy syndrome: Possible aluminum intoxication. N Engl J Med 294:184, 1976.

74. Roth F, Wuthrich H: The clinical importance of hyperkalemia following suxamethonium administration. Br J Anaesth 41:311, 1969.

75. Powell JN: Suxamethonium-induced hyperkalemia in a uremic patient. Br J Anaesth 42:806, 1970.

76. Anderson CB, Codd JR, Graff RA, et al: Cardiac failure and upper extremity arteriovenous dialysis fistulas. Arch Intern Med 136:292, 1976.

77. Fried W: Hematological abnormalities in chronic renal failure. Semin Nephrol 1:176, 1981.

78. Whelchel JD, Shaw JF, Curtis JJ, et al: Effect of pretransplant stored donor-specific blood transfusions on early renal allograft survival in one-haplotype living related transplants. Transplantation 34:326, 1982.

79. Wills MR, Savory J: Aluminum poisoning: Dialysis encephalopathy, osteomalacia and anaemia. Lancet 2:29, 1983.

80. Goldstein DA, Feinstein EI, Chui LA, Pattahiraman R, Massry SG: The relationship between the abnormalities in electroencephalogram and blood levels of PTH in dialysis patients. J Clin Endocrinol Metab 51:130, 1980.

81. Massry SG: Parathyroid hormone as a uremic toxin. In Massry SG, Glassrock R (eds): Textbook of Nephrology. Baltimore, Williams & Wilkins Company, 1983, p 73.

82. Crass MF, Moore PL, Strickland ML, et al: Cardiovascular responses to parathyroid hormone. Am J Physiol 249:E187, 1985.

83. Diethelm AG, Adams PL, Murad TM, et al: Treatment of secondary hyperparathyroidism in patients with chronic renal failure by total parathyroidectomy and parathyroid autograft. Ann Surg 193:777, 1981.

84. Jaeger P, Burckhardt P, Wauters JP, et al: Evidence for a particularly severe secondary hyperparathyroidism in analgesic abuse nephropathy. Am J Nephrol 5:342, 1985.

85. Stanbury SW, Lumb GA, Nicholson WF: Elective subtotal parathyroidectomy for renal hyperparathyroidism. Lancet 1:793, 1960.

86. Diethelm AG, Edwards RP, Whelchel JD: The natural history and surgical treatment of hypercalcemia before and after renal transplantation. Surg Gynecol Obstet 154:481, 1982.

87. Pender JM, Basso LV: Diseases of the endocrine system. In Chernow B (ed): The Pharmacologic Approach to the Critically Ill Patient. Baltimore, Williams & Wilkins Company, 1984.

88. Roizen MF: Perioperative evaluation of patients that require special preoperative and intraoperative management. In Miller RD (ed): Anesthesia. New York, Churchill Livingstone, 1981, p 21.

89. Sutherland DER, Fryd DS, Morrow CE, et al: Kidney transplantation in diabetic recipients: Factors leading to improved results. In Abouna GM (ed): Current Status of Clinical Organ Transplantation. Boston, Martinus Nijhoff, 1984, p 173.

90. Bennett WM, Aronoff GR, Morrison G, et al: Drug prescribing in renal failure: Dosing guidelines for adults. Am J Kidney Dis 3:155, 1983.

91. McMillen MA, Tesi RJ, Baumgarten WB, et al: Potentiation of cyclosporine by verapamil *in vitro*. Transplantation 40:444, 1985.

92. DeLeve LD, Piafsky KM: Clinical significance of plasma binding of basic drugs. Trends Pharmacol Sci 2:283, 1981.

93. Edwards DJ, Lalka D, Cura F, et al: Alpha₁-acid glycoprotein concentration and protein binding in trauma. Clin Pharmacol Ther 31:62, 1982.

94. Jordan ML, Novick AC, Steinmueller D, et al: Renal transplantation in the older recipient. J Urol 134:243, 1985.

95. DiPaolo N, Manganelli A, Strappaveccia F, et al: A new technique for insertion of the Tenckhoff peritoneal dialysis catheter. Nephron 40:485, 1985.

96. Frascino JA: A comparison of self care dialysis modalities. Dial Transplant 14:13, 1985.

97. Sheinfeld J, Linke CL, Talley TE, et al: Selective pretransplant nephrectomy: Indications and perioperative management. J Urol 133:379, 1985.

98. Ochs HR, Greenblatt DJ, Kaschell HJ, et al: Diazepam kinetics in patients with renal insufficiency or hyperthyroidism. Br J Clin Pharmacol 12:829, 1981.

99. Vinik HR, Reves JG, Greenblatt DJ, et al: The pharmacokinetics of midazolam in chronic renal failure patients. Anesthesiology 59:390, 1983.

100. Don HF, Dieppa RA, Taylor P: Narcotic analgesics in anuric patients. Anesthesiology 42:745, 1975.

101. Szeto HH, Inturrisi CE, Honde R, et al: Accumulation of normeperidine, an active metabolite of meperidine, in patients with renal failure or cancer. Ann Intern Med 86:738, 1977.

102. Mostert JW, Evers JL, Hobika GH, et al: Circulatory effects of analgesic and neuroleptic drugs in patients with chronic renal failure undergoing maintenance dialysis. Br J Anaesth 42:501, 1970.

103. Aldrete JA, O'Higgins JW, Starzl TE: Changes of serum potassium during renal homotransplantation. Arch Surg 101:82, 1970.

104. Myers ML, Austin TW, Sibbald WJ: Pulmonary artery catheter infections. A prospective study. Ann Surg 201:237, 1985.

105. Aldrete JA, Clapp NW, Starzl TE: Body temperature changes during organ transplantation. Anesth Analg 49:384, 1970.

106. Virtue RW: Anesthesia for patients involved in renal homotransplantation. In Starzl TE (ed): Experience in Renal Transplantation. Philadelphia, WB Saunders Company, 1964, p 63.

107. Bastron RD, Bailey G, Deutsch S, et al: Anesthesia for patients with chronic renal failure for renal homotransplantation. Anesthesiology 30:335, 1969.

108. Vandam LD: Impressions of anesthetics past. Transplant Proc 13:61, 1981.

109. Linke CA, Merin RG: A regional anesthetic approach for renal transplantation. Anesth Analg 55:69, 1976.

110. Keenan RL, Boyan CP: Anesthesia for organ transplantation. In Chaggerjee SV (ed): Renal Transplantation: A Multidisciplinary Approach. New York, Raven Press, 1980, p 127.

111. Strunin L, Davies JM, Filshie GJ: Anesthesia for renal transplantation. Int Anesthesiol Clin 22:189, 1984.

112. Sear JW: Anesthesia in renal transplantation. In Morris AJ (ed): Kidney Transplantation. New York, Grune & Stratton, 1984, p 219.

113. Christensen JH, Andraeson F, Jansen J: Pharmacokinetics and pharmacodynamics of thiopental in patients undergoing renal transplantation. Acta Anaesthesiol Scand 27:513, 1983.

114. Gulden D, Koehntop D, Rodman J, et al: Fentanyl pharmacokinetics during renal transplantation. Anesthesiology 61:A243, 1984.

115. deTemmerman P, Gribomont B: Enflurane in renal transplantation: Report of 375 cases. Acta Anaesthesiol Scand Suppl 72:24, 1979.

116. Wickstrom I: Enflurane anesthesia in living related donor renal transplantation. Acta Anaesthesiol Scand 25:263, 1981.

117. McArdle B: The serum cholinesterase in jaundice and diseases of the liver. Q J Med 33:107, 1940.

118. Miller RD, Way WL, Hamilton WK, et al: Succinylcholine-induced hyperkalemia in patients with renal failure? Anesthesiology 36:138, 1972.

119. Koide M, Waud BE: Serum potassium concentrations after succinylcholine in patients with renal failure. Anesthesiology 36:142, 1972.

120. Katz J, Kountz SL, Cohn R: Anesthetic considerations for renal transplant. Anesth Analg 46:609, 1967.

121. Walton JD, Farman JV: Suxamethonium hyperkalaemia in uraemic neuropathy. Anaesthesia 28:666, 1973.

122. Nigrovic V: Succinylcholine, cholinoceptors and catecholamines: Proposed mechanism of early adverse haemodynamic reactions. Can Anaesth Soc J 31:382, 1984.

123. Bishop MJ, Hornbein TF: Prolonged effect of succinylcholine after neostigmine and pyridostigmine administration in patients with renal failure. Anesthesiology 58:384, 1983.

124. Miller RD, Matteo RS, Benet RZ, et al: The pharmacokinetics of d-tubocurarine in man with and without renal failure. J Pharmacol Exp Ther 202:1, 1977.

125. Miller RD, Stevens WC, Way WL: The effect of renal failure and hyperkalemia on the duration of pancuronium neuromuscular blockade in man. Anesth Analg 52:661, 1973.

126. Thomson IR, Putnins CL: Adverse effects of pancuronium during high-dose fentanyl anesthesia for coronary artery bypass grafting. Anesthesiology 62:708, 1985.

127. Pinaud MLJ, Souron RJ: Beta-adrenergic effect of pancuronium bromide: Fact or fallacy. Anesthesiology 60:512, 1984.

128. Agoston S, Salt P, Newton D, et al: The neuromuscular blocking action of Org NC 45, a new pancuronium derivative, in anaesthetized patients. Br J Anaesth 52:535, 1980.

129. Rupp SM, Miller RD, Gencarelli PJ: Vecuronium induced neuromuscular blockade during enflurane, isoflurane, and halothane anesthesia in humans. Anesthesiology 60:102, 1984.

130. Krieg N, Rutten JMJ, Crul JF, et al: Preliminary review of the interaction of Org NC 45 with an-

aesthetics and antibiotics in animals. Br J Anaesth 52:33S, 1980.

131. Fahey MR, Morris RB, Miller RD, et al: Pharmacokinetics of Org Nc 45 (Norcuron) in patients with and without renal failure. Br J Anaesth 53:1049, 1981.

132. Meistelman C, Lienhart A, Leveque C, et al: Pharmacology of vecuronium in patients with end stage renal failure. Anesthesiology 59:A293, 1983.

133. Bevan DR, Donati F, Gyasi H, Williams A: Vecuronium in renal failure. Can Anaesth Soc J 31:491, 1984.

134. Hofmann AW: Beitrage zur Kenntniss der fluchtigen basen. Ann Chem 78:253, 1851.

135. Stenlake JB, Waigh RD, Urwin J, et al: Atracurium: Conception and inception. Br J Anaesth 55:35, 1983.

136. Nigrovic V, Auen M, Wajskol A: Enzymatic hydrolysis of atracurium *in vivo*. Anesthesiology 62:606, 1985.

137. Fahey MR, Rupp SM, Fisher DM, et al: The pharmacokinetics and pharmacodynamics of atracurium in patients with and without renal failure. Anesthesiology 61:699, 1984.

138. de Bros FM, Lai A, Scott R, et al; Pharmacokinetics and pharmacodynamics of atracurium under isoflurane anesthesia in normal and anephric patients. Anesth Analg 64:207, 1985.

139. Hunter JM, Jones RS, Utting JE: Use of atracurium in patients with no renal function. Br J Anaesth 54:1251, 1982.

140. Hunter JM, Jones RS, Utting JE: Comparison of vecuronium, atracurium and tubocurarine in normal patients and in patients with no renal function. Br J Anaesth 56:941, 1984.

141. Miller RD, Rupp SM, Fisher DM, et al: Clinical pharmacology of vecuronium and atracurium. Anesthesiology 61:444, 1984.

142. Fisher DM, Canfell C, Miller RD: Stability of atracurium administered by infusion. Anesthesiology 61:347, 1984.

143. Cato AE, Lineburg CG, Macklia AW: Concerning toxicity testing of atracurium. Anesthesiology 62:94, 1985.

144. Shi WZ, Fahey MR, Fisher DM, et al: Increase in minimum alveolar concentration (MAC) of halothane by laudanosine in rabbits. Anesth Analg 64:282, 1985.

145. Ingram MD, Sclabassi RJ, Stiller RL, et al: Cardiovascular effects and electroencephographic effects of laudanosine in "nephrectomized" cats. Anesth Analg 64:232, 1985.

146. Gergis SD, Sokoll MD, Mehta M, et al: Intubation conditions after atracurium and suxamethonium. Br J Anaesth 55:83S, 1983.

147. Foldes FF, Schwarz S, Ilias W, et al: Rapid tracheal intubation with vecuronium: The priming principle. Anesthesiology 61:A294, 1984.

148. Bradley JP, Marsland AR, O'Connor JP: Prolonged neuromuscular blockade after renal transplantation. Anaesth Intensive Care 13:196, 1985.

149. Luciani J, Frantz PL, Thibault PL, et al: Early anuria prevention in human kidney transplantation. Transplantation 28:308, 1979.

150. Carlier M, Squifflet JP, Pirson Y, et al: Maximal hydration during anesthesia increases pulmonary artery pressures and improves early function of human renal transplant. Transplantation 34:201, 1982.

151. Grundman R, Kammerer B, Franke E, et al: Effects of hypotension on the results of kidney storage and the use of dopamine under these conditions. Transplantation 32:184, 1981.

152. Tinker JH, Michenfelder JD: Increased resistance to SNP-induced cyanide toxicity in anuric dogs. Anesthesiology 52:40, 1980.

153. Brezis M, Rosen S, Silva P, et al: Renal ischemia: A new perspective. Kidney Int 26:375, 1984.

154. Baek SM, Brown RS, Shoemaker WC: Early prediction of acute renal failure: II. Renal function response to furosemide. Ann Surg 178:605, 1973.

155. Weimar W, Geerlings W, Bijnen AB, et al: A controlled study on the effect of mannitol on immediate renal function after cadaver donor kidney transplantation. Transplantation 35:99, 1983.

156. Moreno M, Murphy C, Goldsmith C: Increase in serum potassium resulting from the administration of hypertonic mannitol and other solutions. J Lab Clin Med 73:291, 1969.

157. Grodin W, Scantlebury V, Warmington N: Dopaminergic stimulation of renal blood flow and renal function after transplantation. Anesthesiology 61:A129, 1984.

158. Grundman R, Kindler J, Meider J, et al: Dopamine treatment of human cadaver kidney graft recipients: A prospectively randomized trial. Klin Wochenschr 60:193, 1982.

159. Williams GM: Clinical course following renal transplantation. In Morris PJ (ed): Kidney Transplantation. New York, Grune & Stratton, 1984, p 335.

160. Marshland AT, Bradley JP: Anaesthesia for renal transplantation—5 years' experience. Anaesth Intensive Care 11:337, 1983.

161. Chou LM, Beyer MM, Butt KMH, et al: Hypertension jeopardizes diabetic patients following renal transplant. Trans Am Soc Artif Intern Organs 30:473, 1984.

162. Grekas D, Nakos V, Theocharides A, et al: Prophylactic treatment with cimetidine after renal transplantation. Nephron 40:213, 1985.

163. Tilney NL, Collins JJ, Wilson RE: Hemorrhagic pancreatitis: A fatal complication of renal transplantation. N Engl J Med 274:1051, 1966.

164. Lee HM, Mendez-Picon G, Goldman T, et al: The course of long-term survival in kidney transplantation: One center's experience. Transplant Proc 17:106, 1985.

165. Washer GF, Schroter GPJ, Starzl TE, et al: Causes of death after kidney transplantation. JAMA 250:49, 1983.

166. Curtis JJ, Luke RG, Jones P: Hypertension after successful renal transplantation. Am J Med 79:193, 1985.

167. Peters TG, Vaughn WK, Williams JW, et al: Methyldopa therapy and outcome in cadaveric renal transplantation. South Med J 78:1044, 1985.

168. Lundgren G, Wilczek H, Bohman SO, et al: Development of diabetic nephropathy in renal allograft of diabetic patients. Transplant Proc 17:18, 1985.

169. Terasaki PI, Toyotome A, Mickey MR, et al: Patient, graft and functional survival rates: An overview. In Terasaki PI (ed): Clinical Kidney Transplants 1985. Los Angeles, UCLA Tissue Typing Lab, 1985, p 1.

170. Levey AS: The improving prognosis after kidney transplantation. Arch Intern Med 144:2382, 1984.

171. Opelz G: Correlation of HLA matching with kidney graft survival in patients with or without cyclosporine treatment. Transplantation 40:240, 1985.

172. Byer BJ, Hoy WE, May AG, et al: Increased survival time of renal allograft recipients. NY State J Med 85:534, 1985.

173. Ivey GL, Richie RE, Niblack GD, et al: Renal transplantation: A 20-year experience in a Veterans Administration medical center. Arch Surg 120:1021, 1985.

174. Sutherland DER, Goetz FC, Najarian JS: One hundred pancreas transplants at a single institution. Ann Surg 200:414, 1984.

175. Cecka M, Cicciarell J: The transfusion effect. In Terasaki PI (ed): Clinical Kidney Transplants 1985. Los Angeles, UCLA Tissue Typing Lab, 1985, p 73.

176. Gueco IP, Evans DB, Calne RY: Prolonged survival after renal transplantation: A study of 54 patients who lived ten or more years after operation with functioning allografts. Transplant Proc 17:108, 1985.

177. Lau J, Scott JR: Pregnancy following renal transplantation. Clin Obstet Gynecol 28:339, 1985.

# 7

# *Heart and Heart-Lung Transplantation*

JANET WYNER
ELLEN L. FINCH

## ANESTHESIA FOR HEART TRANSPLANTATION

### History

Following many years of laboratory investigation since the early twentieth century, the first clinical heart transplantation was performed in 1967 (Table 7–1). The first experimental work in cardiac transplantation was reported in 1905 by Carrel and Guthrie.[1] They described vascular anastomotic techniques by transplanting a canine heart into the cervical region of another dog. Spontaneous myocardial contractions resumed, which demonstrated that the heart could beat spontaneously without innervation. Further investigations during the 1930's modified and improved the surgical techniques of heterotopic cardiac transplantation.[2] Even after these early experiments, rejection of the graft tissue was rated as a major problem. Subsequently Demikhov performed the first experiments in which the donor heart, transplanted intrathoracically, supported the circulatory load.[3,4] In these experiments the donor heart was placed in parallel with the recipient heart and thus acted as an extra pump. Some centers still use this technique in the performance of their heterotopic cardiac transplantation.[5] The first attempts at orthotopic transplantation of canine hearts was reported by Goldberg et al. in 1958, but the survival was poor, with animals living an average of 117 minutes.[6] In 1960 Lower and Shumway described the first fully successful orthotopic canine cardiac transplantation with recipients surviving 21 days.[7] This success was attributed to surgical improvements, advances in cardiopulmonary bypass, and myocardial preservation by hypothermia. These experiments demonstrated the problem of rejection that was elicited by the donor organ, which, if not controlled, re-

### TABLE 7–1. History of Heart Transplantation

| Year | Event | Ref. |
|------|-------|------|
| 1905 | Heterotopic extrathoracic | 1 |
| 1950 | Heterotopic intrathoracic | 3 |
| 1958 | Orthotopic canine | 6 |
| 1960 | Orthotopic canine | 7 |
| 1964 | Clinical orthotopic chimpanzee heart | 10 |
| 1967 | Clinical orthotopic human heart | 11 |

sulted in graft destruction.[8] Evidence of impending graft rejection was noted to be associated with a decrease in QRS voltage on the ECG, development of atrial or ventricular arrhythmias, and the infiltration of graft tissue with lymphocytes on endomyocardial biopsy.[9]

Hardy and colleagues performed the first clinical orthotopic cardiac transplantation in 1964 at the University Hospital in Mississippi.[10] The recipient was a 68-year-old man with end-stage cardiac disease whose heart was replaced with a chimpanzee heart. This heart was too small and could not support the circulation; the patient died soon after cardiopulmonary bypass. In 1967 Barnard and colleagues transplanted a donor heart from a patient with irreversible brain death into a patient with end-stage cardiomyopathy.[11] The recipient did well until developing pneumonia and died on the 18th postoperative day. After this initial procedure there was a plethora of transplantations done around the world (Fig. 7–1). Within the first year more than 101 transplantations were performed, but with the attending poor survival rates enthusiasm for the procedure decreased.

In 1968 the clinical heart transplantation program at Stanford University Medical Center was initiated. It has continued to be active, with a gradual increase over more recent years. The success as a treatment method for selected patients with end-stage cardiomyopathy has encouraged the re-establishment of a number of centers throughout the world (Fig. 6–1). By January 1982, 664 patients had undergone cardiac transplantation throughout the world, with one third of these having been performed at Stanford University Medical Center.[12] Alternative therapy for the terminally sick cardiac patient is either the insertion of a total artificial heart or the left-ventricular assist device; both are still in the experimental phase.[13,14] These devices, however, have been used as interim treatment in patients waiting for a human heart.

Since the inception of the Stanford clinical program, several major advances have been made both clinically and in the laboratory (Table 7–2). These include refinement of recipient selection criteria, perfection of the operative technique, improvement of cardiac preservation, and better diagnosis and treatment of graft rejection.[15,16,17] In 1973 rabbit antithymocyte globulin was introduced for immunosuppression, transvenous endomyocardial biopsies were done for the diagnosis of rejection, and methods to monitor the immunological status were established.[18,19,20] The development of graft atherosclerosis was noted soon after transplantation began, and measures to minimize its development were undertaken.[21] More recently, in 1978, investigational work with cyclosporine began and was incorporated into the clinical treatment for immunosuppression in December 1980.[22–24] Currently, laboratory and clinical

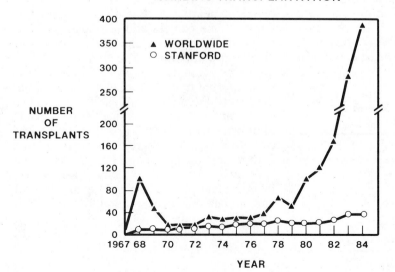

**Figure 7–1.** Cardiac transplantation worldwide, 1968 to 1984.

**TABLE 7–2.  Stanford Cardiac Transplantation: Principal Developments in Clinical Program**

| | |
|---|---|
| 1968 | Inception of clinical program |
| 1970 | Refinement of recipient selection criteria |
| 1971 | Institution of measures to minimize graft arteriosclerosis |
| 1972 | Endomyocardial biopsy |
| 1973 | Rabbit antihuman thymocyte globulin |
| 1974 | Immunological monitoring |
| 1975 | Cardiac retransplantation |
| 1977 | Distant donor heart procurement |
| 1980 | Cyclosporin A immune suppression |
| 1981 | Combined heart and lung transplantation |

Data from Pennoch JL, Oyer PE, Reitz BA, et al: Cardiac transplantation in perspective for the future. J Thorac Cardiovasc Surg 83:168, 1982, with permission of the authors and publisher.

efforts are directed toward perfection of immunosuppressive treatment and prevention of its complications.

## Survival

The one-year survival of patients undergoing heart transplantation during 1968 (the first year of the program at Stanford) was 22 per cent. The survival rate at one year has steadily increased, with substantial improvement over the past six years. This improvement in survival has been attributed to refinement in patient selection, improved postoperative care, and the introduction of cyclosporine.[16] Approximately 80 per cent of patients currently undergoing cardiac transplantation

may be expected to survive one year, and between 60 and 65 per cent of patients survive for three years[12] (Fig. 7–2). Survival statistics are much poorer for patients accepted as candidates for transplantation for whom an acceptable donor heart cannot be found quickly. Only 10 per cent of accepted candidates who have not undergone transplantation within three months of selection survive to undergo surgery. After transplantation approximately 85 per cent of recipients are considered rehabilitated and are able to return to work or other comparable activities.[25] Inability to do so has generally resulted from complications of immunosuppression such as corticosteroid therapy.

## Physiology of the Denervated Heart

In orthotopic heart transplantation the operative technique results in retention of a small section of the posterior walls of the left and right atria. This portion includes the sinoatrial nodal tissue, which retains both sympathetic and parasympathetic innervation. The donor heart has its own sinoatrial node, which is not innervated. This sinoatrial node controls the allograft heart rate, which is persistently higher than the recipient rate.[26] On the ECG two P waves from the recipient's atrial remnant and the donor atrium may be recorded. Following the administration of atropine, an increase in the recipient's P wave occurs with no change in the donor and effective heart rate. Amyl nitrate induces ar-

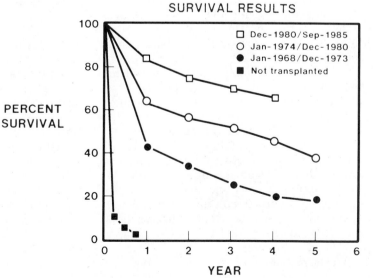

**Figure 7–2.** Survival of patients accepted for transplantation. Patients who have died before operation contrasted to transplant survival: Stanford experience.

**TABLE 7–3.    Effects of Drugs on the Denervated Heart**

| Agent | Sinus Rate | Atrioventricular Conduction | Intraventricular Conduction |
|---|---|---|---|
| Atropine | – | – | |
| Pancuronium | – | – | |
| Endrophonium | – | – | |
| Propranolol | ↓ | ↓ | – |
| Isoproterenol | ↑ | ↑ | |
| Norepinephrine | ↑ | ↑ | |
| Methoxamine | – | | |
| Acebutolol | ↓ | ↓ | – |
| Digoxin acute | – | – | |
| Digoxin chronic | – | ↓ | |
| Quinidine | ↓ | ↓ | ↓ |
| Amyl nitrate | – | | |

– = no effect; ↓ = decrease; ↑ = increase.

terial hypotension, but fails to increase donor heart rate. Intravenous tyramine, which causes a rise in blood pressure, produces a decrease in the recipient's heart rate, but no change in donor heart rate (Table 7–3). Also, stimuli such as hand grip, Valsalva maneuver, or carotid sinus massage, which normally act through autonomic innervation, produce no change in donor sinus rate.[27] To date, no evidence of reinnervation of the transplanted human heart as long as 12 years after surgery has been demonstrated.[28,29]

Following cardiac transplantation the majority of survivors (85 per cent) return functionally to NYHA Class I by one year.[25] Late postoperative studies have demonstrated normal or near-normal resting hemodynamics.[29,30] The right- and left-sided filling pressures are normal, and the cardiac output is slightly decreased. The denervated heart retains its intrinsic control mechanisms, which include: a normal Frank-Starling effect demonstrated with volume loading; normal impulse formation and conductivity; and intact alpha and beta adrenergic receptors without evidence of denervation hypersensitivity.[26,27,31,32] The beta adrenergic receptor density increases twofold in transplanted animal hearts four weeks following transplantation. This is presumably due to denervation up-regulation.[33] This increase in receptor concentration may result in a heightened response in the transplanted heart to catecholamines.[34] However, this has not been demonstrated in humans.

The transplanted heart responds atypically to exercise, stress such as hypovolemia or hypotension, and certain drugs as a result of the lack of autonomic neural control of the sinoatrial node.[31] Initially during exercise, the cardiac output increases as venous return (preload) increases secondary to muscular activity. Subsequently after several minutes, the increase in cardiac output is due to augmentation of myocardial activity and heart rate, following rises in circulating catecholamine levels. Systolic blood pressure continues to increase, suggesting that peripheral reflexes are intact. Following exercise there is a more gradual decrease in heart rate and inotropism in these patients as plasma catecholamine levels decrease. Accordingly, increase in cardiac output is dependent upon increases in venous return until circulating catecholamine levels rise sufficiently to increase heart rate and contractility. Therefore, in management of transplant patients the delayed response to stress and a poor tolerance to intravascular volume depletion must be appreciated.

The effects of various drugs on the transplanted heart have been investigated (Table 7–3). Only drugs acting on the heart directly, without involvement of the autonomic nervous system, can be expected to affect the donor heart. Electrophysiological studies using norepinephrine, epinephrine, isoproterenol, and adrenergic antagonists produce responses similar to those in normal patients.[30] Contrariwise, agents, such as pancuronium, cholinergic antagonists, and anticholinesterases, that exert their effects on the heart indirectly through the autonomic nervous system have no effect on heart rate.

Drugs, such as digoxin and quinidine, that act through mixed autonomically mediated and direct mechanisms will manifest only their direct cardiac effects. For example, short-term administration of digoxin to transplant patients has no effect on the donor sinus heart rate, which suggests that digoxin's short-term effects are autonomically mediated. However, long-term administration of digoxin to these patients depresses atrioventricular conduction and decreases donor heart rate, which suggests that long-term administration of digoxin acts directly on the heart.[35] Quinidine also has both direct and indirect autonomically mediated effects on the heart that may oppose each other, particularly in the normal patient. In the transplanted heart quinidine slows intraventricular conduction (as in the innervated heart), atrioventricular conduction, and sinus rate; the last two effects being opposite from its vagolytic effects in the intact heart.[28]

Atrial, junctional, and ventricular dysrhythmias are common in the denervated heart, especially during the first six months following transplantation, with the incidence increasing during episodes of rejection.[36,37] These dysrhythmias respond to treatment of rejection and, if hemodynamically significant, can be treated with electrical cardioversion or antiarrhythmic drugs that act directly on the conduction system. Free from vagal tone, the transplanted heart has a resting rate of 90 to 120 beats per minute. The coronary vasculature retains its response to changes in metabolic demand, but loses its basal alpha adrenergic tone, and therefore resting coronary blood flow is increased.[38] The coronary arteries also remain responsive to adrenoreceptor agonists and antagonists. During coronary angiography, transient bradycardia is usually seen when radiographic contrast agents are injected into either the right or left coronary artery. In transplanted hearts, slight bradycardia may occasionally occur with injection of the right coronary artery, suggesting that this effect is mediated by autonomic reflexes. Occlusive coronary atherosclerosis and myocardial infarction may occur in transplanted hearts without any angina, which supports the fact that the transplanted heart remains devoid of autonomic innervation.

## Recipient Selection

All patients accepted for heart transplantation have advanced cardiac disease not amenable to medical or surgical treatment and have a prognosis for survival of several weeks or months.

The guidelines that are followed to select suitable patients for transplantation have evolved from the initial five years of clinical experience. Assessment of potential recipients includes a history and physical examination, biochemical and hematological investigation, and cardiac catheterization with hemodynamic and angiographic studies. In addition, a careful psychosociological evaluation is performed, as the candidate must be in a stable and supportive home environment.

Several contraindications to acceptance have evolved, including: (1) age over 55 years, (2) presence of active infectious disease process, (3) systemic disease that may compromise survival or increase morbidity (such as insulin-dependent diabetes mellitus, irreversible renal or hepatic disease, severe peripheral vascular disease, or malignant disease), (4) recent unresolved pulmonary infarction, and (5) markedly elevated pulmonary vascular resistance (greater than 8 Wood units) unresponsive to vasodilator therapy; this last contraindication has been instituted, since the normal donor right ventricle may not perform efficiently against high pulmonary resistance.[16,39] If the recipient has elevated pulmonary vascular resistance an effort is made to obtain a large heart and, if possible, to transport the donor body to the same hospital to decrease ischemic time of the donor heart.

In the Stanford transplant population the primary diagnosis is either ischemic heart disease or idiopathic cardiomyopathy. Patients with other pathological disease states such as valvular or congenital heart disease also undergo heart transplantation, but much less frequently, since these patients often have excessively high pulmonary vascular resistances (Table 7–4).

## Donor Selection

An important development in clinical heart transplantation was the establishment of a legal definition of irreversible brain death in the presence of normal respiratory and cardiac function.[40,41] The neurological catastrophes that provide organ donors include motorcycle or automobile accidents, falls, intracranial hemorrhage, gunshot wounds, and brain tumors.

Potential donors for cardiac transplanta-

**TABLE 7–4.  Stanford Cardiac Transplantation: Recipient Diagnosis**

| Diagnosis | No. Patients |
|---|---|
| Coronary artery disease | 152 |
| Cardiomyopathy | 171 |
| Valve disease with cardiomyopathy | 19 |
| Congenital heart disease | 5 |
| Coronary artery emboli | 2 |
| Cardiac tumor | 1 |
| Post-traumatic aneurysm | 1 |
| Myocarditis | 1 |
| Sarcoid | 1 |
| Total | 353 |

tion must be less than 35 years of age, since a positive correlation has been demonstrated between the development of coronary atherosclerosis in the graft tissue and age of the donor.[21,42–44] The heart must be assessed as normal with a negative history of heart defects and a normal ECG. Abnormalities in ST segments and atrial premature contractions are often present in the neurologically dead, but must be differentiated from pathological processes. The donor must also be free from infection, chest trauma, and malignant disease. If cardiac disease is suspected, cardiac catheterization, coronary angiography, or echocardiography should be performed to define the extent of the pathological process. At Stanford, if a male donor is over 35 years or a female is over 40 years, coronary angiography is performed. In 37 potential cardiac donors who were over the accepted age limit, coronary arteriography demonstrated significant coronary artery disease in 10 patients and mitral regurgitation in 3 patients.[42]

Since the improvement in myocardial preservation, distant heart procurement has now become routine by most centers performing cardiac transplantation.[44,45] Donor hearts harvested at distant hospitals are arrested by 500 ml hypothermic electrolyte solution infused into the aortic root. The hypothermic cardioplegic solution used at Stanford contains 5 per cent dextrose in 500 ml water with 15 mEq of potassium chloride, 12.5 gm of mannitol, and 12.5 mEq of sodium bicarbonate, providing an osmolarity of 440 mOsm and a pH at 4°C of 8.1 to 8.4. The donor heart is then excised and packed sterilely in a transport bag containing cold normal saline (4°C) and then placed into an ice chest filled with ice during the transfer.[45] The longest is-

chemic period for the donor heart at Stanford has been 3.5 hours, although up to 4.5 hours' duration has been reported by others with subsequent good graft function. Billingham and colleagues demonstrated on endomyocardial biopsy that damage to capillary endothelial cells occurs in human heart transplants one year after transplantation with distant heart procurement but not in on-site donors.[46] Experimentally, in rat cardiac isografts, apart from fibrosis, no functional or ultrastructural changes have been shown after 4, 8, and 12 hours of pretransplantation preservation with hypothermic cardioplegic solution. The conclusion from this study was that chronic fibrosis may be the limiting factor for prolonged hypothermic cardiac preservation.[47] A difference between the function of hearts from on-site and from distant donors (either by immediate cardiac function or by light and electron microscopical examination of ventricular biopsy specimens at the time of surgery) has not been demonstrated.[12]

Matching a potential cardiac donor for a recipient is determined by compatible body mass, ABO blood group compatibility, and a negative lymphocyte crossmatch (lack of cytotoxic effect of recipient's serum on donor lymphocytes).[42,48–50] Recently compatibility for the human lymphocyte antigen HLA-A2 has been attempted, as an increase in coronary atherosclerosis has been observed in the transplanted heart when this antigen is not similar in donor and recipient.[42,43]

## Surgical Procedure

The operative technique used for orthotopic cardiac transplantation has not changed much since the initial description by Lower and Shumway in 1960[7] (Fig. 7–3).

Through a median sternotomy the recipient heart is exposed, and after heparin is administered central cannulation for cardiopulmonary bypass is carried out in the usual manner. Extensive manipulation of the heart is avoided until the heart is emptied during cardiopulmonary bypass, as a loosely attached thrombus may be present in the dilated ventricles of the recipient. Once cardiopulmonary bypass is established the recipient diseased heart is excised, leaving a cuff of atria and adequate remains of the aorta and pulmonary artery. The donor heart is then examined, trimmed appropriately, and inserted into the recipient's chest. Intraoperative myocardial protection is provided

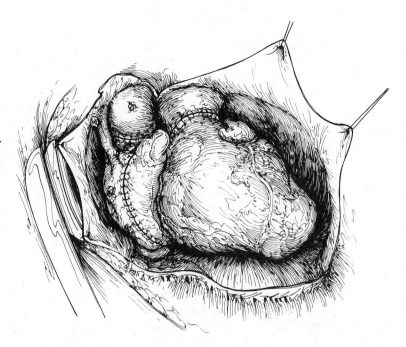

**Figure 7–3.** Surgical procedure of heart transplantation showing sites of anastomosis. (From Jamieson SW: Operative Surgery, 4th ed. Surrey, England, Butterworths, 1986.)

by continuous irrigation of the chest cavity with topical hypothermic solution and strict avoidance of left ventricular distension. The anastomoses of the left and right atria are performed first. An air-free line is then secured into the left atrial appendage that continuously irrigates the left ventricular cavity with cold saline, thus eliminating air in the heart and providing myocardial cooling. During this time the aortic anastomosis is completed, and after air is removed from the heart the aortic cross-clamp is removed. Ischemic time of the transplanted heart begins with aortic cross-clamping of the donor heart and ends when the recipient's aortic cross-clamp is removed. Finally, the pulmonary artery anastomosis is performed. Generally the heart resumes electrical activity spontaneously, although occasionally direct current shock may be necessary.

A variable period of resuscitation is required during which all air is removed and the core temperature reaches at least 36°C. An isoproterenol infusion is often started to maintain heart rate at 100 to 120 beats per minute, and if cardiovascular function is adequate, cardiopulmonary bypass is discontinued. Two temporary pacing wires are placed on the donor right atrium, and the surgical incision is closed in the routine manner.

The patient is then transferred to the intensive care unit where reverse isolation techniques are used.

Timing of the surgical procedure is crucial because avoidance of long ischemic times is highly desirable. If the donor heart is harvested from a distant hospital, the recipient, who is ready with intravascular catheters in place, is not anesthetized until the donor heart has been visually examined as macroscopically normal.

### Anesthetic Management

For the anesthetic care of the transplant patient the operating room team requires the services of an experienced cardiac anesthesiologist who is familiar with the anesthetic management of patients with terminal cardiac disease. These patients have severe ventricular dysfunction and associated pathophysiological changes in other organ systems that have to be considered during their care. Strict attention to detail and close observation and treatment of physiological trends is mandatory.

Several anesthetic techniques and agents have been used for this procedure.[51–55] However, the literature addressing the most appropriate anesthetic management of heart transplantation for both the initial and subsequent operation is sparse. The anesthetic techniques described here are based on our clinical experience gained over the years.[56]

### Heart Donors

Management of the cardiac donor is crucial to the success of heart transplantation, and the anesthesiologist must protect the donor heart from injury until it is harvested. Periods of hypotension before the heart is removed may be associated with poor postoperative graft function. All donors have irreversible brain injury with inherently unstable cardiovascular system. Many have raised intracranial pressure that has been treated with diuretics, further complicating cardiovascular stability through intravascular hypovolemia. In addition, diabetes insipidus is common in the majority of neurologically dead patients; therefore, vasopressin, 5 to 10 units intravenously, may have to be administered to limit the diuresis. Hypotension and hypovolemia must be vigorously treated first with fluid replacement and, if necessary, with supplemental doses of vasopressor agents such as metaraminol. Hypertension may occur in response to surgical stimulation and may have to be treated with a vasodilator such as sodium nitroprusside.[57] The explanations given for the pressor response in brain-dead patients are either the existence of peripheral or spinal vasoconstrictor responses or humoral responses such as adrenal medullary stimulation by reflex spinal arc.[58,59] Pulmonary insufficiency may occur as a consequence of neurogenic pulmonary edema,[60] and hypothermia may develop through disruption of thermoregulatory mechanisms.[42] Therefore, when the anesthesiologist visits the donor before surgery, all the physiological changes that may be associated with the neurologically dead patient must be carefully considered and the necessary preparations made (Table 7–5).

After the donor is transferred to the operating room, monitors, including ECG, temperature, urine output, oxygen saturation, arterial pressure, and central venous pressure, are established and maintained. Good venous access should be established in the event that massive fluid transfusions are required. Vasoactive drugs such as calcium, ephedrine, and epinephrine and an infusion set of metaraminol (50 mg in 250 cc 5 per cent dextrose in water) should be available to respond emergently to acute changes in cardiovascular function. The donor trachea is already intubated; the position of the endotracheal tube should be verified after transport to the operating room. Ventilation with 100 per cent oxygen, tidal volume of 12 to 15 $cc \cdot kg^{-1}$ and positive end-expiratory pressure (PEEP) 2.5 to 5 cm is routinely applied. The mean arterial pressure is maintained between 70 and 90 mm Hg with either metaraminol or nitroprusside, if necessary. The central venous pressure is maintained at 10 to 15 mm Hg with Ringer's lactated solution (approximately 75 to 125 $cc \cdot hr^{-1}$ plus previous hour's urine output). Arterial blood gases, serum potassium, and hematocrit should be measured at the start of the procedure. If the hematocrit is less than 30 per cent, readily available cross-matched blood is usually transfused. Anesthesia is not required even though marked hypertension may occur with surgical stimulation. Muscle relaxants (pancuronium) may be administered to avoid extensive muscle twitching. If other organs are to be harvested, the anesthesiologist should be familiar with the special needs of the other surgical teams. It is the responsibility of the anesthesiologist to give the cardioplegia solution, avoiding air bubbles.

Distant heart procurement is now routinely used by most heart transplant centers.[45,61] If an anesthesiologist accompanies the surgical team to an unfamiliar hospital, it is crucial

---

**TABLE 7–5.   Guidelines for Donor Management**

| Donor Trait | Clinical Problem | Treatment |
|---|---|---|
| Loss of respiratory mechanics | Apnea | Control ventilation |
| Neurogenic pulmonary edema | Hypoxia, hypercarbia | Diuretics, PEEP |
| Pituitary gland dysfunction | Diabetes insipidus | Vasopressin, fluids |
| Loss of vasomotor tone | Decrease in blood pressure | Hydration, vasopressors |
| Thermoregulatory dysfunction | Hypothermia | Warming blanket, humidifier, warm intravenous fluids |

that the anesthesiologist is comfortable with the new setting and has all the necessary equipment.

### Heart Recipient

**Preoperative Evaluation.** During the preoperative evaluation of the recipient, apart from the usual anesthetic history, some special concerns need to be addressed. Patients accepted for heart transplantation have advanced cardiac disease and are classified as NYHA Class IV and ASA Class IV or V. Physical signs of congestive heart failure may be present as well as mild to moderate renal or hepatic dysfunction secondary to cardiac failure. Preoperative ventricular arrhythmias are often present, particularly in patients suffering from idiopathic cardiomyopathy. Cardiac catheterization data confirm severe left ventricular dysfunction as evidenced by low cardiac output and ejection fraction. If pulmonary hypertension and elevated pulmonary vascular resistance are documented, the response to vasodilators should be established. Evaluation of any recent changes in physical status must be attained as well as current medication, especially cardioactive drugs, diuretics, and antithrombotic agents. Although these patients are very anxious, heavy premedication is avoided until the patient arrives in the operating suite. A small oral dose of diazepam (5 to 10 mg) may be given, if necessary, on call to the operating room.

**Equipment and Monitoring.** Since all recipients are to be immunosuppressed, strict adherence to aseptic techniques is mandatory. All airway equipment, including tubing in the anesthesia circle system, must be sterile and handled with gloves. Bacterial filters are routinely used in both limbs of the circle system. In our institution we have a number of trays available with essential airway equipment that has been gas sterilized. Standard monitors include electrocardiograph, arterial and central venous cannulas, rectal or bladder and nasopharyngeal temperature probes, esophageal stethoscope, and oxygen saturation monitor. Initially, when the program started, a urinary catheter was not routinely inserted; instead a suprapubic catheter was placed at the end of surgery.[56] The reason for avoiding transurethral catheterization was to decrease any possible bacteremia that may be associated with this procedure; since this theoretical consideration has not been substantiated, at present a transurethral cath-

eter is placed after anesthesia induction prior to surgery. All intravascular catheters are sited, using strict aseptic techniques. Central venous catheters are inserted via the left internal jugular vein, thereby preserving the right internal jugular vein for future postoperative cardiac biopsies.[20] Arterial cannulas are placed percutaneously in a radial artery, avoiding direct surgical arterial placement because of the enhanced risk for infection by an open procedure. Pulmonary artery catheters have not been used for routine monitoring, as they would have to be removed from the surgical field when the diseased heart is excised. Furthermore, the catheter represents a potential source of infection to the recipient. If a pulmonary artery catheter has previously been placed for medical treatment prior to surgery, it is used during anesthesia induction and left in place until the onset of bypass.

**Anesthetic Techniques and Drugs.** During the early period of cardiac transplantation at Stanford, the preferred anesthetic agent was methoxyflurane. However, following the documentation of methoxyflurane nephrotoxicity, its use was abandoned.[62] About that time, high-dose narcotic anesthesia technique was being introduced into cardiac anesthetic practice, and this method rapidly became popular for cardiac transplantation.[63] Recently there has been a trend toward using fentanyl or sufentanil rather than hydromorphone, morphine, or meperidine.[64] As each of the volatile agents, including halothane, enflurane, and isoflurane, has the potential to depress myocardial contractility, they are best avoided as primary agents.[65,66] However, there may be instances when low concentrations of volatile anesthetics can be safely used to supplement narcotics in transplant recipients. Narcotics produce less myocardial depression, but are eliminated slowly, particularly in patients with impaired liver and kidney functions, which may necessitate prolonged ventilatory support with its attendant higher risk of pulmonary infection in immunosuppressed patients. Therefore, lower doses of narcotics are used than may be employed for other open heart cases. Cardiac transplantation is performed when a donor heart becomes available; consequently the surgery is done on an emergency basis and patients are assumed to have full stomachs. Furthermore, cyclosporine A is administered orally preoperatively, and although the volume of the vehicle in which the drug is administered is small (20 ml), even in patients who have otherwise been fasting several hours, the intragastric volume will be greater than 25 ml. For these reasons a rapid-sequence induction technique is used. After preoxygenation, anesthesia is induced using cricoid pressure to decrease the probability of pulmonary aspiration. Agents to increase the pH of gastric contents (e.g., ranitidine) or to decrease gastric volume, (e.g., metoclopramide) may be given prior to anesthesia induction. Anesthesia drugs vary, but may include etomidate (0.1 to 0.2 mg·kg$^{-1}$), low-dose ketamine (0.1 mg·kg$^{-1}$ repeated if necessary), or diazepam (0.1 to 0.2 mg·kg$^{-1}$). Relaxation for intubation is most efficiently and safely achieved with either a combination of pancuronium (0.05 mg·kg$^{-1}$) and metocurine (0.2 mg·kg$^{-1}$) or vecuronium (0.1 mg·kg$^{-1}$). Occasionally inotropic support may be appropriate during anesthesia induction. Usually a high preload is required because of the severely depressed ventricular function and fixed stroke volume. Since most of these patients have been treated with diuretics, the loss of sympathetic tone during anesthesia induction may result in a fall in arterial pressure. Our current anesthetic regimen consists of fentanyl 30 to 50 μg·kg$^{-1}$, or sufentanil 10 to 15 μg·kg$^{-1}$, muscle relaxant, diazepam 0.1 to 0.3 mg·kg$^{-1}$, and controlled ventilation with 100 per cent oxygen. Nitrous oxide is avoided because of its potential myocardial depression, ability to further increase pulmonary vacular resistance, and propensity to enlarge an inadvertent air embolus.[67,68]

**Intraoperative Management.** During the precardiopulmonary bypass period the anesthetic management is similar to that employed in any severely compromised patient having cardiac surgery with the overall aim of maintaining major organ perfusion. To achieve this, inotropes and/or large amounts of volume may be required. In patients who have previously had cardiac surgery, hemodynamic instability should be anticipated, particularly during dissection and manipulation of the heart. With respect to the period of cardiopulmonary bypass, there are no specific requirements. No attempt to terminate bypass is made until the patient has warmed to a core temperature greater than 36°C and until the ECG has returned to its normal configuration. Since the donor heart is denervated, junctional rhythms secondary to acute denervation or to surgical trauma are com-

mon. Therefore, prior to termination of bypass an isoproterenol infusion is started to maintain a heart rate of 100 to 120 beats·min$^{-1}$. Infusion of dopamine may be required if the donor heart appears to be contracting poorly. Sodium nitroprusside is used after cardiopulmonary bypass to decrease afterload and to provide controlled venodilation, which permits intravascular volume expansion in the hypothermic patient. After cardiopulmonary bypass has successfully been terminated, methylprednisolone (500 mg) is administered intravenously. Most patients undergoing cardiac transplantation have abnormal coagulation indices either secondary to congestion of the liver or because of treatment with anticoagulants. These abnormalities are further aggravated by cardiopulmonary bypass, and thus most patients require replacement of coagulation factors with fresh frozen plasma and platelet transfusion. At the end of the procedure the patient is transferred to the intensive care unit; ventilation is provided with 100 per cent oxygen using a sterile transport circuit.

**Postoperative Course and Management.** Reverse isolation is maintained in the intensive care unit, with meticulous attention being paid to sterility of all airway equipment. Mechanical ventilation is usually required for 18 to 24 hours, with the goal to remove the endotracheal tube as soon as possible to minimize pulmonary contamination. Apart from immunosuppression and the maintenance of an isoproterenol infusion until the recipient heart can spontaneously maintain an adequate rate, postoperative care is similar to that of routine cardiac surgery patients. Deterioration in liver and renal function often occurs postoperatively, as preoperative organ failure is exacerbated after the insult of surgery and bypass. After cardiac transplantation, suppression of the immune response is required indefinitely. Acute rejection episodes usually occur during the first three postoperative months with 90 per cent of patients experiencing at least one episode of rejection in this period. After 12 months the frequency of acute rejection is markedly decreased.[12,69] Maintenance of a stable graft-host relationship depends on various combinations of immunosuppressants.[70,71] These have included steroids, azathioprine, antihuman thymocyte globulin derived from rabbits or horses, and since 1980, cyclosporine.[22–24] Presently there is no one treatment regimen. Protocols change frequently, depending on specific patient needs and ongoing research protocols. Irrespective of the treatment protocol, all patients receive cyclosporine (12 to 16 mg·kg$^{-1}$) and azathioprine (4 mg·kg$^{-1}$) preoperatively. Immediately after bypass is terminated, all patients receive 500 mg methylprednisolone intravenously followed in the postoperative period by 125 mg for three further doses. Oral prednisone is then started in some patients, depending on the treatment protocol, at a dose of 1.5 mg·kg$^{-1}$·day$^{-1}$, tapered to a maintenance dose of 0.1 mg·kg$^{-1}$ by the time of discharge from the hospital. Oral azathioprine (1 to 2 mg·kg$^{-1}$) is begun on the first postoperative day and maintained at the highest dose compatible with normal leukocyte and thrombocyte counts. Cyclosporine administration is resumed postoperatively, 9 mg·kg$^{-1}$·day$^{-1}$, and the dose adjusted to achieve cyclosporine blood levels of 200 to 300 ng·ml$^{-1}$ for the first 30 postoperative days and of 50 to 150 ng·ml$^{-1}$ after 30 days. Horse antihuman thymocyte globulin is administered intravenously 10 mg·kg$^{-1}$·day$^{-1}$ for seven days, and its effect is monitored by circulating T lymphocytes and erythrocyte rosette formation.[12,72] Clinical indications of graft rejection include a voltage decrease of 15 per cent on the surface ECG, development of an S$_3$ gallop, and fever.[9,12] Confirmation of this diagnosis includes tests of immunological reactivity by measurement of rosette counts, determination of serum globulin levels, and histology of endomyocardial biopsy specimens.[19,20,71] Since the introduction of cyclosporine, the diagnosis of rejection depends mainly on histological examination of the endomyocardial tissue.[73] Therefore, regular biopsies are important in the management and prevention of rejection in cyclosporine-treated patients. Percutaneous endomyocardial biopsy is performed under local anesthesia via the right internal jugular vein; under fluoroscopic control three or four biopsy specimens are obtained. Graft biopsies are obtained initially on the sixth postoperative day, weekly for the first two months, and then every three to four months for an indefinite period. This technique for monitoring rejection is unique for cardiac transplantation. The histological features of acute rejection include infiltration by mononuclear cells, which involves the perivascular structures first and a more diffuse interstitial distribution later. More advanced injury includes interstitial edema, hemorrhage, and frank necrosis.[73] The histological appearance of biopsy specimens from patients treated with cyclosporine[74] is different from those patients treated conventionally with azathioprine and steroids.[75] During rejection in patients treated with cyclosporine, moderate to severe lymphocytic infiltration is present, edema is rarely seen, and myocyte necrosis usually is seen.[12,24] Since the introduction of cyclosporine the incidence and severity of rejection are less and appear easier to control. The assumption that uniform rejection occurs within all areas of the myocardium has been discredited. In animal experiments increased severity of rejection has been found in tissue taken from the right ventricle as compared to the left ventricle.[76] Recently, noninvasive assessment by M-mode echophonocardiography of cardiac rejection has been useful in patients treated with azathioprine. During rejection proven by endomyocardial biopsy there is a reduction in isovolemic relaxation period and changes in left ventricular mass.[77,78] The association between positive endomyocardial biopsy and indices of left ventricular systolic function and left ventricular mass has not been a reliable indicator of rejection in patients treated with cyclosporine.[79] Treatment of acute rejection includes methylprednisolone, 1 gm bolus for three days, then an increase in oral prednisone to 1.5 mg·kg$^{-1}$·day$^{-1}$. Antihuman thymocyte globulin, 2.5 mg·kg$^{-1}$·day$^{-1}$, is usually reserved for the third or subsequent episodes of rejection; 95 per cent of all acute rejection episodes are successfully reversed.[12,75]

The development of graft atherosclerosis is a major factor limiting long-term survival.[44] This phenomenon is probably related to immunological injury to the donor endothelium with subsequent platelet adhesion and plugging. Occlusive coronary artery disease may subsequently develop, resulting in myocardial ischemia. Factors positively correlated with the development of postoperative graft atherosclerosis include donor age over 35 years, persistent hypertriglyceridemia, and incompatibility for HLA-A2 antigen. The development of this process is not related to the recipient's age or the pretransplant cardiac disease. Prophylaxis against this complication has included dipyridamole and warfarin, which have decreased the incidence of graft atherosclerosis from nearly 100 per cent at three years to the current incidence of 38 per cent at five years. Antiplatelet therapy with dipyridamole has largely replaced warfarin as the routine prophylaxis. Other therapeutic manipulations include low-fat, low-cholesterol diet, regular exercise, and abstinence from smoking. The onset of atherosclerosis in the coronary vessels is not associated with angina, since the donor heart is denervated. Diagnosis is usually made on coronary arteriography performed at yearly intervals, and if the disease is significant, retransplantation is usually advised.

## Immunosuppression

The most common major complication and cause of death following cardiac transplantation is infection[80] (Table 7–6). An analysis of the primary cause of death in cardiac recipients from 1968 until 1980 revealed that 34 per cent died of infections. The causative infective agents included bacterial (55 per cent), viral (22 per cent), fungal (13 per cent), protozoal (6 per cent), and nocardial (4 per cent).[12] Since the dose of immunosuppressants required for graft maintenance is high, especially during the early postoperative months, cardiac recipients are highly susceptible during this time to opportunistic microorganisms. The most common site of infection is the lung, resulting in pneumonias, empyemas, and cavitating pulmonary abscesses, especially from organisms such as *Aspergillus* and *Nocardia*. Although the highest mortality has been associated with fungal infections, these can be successfully treated if diagnosed before systemic dissem-

ination. Other infectious episodes may occur as a result of septicemia, urinary tract infection, central nervous system infection, retinitis, or osteomyelitis. Early diagnosis and aggressive treatment of infection have resulted in a successful outcome in the majority of patients, irrespective of the severity of the infection. Routine postoperative management includes daily physical examination, chest roentgenogram, and frequent sputum and urine cultures for the prompt diagnosis of this complication. If a recipient is symptomatic with radiographic changes and positive sputum cultures, immediate transtracheal aspiration is undertaken for culture and Gram stain. If the diagnosis is not obtained by this method, bronchial aspiration of the lung is performed. Bacterial infections are treated with broad-spectrum antibiotics; fungal infections with amphotericin B, sometimes in conjunction with 5-fluorocytosine; nocardial and protozoal infections with sulfa derivatives, in combination with trimethoprim in the case of the latter organism. Viral infections, especially herpes simplex, herpes zoster, and cytomegalovirus, occur quite commonly. Treatment with the antiviral agent acycloguanosine has been successful with minimal drug toxicity. In the cyclosporine-maintained patients there is less infection and a better therapeutic response to anti-infection measures compared to those maintained with azathioprine.[24] The issue of post-transplantation infectious complications is also addressed in Chapter 5.

Cardiac transplant recipients share the same propensity for the development of malignant transformations as other immunosuppressed patients, such as renal transplant recipients.[81,82] Lymphomas have been diagnosed in 15 patients at Stanford.[83] Other malignant states include skin cancer, adenocarcinoma of the colon, and acute myelogenous leukemia. The high incidence of lymphomas in patients treated with cyclosporine, corticosteroids, and rat antithymocytic globulin is a major concern. Recent evidence has supported the contention that these tumors are associated with the Epstein-Barr virus (EBV). Reactivation and development of the EBV disease appears to be enhanced by antithymocytic globulin treatment and further aggravated by cyclosporine, which inhibits T-cell responses to EBV-infected autologous B cells.[84] Therefore, current treatment regimens of immunosuppres-

**TABLE 7–6. Stanford Cardiac Transplantation: Primary Cause of Death (n = 353 patients)**

| Cause of Death | No. |
| --- | --- |
| Infection | 100 |
| Acute rejection | 34 |
| Graft arteriosclerosis | 20 |
| Malignant disease | 12 |
| Pulmonary hypertension | 7 |
| Sudden death | 6 |
| Cerebral vascular accident | 4 |
| Pulmonary embolus | 2 |
| Cerebral edema | 1 |
| Myopathy | 1 |
| Suicide | 1 |
| Acute graft failure | 3 |
| Hepatic failure | 1 |
| Other | 1 |
| Total | 193 |

sion have been modified to decrease the use of antithymocytic globulin. Observations for and early diagnosis of malignant transformation are an important part of the long-term management of transplant recipients.

Other complications associated with chronic corticosteroid administration include aseptic necrosis of the femoral head, cataracts, and cytomegalovirus retinitis. Side effects of cyclosporine therapy include renal dysfunction, arterial hypertension, hirsutism, and mild tremors.[24,85] In the majority of cyclosporine-treated patients renal dysfunction has been observed, sometimes requiring either termination of the drug or temporary renal dialysis. Renal biopsies performed late postoperatively have demonstrated renal fibrosis. Arterial hypertension may occur as soon as one month postoperatively and is usually severe, requiring aggressive medical therapy. The mechanism by which cyclosporine causes hypertension is not known.

## Anesthesia for Operations in Cardiac Transplant Recipients

Heart transplant recipients may require surgery for complications secondary to post-transplantation therapy or unrelated surgical problems (Table 7–7). These procedures are either elective (hip replacement for aseptic necrosis or cataract surgery) or emergent ("acute abdomen"). General anesthesia has been the preferred technique, but more recently regional anesthesia has been employed if no contraindications are present. Nineteen total joint replacements for steroid-induced osteonecrosis were performed between February 1976 and October 1984 at Stanford University. General anesthesia was utilized in 16 of these procedures, and regional anesthesia, either subarachnoid block or epidural analgesia, in the remaining 6. There were no intraoperative or postoperative complications related to anesthesia in these patients.[86]

### Anesthetic Management

Experience with subsequent anesthesia for both emergency and elective procedures in cardiac transplant recipients has demonstrated that a variety of techniques can be used safely.[55,87,88] Functional impairment of the transplant heart is usually not present unless acute rejection is taking place. However, certain considerations must be observed when anesthetizing these patients.

Transplant recipients are compromised hosts undergoing long-term immunosuppressive therapy, and as infection is still the major cause of morbidity and mortality, strict aseptic precautions must be maintained. As with the primary procedure for all subsequent operations, intravascular monitoring, drug administration, and airway manipulation should be performed as aseptically as possible. Routine monitoring should include heart rate, oxygen saturation, and blood pressure and an ECG. Invasive arterial and central venous pressure monitoring is undertaken only if the patient is hemodynamically unstable (i.e., rejecting) or if required by the surgical procedure. Postoperative mechanical ventilation should be avoided if possible, to decrease the risk of pulmonary infection. The specific immunosuppressants these patients are taking must be considered preoperatively. The problems of anesthetizing patients who have been receiving long-term steroid treatment are well documented.[88,89] Azathioprine may cause hepatic dysfunction and thus interfere with the action and metabolism of various anesthetics.[90] Cyclosporine A is a known potent nephrotoxic agent and may result in an increase of serum potassium to near pathological concentrations.[91] A further renal insult from drugs or low cardiac output may result in anuria.

Since the transplanted heart remains autonomically denervated, qualitatively abnormal responses to volume manipulation and pharmacological interventions can occur.

---

**TABLE 7–7. Surgical Procedures Performed After Cardiac Transplantation**

Emergency exploration for mediastinal bleeding
Complications caused by infection (usually abscess drainage)
  Laparotomy
  Craniotomy
  Mediastinotomy/thoracotomy
  Extremity abscess drainage
  Bronchoscopy
  Vitrectomy
  Scleral buckle
Complications caused by steroid treatment
  Total hip arthroplasty or pinning
  Laparotomy for perforated viscus
  Cataract excision
Vascular surgery
  Aortic
  Peripheral
  Amputations
Elective cholecystectomy

The denervated heart lacks the ability to respond acutely to hypovolemia or hypotension with reflex tachycardia. Increases in cardiac output are dependent upon increases in venous return until circulating catecholamine levels rise sufficiently to increase heart rate and contractility. Therefore, intravascular volume depletion may be poorly tolerated, particularly when anesthetics that suppress the sympathoadrenal system are used. Preload manipulation is important with any anesthetic technique, particularly with major conduction anesthesia, which is often associated with hypotension secondary to sympathetic blockade. If spinal or epidural anesthesia is chosen, prophylactic ephedrine should be administered. Only drugs acting on the heart directly, without involvement of the autonomic nervous system, affect the donor heart. Therefore, when these patients are being anesthetized a direct-acting chronotropic drug (isoproterenol), an inotropic drug (epinephrine or dopamine), and a direct vasoconstrictor (phenylephrine) should be available. Agents such as pancuronium, anticholinergics, and anticholinesterases have no effect on the denervated heart. Drugs that exhibit ganglionic blockade (d-tubocurarine) may cause arterial hypotension and should be avoided. If one remembers the specific considerations discussed, a number of anesthetic techniques can be used safely; however, it is advisable to avoid drugs that cause myocardial depression.

## ANESTHESIA FOR HEART-LUNG TRANSPLANTATION

Combined heart and lung transplantation is presently the only corrective therapy for patients with end-stage cardiopulmonary disease.[92] Donor organ availability is limited, perioperative mortality remains high, and long-term complications occur, but potential recipients add their names daily to growing lists of those awaiting the operation. The anesthesiologist is called upon to assess a patient with severe right ventricular failure, pulmonary hypertension, and hypoxemia for surgery to occur within hours. Appropriate anesthetic management, both before and after transplantation, requires an understanding of the altered physiology of these patients and the special requirements of the heart and lung transplantation operation itself. Although there are many similarities to isolated heart transplantation, transplanta-

tion of the lungs in addition to the heart involves certain special considerations for the anesthesiologist. This section will discuss the unique aspects of the pathophysiology and anesthesia of heart-lung transplantation, and attempt to avoid repetition of issues covered in the section on heart transplantation, many of which are of obvious relevance to the combined cardiopulmonary transplant situation.

### History

The first human heart-lung transplantation was performed by Cooley in 1968.[93] Lillehei and Barnard both performed heart-lung transplantation several years later.[94,95] None of these early patients survived the perioperative period, but an important discovery was made—patients could resume normal respiration. Previous experimental work on primates suggested that denervated lungs could continue normal respiration,[96] but heart-lung transplants in dogs had been unsuccessful because of respiratory function abnormalities in the postoperative period.[97] Long-term survival of primates after heart-lung transplantation was first achieved with the use of the immunosuppressant drug cyclosporine.[98] Nearly 20 years of extensive laboratory experimental work on heart and heart-lung transplantation, as well as the success of clinical heart transplantation, permitted initiation of the clinical heart-lung transplantation program at Stanford in 1981.

### Survival

Twenty-seven patients have undergone 28 combined heart and lung transplantations to date at Stanford (Table 7–8). Fifteen are currently alive, including one patient who had retransplantation 37 months following his initial operation.[99] Approximately 100 heart-lung transplantations have been performed world wide since 1981; the majority at three centers in the United States and Great Britain (Stanford University Hospital, the Univer-

**TABLE 7–8.   Stanford Heart-Lung Transplantation: Summary**

| | |
|---|---|
| Number | Patients 27 (Transplants 28) |
| Age | 20–45 Years (av. 33 years) |
| Sex | Female 10, males 17 |
| Diagnosis | Primary pulmonary hypertension 14 |
| | Eisenmenger's syndrome 13 |
| Outcome | Alive: 15 patients (1 month–53 months) |
| | Deaths: 8 hospital; 4 late |

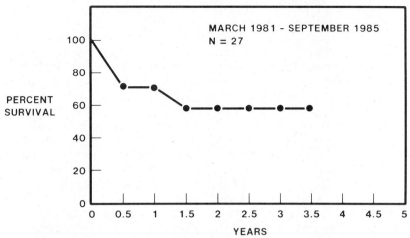

**Figure 7–4.** Survival rates of patients having heart-lung transplantation.

sity of Pittsburgh Hospital, and Harefield Hospital in England).[100] At Stanford, one- and two-year survivals are 74 per cent and 59 per cent, respectively (Fig. 7–4).[101] The relatively large series at Stanford has allowed both surgeons and anesthesiologists to better understand the optimal perioperative management, complexities of postoperative care, and long-term complications associated with this uncommon operation.

## Physiology of the Transplanted Heart and Lungs

Understanding of the pathophysiology of the transplanted heart and lungs is incomplete. The much greater clinical experience with isolated heart transplantation has permitted extensive investigation of the physiological consequences of cardiac denervation, as reviewed in the previous section on heart transplantation. The smaller series of patients undergoing combined heart and lung transplantation has limited observations and data collection, and therefore many physiological and pharmacological considerations of interest to the anesthesiologist remain speculative.

The transplanted lung is denervated and also deprived of lymphatic drainage and bronchial blood flow. Perhaps the most remarkable aspect of denervation of the lungs is the apparent absence of immediate consequences. Patients awaken from anesthesia in the anticipated manner and resume normal respiratory patterns and gas exchange. They can be seen riding exercise bicycles by the bedside. However, there are subtle changes in pulmonary function resulting from surgical denervation, and the long-term consequences may be of extreme significance. Vagal innervation of the lungs is lost during this operation. Bilateral vagotomy in awake humans causes an increase in end-tidal $CO_2$ after maximal breath holding, but resting tidal volume and respiratory rate remain normal.[102] Vagal efferent fibers innervate the pulmonary vasculature, respiratory tract mucous glands, and cilia, as well as the larynx and bronchi. Pulmonary stretch receptors, which are present in the smooth muscle of the respiratory tract from the trachea to the bronchioles,[103] send information regarding airway distension via vagal pathways to the medullary respiratory center. The Hering-Breuer inflation reflex causes apnea after a period of lung distension, and indicates intact vagal afferents. This reflex is absent in monkeys immediately after heart-lung transplantation,[104] but has not been studied in the transplant patients. The Hering-Breuer reflex may play a part in the central integration of ventilatory control, possibly by selecting the respiratory pattern that reduces the work of breathing in the presence of pulmonary pathology. The tachypnea frequently seen with inhalation of halothane is thought to be caused by stimulation of pulmonary stretch receptors and will probably be absent in the heart-lung recipients.[103] Vagotomy may explain the subtle alterations in the ventilatory pattern seen in transplant patients. Some patients have a resting $Pa_{CO_2}$ of 45 to 50 mm Hg in the early postoperative period, but remain alert with normal oxygenation. Of note, the ventilatory response to hypercapnia in vagotomized dogs is abnormal.[105] Respiratory depressant effects of narcotics or sleep may not be followed by increased ventilation upon awakening in these patients, which is of obvious concern to the anesthesiologist. In the later postoperative period, patients have a resting mean $Pa_{CO_2}$ of 31 mm Hg,[106] but the mechanism for this later post-transplant alveolar hyperventilation remains unclear.

The cough reflex is also lost following transplantation. This reflex occurs with stimulation of the subepithelial mechanoreceptors of the trachea, bronchi, and bronchioles. The cough reflex may include tachypnea and reflex bronchoconstriction as well as cough. The post-transplant patient can consciously produce a cough, but stimulation below the tracheal anastomosis has no reflex effect. The patient has no awareness of pulmonary secretions. The anesthesiologist must delay extubation of the trachea in these patients until a verbal suggestion to cough can be understood; the heart-lung recipient can only "protect his airway" when he is fully awake.

Bronchomotor tone is primarily related to vagal efferent control.[107] Vagotomy results in bronchodilatation, and vagal stimulation causes bronchoconstriction.[108] Vagotomy appears to prevent reflex bronchoconstriction related to stimulation of small airway irritant receptors,[109] analogous to the loss of the cough reflex. Bronchospasm can still occur in the transplant patient and was severe during anesthesia in one patient having apparent late lung rejection at Stanford. Vagotomy appears to remove the bronchoconstriction resulting from dust or irritant gas inhalation which may have a protective function. Since vagal innervation to mucous glands and cilia is lost, removal of inhaled foreign materials also is thought to be affected. Late post-transplant pulmonary disease may be related to these processes.[109]

Reinnervation of the transplanted lung has not been found to occur in humans, presumably because immunosuppressants inhibit regrowth of preganglionic nerve fibers. Autotransplantation of the lung in the dog, requiring no immunosuppressant treatment, results in reinnervation after three to six months.[110]

Absence of lymphatics in the transplanted lungs has direct consequences for fluid management. Heart-lung transplant recipients tolerate volume loads poorly; pulmonary edema occurs readily and may be difficult to resolve because of the loss of lymphatic drainage. The filtration function of the lymphatics is also lost, and particulate matter, such as platelet aggregates in transfused blood, are filtered by the lungs but not removed by the reticuloendothelial system. Persistent hypoxemia may result from injudicious administration of fluid and blood products. The role of the lymphatics in prevention and resolution of pneumonia is unclear, but recurrent pulmonary infections have occurred in long-term survivors of this operation.[109] Experimental work suggests that lymphatic connections may re-form after several weeks,[111] so the chronic implications may be insignificant.

The transplanted lungs undergo a period of complete ischemia averaging about one hour. The suggestion that reperfused ischemic tissues have increased susceptibility to oxygen toxicity is based on experimental work on organs other than the lung.[112] However, there is growing concern that oxygen-free radicals may be responsible for pulmonary injury,[113] and their toxicity may be enhanced by a period of ischemia. To avoid the possible development of an alveolar-capillary leak, typical of hyperoxic lung injury, the lowest inspired oxygen concentration compatible with maintaining a $Pa_{O_2}$ of at least 70 mm Hg is routinely used.

The long-term consequences of heart and lung transplantation are thought to represent a sum of effects from chronic rejection, recurrent pulmonary infection, pulmonary denervation, and immunosuppressant drugs. Although patients who leave the hospital initially lead a nearly normal life, late survivors have experienced an increasing incidence of serious complications.

Hemodynamic evaluation at one year following surgery has demonstrated a marked fall in mean pulmonary artery pressure (73 ± 19 mm Hg to 9 ± 3 mm Hg) and mean pulmonary vascular resistance (18.3 ± 10.8 Wood units to 1.0 ± 0.56 Wood units).[99] Left ventricular cineangiography appears normal. Cardiac index doubles over pretransplantation values.[106] Coronary arteriography shows collateral vessels from the right and left coronary arteries flowing to the area of the tracheal anastomosis in all patients studied.[99] Although coronary artery disease can be recognized at angiography after transplantation, one patient with a recent normal coronary arteriogram who underwent retransplantation for pulmonary rejection was found to have diffuse coronary artery disease on pathological examination.[111] The diffuse, distal, concentric three-vessel coronary artery disease of graft atherosclerosis can be difficult to visualize with the arteriogram.[114] The anesthesiologist must be aware of the likelihood of significant coronary artery disease in the heart-lung transplant recipient despite the absence of angina and a recent normal coronary arteriogram. Proliferative coronary atherosclerosis may cause sudden death in heart-lung transplant patients, as well as in heart transplant recipients; the mechanism is thought to involve immune-mediated vascular injury of chronic rejection. Intimal proliferation has also been seen in small pulmonary arterioles of the transplanted lung.[99]

Immediately following heart-lung transplantation there is a significant fall in most measured lung volumes, which results in a restrictive ventilatory defect lessening with time.[115] At one year after transplantation, oxygenation is normal (mean $Pa_{O_2}$ 86.9 ± 9 mm Hg), and the alveolar-arterial gradient for oxygen is slightly elevated.[99]

Nearly half of those who survive more than one year after heart-lung transplantation have developed late pulmonary complications.[101,116] The late symptoms include worsening dyspnea and recurrent pulmonary infections, often with chronic bronchitis. Pathological examination has revealed diffuse, low-grade pulmonary vascular disease, bronchiectasis, and bronchiolitis obliterans. The $FEV_1/FVC$ decreases from 92 per cent to 55 per cent over one year after transplantation,[101] and the $FEV_{25-75}$ falls from 73 per cent to 8.8 per cent of predicted value over the same period.[116] One patient developed worsening bronchiolitis obliterans, unresponsive to increased immunosuppressant therapy, and required reintubation and later retransplantation. Another patient developed severe chronic bronchitis with respiratory failure and died 15 months following transplantation.[111] Obliterative bronchiolitis has been diagnosed as early as 14 months after transplantation. Fibrosis related to cyclosporine therapy has been suggested as a possible cause of these late pulmonary changes, but chronic rejection and the effect of de-

nervation on mucociliary function and cough reflex remain the most likely causes.[117] Now, decreases in airflow are recognized as a probable early sign of pulmonary rejection; therefore, pulmonary function tests are obtained for all patients regularly, and steroid treatment is started early for signs of airway obstruction.[116] The consequences of transplantation of the heart and lungs are an evolving process and require continuing vigilance from the anesthesiologist involved in the treatment of these patients.

## Recipient Selection

A wide range of diseases results in end-stage cardiopulmonary disease, but heart-lung transplantation at Stanford has been limited to young adults with either primary pulmonary hypertension or Eisenmenger's syndrome. These patients are generally well except for their cardiopulmonary disease, and the tracheobronchial tree remains sterile. Patients with other systemic diseases involving heart-lung failure, such as rheumatoid arthritis or cystic fibrosis, might have recurrence of their disease in the transplanted organs. Patients with chronic pulmonary infection with cor pulmonale might be expected to have early postoperative infection of the graft. Because of the severe shortage of suitable donor organs, transplantation must be limited to those judged to have the greatest chance of a successful outcome. The average age of recipients at Stanford is 33 years (range 20 to 45 years). Patients who are expected to live only one to two more years are chosen for transplantation, yet moribund patients are unlikely to survive the stress of surgery, so timing of recipient selection can be difficult.[99]

Eisenmenger's syndrome is characterized by increased pulmonary blood flow, usually as a result of congenital intracardiac left-to-right shunt. These cyanotic patients have severe pulmonary hypertension and right ventricular hypertrophy, often with right ventricular failure. Systemic vasodilation causes increased right-to-left shunt and decreases pulmonary blood flow, a phenomenon well known to the anesthesiologist who works with pediatric patients undergoing repair of cyanotic cardiac lesions. Arterial hypoxemia may be profound; mean $Pa_{O_2}$ of 38 ± 13 mmHg was found in pretransplant patients with Eisenmenger's syndrome at Stanford.[99] The chronic hypoxemia results in polycythemia, often requiring periodic phlebotomy. Although red cell number is increased, the total body hemoglobin level remains normal, a state termed "relative anemia" when observed in infants with cyanotic heart disease.[106] This disparity between hematocrit and hemoglobin concentration (probably on the basis of iron deficiency) suggests that phlebotomy should not immediately precede surgery in these patients. In spite of profound hypoxemia, the cardiac index remains normal in these patients. The relationship between $Sa_{O_2}$ and $Pa_{O_2}$ also remains normal, indicating no decrease in the affinity of hemoglobin for oxygen.[106] Transcutaneous oxygen saturation monitoring remains an accurate reflection of arterial oxygenation. The normal mentation and moderate exercise capability of these severely hypoxic patients appears extraordinary, but any decrement in $Pa_{O_2}$ during anesthesia is unlikely to be well tolerated.

The patients with primary pulmonary hypertension have a mean preoperative $Pa_{O_2}$ of $76 \pm 14$ mmHg,[99] but pulmonary artery pressures approach values of systemic arterial pressures, cardiac output is reduced, and right ventricular failure with tricuspid regurgitation develops. Sudden death often occurs within several years of diagnosis.[118] The lungs show progressive changes of fibrinoid necrosis and peripheral vascular thrombotic occlusions. Dyspnea occurs out of proportion to the degree of hypoxemia, and the ability to exercise is severely limited. Progressive ventilation-perfusion abnormalities and hypoxemia are accompanied with peripheral cyanosis; central cyanosis occurs when a patent foramen ovale allows a right-to-left shunt. Pulmonary function tests may show a restrictive pattern,[119] presumably because of decreased lung compliance resulting from arteriolar hypertrophy. This mild restrictive pattern is present in 33 per cent, and an obstructive pattern is discernible in 50 per cent of those awaiting transplantation.[115] A variety of vasodilators have been used, with little success, to treat these patients. Patients awaiting transplantation are typically anticoagulated, use nasal oxygen continually, and may take nitroglycerin, hydralazine, or nifedipine. Attempts to suddenly manipulate pulmonary artery pressure in the individual patient are unwise; systemic hypotension is very poorly tolerated. Refractory bradycardia may result from a decrease in systemic

blood pressure and cause a marked fall in cardiac output that is difficult to restore. An episode of hypotension followed by sinoatrial and atrioventricular node ischemia has been associated with sudden death in these patients.[120]

Dilation of the left pulmonary artery may cause dysfunction of the left recurrent laryngeal nerve, increasing the risk of aspiration of gastric contents in these patients. Left recurrent nerve palsy is characterized by hoarseness and may be a consequence of the transplantation as well as a sign of the pretransplantation pulmonary hypertension.

Few anesthesiologists have occasion to anesthetize patients with Eisenmenger's syndrome or primary pulmonary hypertension; anesthetic and surgical risk is generally considered prohibitively high. Safe anesthetic management for the transplantation is simply based upon maintaining the patient's cardiac and pulmonary hemodynamic stability under anesthesia until the affected organs can be removed. Techniques that increase pulmonary artery pressure (light anesthesia, airway obstruction, hypoxia, nitrous oxide, ketamine administration) and decrease systemic vascular resistance (vasodilators, acidosis, histamine-releasing drugs) are carefully avoided.

These patients have frequently had previous thoracic surgery, either a palliative cardiac operation or lung biopsy, resulting in adhesions and increased surgical bleeding. Hepatic congestion from right-sided cardiac failure as well as anticoagulant medication also increases the likelihood of bleeding.

Recipients and donors are matched for ABO blood group and lymphocyte compatibility as well as height and weight. Chest size is approximated by superimposition of donor and recipient chest radiographs.

## Donor Selection

Only approximately 20 per cent of heart donors have lungs suitable for transplantation.[92] Potential donors often have neurogenic pulmonary edema, pneumonia, or chest trauma. Prolonged endotracheal intubation increases the likelihood of tracheobronchial infection, pulmonary barotrauma, or oxygen toxicity. The suitable donor is treated with pulmonary ventilation, using 40 per cent oxygen. At the present time, donors must be transported to the site of the transplant operation, although research on lung preservation promises that distant organ procurement may soon be possible for the heart-lung bloc as well.[121] The anesthesiologist must accompany the donor in transit, using manual controlled ventilation. Increased intracranial pressure from head trauma may cause diabetes insipidus and require vasopressin and judicious fluid management.

Acceptable donors must have a $Pa_{O_2}$ of at least 100 mm Hg using 40 per cent oxygen and peak inspiratory pressure of less than 30 mm Hg with a normal tidal volume.[92] Chest radiographs are obtained every six hours, with the final x-ray film determined to be clear within one to two hours of surgery.

## Surgical Procedure

The donor operation removes the heart and lungs as a single unit. When the chest has been opened, heparin, 300 units·kg$^{-1}$, is given into the right atrium, and cold potassium cardioplegia solution is infused into the cross-clamped aorta to arrest the heart. The cardioplegia solution used at Stanford contains potassium chloride, 30 mEq·L$^{-1}$. The main pulmonary artery is then cannulated, and 20 ml·kg$^{-1}$ of cold potassium solution is infused through tubing containing a 5 $\mu$ filter. The lung perfusate is modified Collins' II solution, containing potassium chloride, 115 mEq·L$^{-1}$. Gentle ventilation of the lungs during infusion of the cold solution allows even distribution of the perfusate. The chest cavity is filled with cold solution (PhysioSol Irrigation). The trachea, aorta, and venae cavae are incised, and the heart and lungs are removed to a sterile basin of cold solution for transport to the adjoining operating room where the recipient awaits implantation.

After initiation of cardiopulmonary bypass and cooling, the recipient aorta is cross-clamped and the heart excised, leaving a cuff of right atrium. The left lung and then the right lung are removed. Care is taken to preserve the phrenic, vagus, and recurrent laryngeal nerves. The bronchial arteries in cyanotic patients tend to be large, and the surgeon must effect hemostasis of these vessels while the chest is empty. The donor organs are placed in the chest and the tracheal anastomosis performed. The atrial anastomosis follows, with the suture line avoiding the sinus node of the graft atrium. Air removal maneuvers follow completion of the aortic anastomosis. The aortic cross clamp is removed, and the patient is warmed in preparation for discontinuation of cardiopulmonary bypass.[122]

## Anesthetic Management

The anesthesiologist must be in close communication with the transplant surgeon regarding the timing of the donor and recipient operations. An adequate interval for assessment and preoperative preparation of the recipient must be anticipated and consideration given to factors that may delay the start of the donor operation, such as previous chest surgery in the recipient. Heart-lung donors often also donate kidneys, corneas, and other organs, frequently necessitating the involvement of several surgical teams.

### Heart-Lung Donors

The donor is transported to the operating room using a gas-sterilized Jackson-Rees system and maintained with a 40 per cent inspired oxygen concentration with 5 cm $H_2O$ positive end-expiratory pressure. Sterile technique is used for any intravenous line placement. Patients usually have a central venous catheter in place; a left-sided radial artery catheter is necessary, since the right subclavian artery may be clamped during the dissection.

ECG, central venous pressure, and arterial pressure are continuously monitored. The donor mean arterial pressure is maintained between 70 and 80 mm Hg, which may require administration of nitroprusside or metaraminol. Central venous pressure should be maintained at 5 to 10 cm $H_2O$; crystalloid solution is administered at a rate of 100 ml·hr$^{-1}$ or as required. Serum potassium and arterial blood gases are determined every 30 minutes. Methylprednisolone, 30 mg·kg$^{-1}$, is given before the incision is made. Muscle relaxation is achieved with pancuronium, if necessary.

The anesthesiologist must be certain that the heparin has been administered to maintain adequate anticoagulation, which is verified by means of the activated clotting time test. Administration of the cold cardioplegia and lung preservation solution are the responsibility of the anesthesiologist; one 500 ml pressurized bag and two 1000 ml pressurized fluid administration bags are needed. Constant communication between the donor and recipient operating teams prevents premature harvesting of the donor organs, thereby lessening the ischemic time of the graft.

### Heart-Lung Recipient

Preoperative assessment of the recipient frequently is made just prior to surgery. The anesthesiologist is often informed of the impending transplantation while the recipient is still being reached by his beeper in the community. The recipient usually has a full stomach and will also receive oral cyclosporine solution before surgery.

Laboratory evaluations include hematocrit, serum potassium, and blood coagulation studies, in addition to the cross-match tests. An elevated hematocrit value will allow removal of one or two units of autologous fresh blood just before bypass for later retransfusion. An increased prothrombin time, a frequent finding, is treated with vitamin K and slow infusion of fresh frozen plasma. A low level of serum potassium is not corrected. Potential recipients are selected for emotional stability and motivation, and premedication is neither necessary nor desirable in view of the potential for hemodynamic instability. The anxious patient can be given small incremental doses of diazepam upon arrival in the operating room when the anesthesiologist is in constant attendance.

The operating room is set up with a gas-sterilized circle system and sterile airway equipment. It is most useful to have always sterilized and ready a tray containing several sizes of endotracheal tubes, a selection of laryngoscope blades, stylet, esophageal stethoscope, temperature probe, oral airway, mask, ventilation bag, and PEEP valves. The anesthesiologist, wearing sterile gloves and leaving the work surfaces covered with a sterile towel, arranges the airway equipment and checks the circuit. A full air tank is added to the anesthesia machine.

The recipient is placed on a warming blanket on the operating table, electrocardiograph leads are secured, and nasal oxygen is given. All intravenous tubing is carefully examined for retained air bubbles before connection to the patient. Skin sites for intravenous placement are prepared with povidone-iodine, and all lines are placed by the anesthesiologist while wearing sterile gloves. Puncture sites are covered with antibacterial ointment and a sterile dressing. Two 14-gauge peripheral intravenous catheters, a radial artery catheter, and a left internal jugular central venous catheter (double or triple lumen) are used. The right internal jugular vein is avoided to permit postoperative endomyocardial biopsies. A pulse oximeter probe to measure continuous arterial oxyhemoglobin saturation is placed on the bridge of the nose where it consistently detects a pulse during the post-bypass period.

A modified rapid-sequence anesthesia induction technique is used. The patient is preoxygenated, and cricoid pressure is applied. Fentanyl or sufentanil combined with diazepam or etomidate with pancuronium forms the basis of the anesthetic technique. Etomidate is especially useful because of rapid loss of awareness and maintenance of hemodynamic stability, allowing tolerance of early muscle relaxation and avoidance of narcotic-induced chest wall rigidity. The adrenal-suppressant effects of etomidate[123] are of little concern because these patients receive large doses of steroids during the perioperative period. Lidocaine (1 mg·kg$^{-1}$) may be administered before intubation. If hemodynamically tolerated, large doses of narcotics (fentanyl, 10 to 40 μg·kg$^{-1}$) are administered before intubation to avoid pulmonary hypertension with airway manipulation. If a small initial dose of narcotic causes hypotension, incremental doses of etomidate (0.1 mg·kg$^{-1}$) provide adequate conditions for intubation. Respiratory or metabolic acidosis causes pulmonary vasoconstriction and systemic vasodilation, which may be heralded by a fall in the oxygen saturation value. In patients with Eisenmenger's syndrome, resting baseline $Sa_{O_2}$ may be as low as 24 per cent,[106] so relative changes are of importance. Mild respiratory alkalosis promotes pulmonary arterial dilation.

A large endotracheal tube is selected (8 or 9 mm ID), since postoperative fiberoptic bronchoscopy may be needed. The endotracheal tube cuff is passed just beyond the vocal cords under direct vision and inflated only to prevent an air leak. Cuff pressures are rechecked periodically during the procedure to prevent excessive pressure on the mucosa near the tracheal anastomosis. An oral nasogastric tube is passed, but the stomach contents should not be aspirated because the recently administered oral cyclosporine solution would be lost. A Foley catheter is placed using sterile technique. Intramuscular antithymocyte globulin and intravenous antibiotics (nafcillin and erythromycin) are administered. Although many patients have received diuretics and are relatively hypovolemic, crystalloid administration should be limited at all times to avoid lung edema and to allow later blood product administration.

Inhalational anesthetics are best avoided during the induction and pre-bypass management of these patients. Although pulmonary artery pressure may decrease with inhalation anesthesia, systemic arterial hypotension frequently develops, and intracardiac shunting may increase. Myocardial depression is also an undesirable effect of these drugs. Nitrous oxide is clearly contraindicated, since decreased inspired oxygen concentration would exacerbate hypoxemia. In patients with pulmonary hypertension, nitrous oxide may increase pulmonary vascular resistance with subsequent hemodynamic decompensation.[68,124] In patients with intracardiac shunts, nitrous oxide also increases the likelihood of significant air embolism.

Arterial blood gases, potassium, and baseline activated clotting time are determined. Supplemental potassium is not administered or added to the extracorporeal circulation prime because of the high potassium concentration ($115 \ mEq \cdot L^{-1}$) of the donor lung perfusate that is washed out from the graft. Heparin is administered, and adequate prolongation of the activated clotting time assured before cardiopulmonary bypass is begun. A Y attachment on the venous inflow line of the bypass pump allows removal of heparinized autologous blood for post-bypass transfusion.

During bypass, these patients often require nitroprusside infusion into the venous reservoir to maintain the mean arterial pressure at 45 to 55 mm Hg. During formation of the tracheal anastomosis, the endotracheal tube may have to be withdrawn slightly. When the tracheal suture line is completed, occasional lung inflations are provided with air (four to six times per minute). When the aortic anastomosis is complete, controlled ventilation using 5 cm $H_2O$ PEEP is provided with 40 per cent oxygen in air. The patient is placed in the Trendelenburg position, and air removal maneuvers requiring sustained lung inflations are performed.

The mean arterial pressure is raised to 60 to 70 mm Hg after unclamping of the aorta. Isoproterenol infusion is begun, usually at a rate of 0.5 to 1.0 $\mu g \cdot min^{-1}$, to achieve a heart rate of 110 beats per minute. Even in the presence of tachycardia, isoproterenol is usually continued for inotropic effect. Dopamine (2.5

to 3 $\mu g \cdot kg^{-1} \cdot min^{-1}$) is added to promote renal blood flow. Other inotropic drugs are rarely necessary.

If surgical hemostasis is adequate, bypass is generally discontinued uneventfully. Nitroprusside is added to accommodate blood volume transfer from the bypass pump reservoir. On occasion, severe bleeding occurs during this period, prompting temporary resumption of bypass. When all required pump volume has been given, furosemide (20 mg), mannitol (25 gm), methylprednisolone (500 mg), and additional antibiotics are given. Relatively long bypass periods (ranging from one and one-half to nearly six hours) and preoperative coagulopathies often result in significant hemostatic problems after the heparin effect is antagonized. Autologous blood has been useful in many patients and should be transfused before stored blood. The average patient requires 2 to 4 units of homologous blood, but some patients need more than 20 units of blood and continuous use of an autotransfusion device. Most require 8 to 10 units of platelets, 2 units of fresh frozen plasma, and 8 to 10 units of cryoprecipitate. Epsilon aminocaproic acid and Factor IX concentrates have been occasionally useful. Bleeding with subsequent clot formation at the tracheal anastomosis may occlude the tracheal lumen. The anesthesiologist must be alert to this possibility in the bleeding patient who develops what appears to be rapidly decreasing lung compliance. Suctioning or immediate fiberoptic bronchoscopy may be necessary.

Oxygenation is usually adequate with 40 per cent inspired oxygen after bypass, but addition of PEEP may be necessary in some patients. Arterial blood gases are determined every 30 minutes. Patients needing large amounts of blood and blood products may exhibit a progressive fall in oxygenation as colloid and platelet-fibrin aggregates accumulate in the alveoli. Increased inspired oxygen concentration and restriction of the use of further blood products may be necessary.

The recipient is transported to the intensive care unit with manual controlled ventilation and continuous monitoring of mean arterial pressure. A sterile Jackson-Rees system is used for ventilation, and PEEP is approximated by end-expiratory bag pressure. Sterile gloves and mask are worn by all persons assisting with the transport of the patient.

## Postoperative Care

Transplant patient intensive care unit rooms are isolated from those for other surgical patients. Gown, mask, and gloves are worn by those entering the isolation rooms in the immediate postoperative period. Skilled ICU nurses remain at the bedside 24 hours a day. During the first 8 to 12 hours after surgery, the patient usually receives sodium nitroprusside infusion to assist rewarming. Isoproterenol is often useful during this period, since the transplanted heart cannot suddenly respond to changes in afterload associated with rewarming. The patient with continuing chest tube blood loss is kept sedated, but most are allowed to gradually awaken from the anesthesia and narcotics. During this period, several of the heart-lung transplant patients at Stanford have required re-exploration for bleeding. Most patients are weaned uneventfully from the ventilator and are extubated at 12 to 18 hours after arrival in the ICU. When necessary, the patient must be reintubated with sterile technique and with great care for the tracheal anastomosis. Endotracheal tube cuff pressure should be routinely measured and should not exceed 20 cm $H_2O$ because of the potential for ischemia in this poorly vascularized area. All sedative and analgesic drugs are carefully titrated with consideration for the frequent hepatic dysfunction in these patients with preoperative right-ventricular failure. Soon after extubation, training for cough and clearing of secretions is initiated. A program of physical therapy and nutrition is carefully followed. Most patients remain in the hospital for four to six weeks before being discharged home.

Immunosuppression begins before surgery with oral cyclosporine (18 mg·kg$^{-1}$) and rabbit antithymocyte globulin. Oral cyclosporine (1.5 mg·kg$^{-1}$·day$^{-1}$) is continued after surgery, adjusted for cyclosporine levels. Methylprednisolone, 500 mg, is administered during surgery, then continued for three doses of 125 mg over 24 hours. Rabbit antithymocyte globulin is continued for a three-day course, until the measured level of circulating T lymphocytes (rosette test) falls below 10 per cent. Azathioprine is given daily for two weeks to avoid steroid treatment during the period of tracheal healing. Thereafter, azathioprine is discontinued, and immunosuppression is maintained with prednisone (0.2 mg·kg$^{-1}$·day$^{-1}$) and cyclosporine.[92,125]

Endomyocardial biopsy is performed weekly for diagnosis of cardiac rejection. Rejection episodes in the first four weeks are treated with methylprednisolone, 1 gm·day$^{-1}$, for three days, and with increased oral steroids after the first month. Rabbit antithymocyte globulin is added for resistant rejection episodes. Rejection episodes are most frequent in the first nine weeks after transplantation.[92]

Pulmonary rejection does not always occur in conjunction with cardiac rejection.[126] Diagnosis of pulmonary rejection is often presumptive, and differentiation between an acute rejection episode and sudden severe pneumonia can be very difficult. Consideration has been given to more frequent use of lung biopsy in the future. Bronchoalveolar lavage has not yet been useful in the diagnosis of rejection.[127] Chest radiographic evidence of pulmonary edema appearing within the first weeks after transplantation has been termed the implantation response[111] and has occurred after heart-lung and unilateral lung transplantation.[92] It is associated with fevers and mild respiratory insufficiency. The syndrome has responded to increased steroid treatment and probably represents isolated pulmonary rejection.[111]

Infection remains the greatest threat to the heart-lung transplant patient in the postoperative period. Surveillance cultures are routine. The donor trachea is cultured before implantation. Transtracheal aspirations are performed and blood cultures are obtained for any episode of fever, leukocytosis, hypotension, or radiographic change. Most patients develop some infectious episode during their ICU course, usually of an opportunistic type. The range has included cytomegalovirus, herpes, bacteroides, enterococcus, and *Serratia*, *Legionella*, and *Candida* organisms and others.[125] One patient developed sudden dehiscence of the aortic anastomosis weeks after surgery, resulting from a candidal fungal infection of the aortic suture line. The donor trachea culture had grown *Candida* in that case. The importance of a high index of suspicion regarding occult infection cannot be overemphasized. Acute pancreatitis, often not recognized clinically, has been found to occur in some post-transplant patients.[128] Infection, steroids, cardiopulmonary bypass, rejection, renal failure, and azathioprine may all contribute to the development of pancreatitis. Cyclosporine is both hepatotoxic and nephrotoxic. It is metabolized by the liver, and doses must continually be adjusted for variations in hepatic metabolism. Hepatic dysfunction is especially common in patients with preoperative tricuspid regurgitation and primary pulmonary hypertension.[125] Renal insufficiency has prompted periods of hemodialysis in some patients. Chronic nephropathy associated with cyclosporine treatment is a significant problem.[85] Renal biopsies have shown fibrosis.[111] All patients eventually develop systemic arterial hypertension, which can be very difficult to control medically.

Mild normocytic anemia (hemoglobin concentrations $11.0 \pm 0.8$ gm·dl$^{-1}$) occurs several months after transplantation.[106] Although recurrent infections and immunosuppressions may explain this anemia, a blunted erythropoietin response resulting from the pretransplant intense hypoxic stimulus to erythropoiesis has been postulated.

Post-transplant patients have needed a variety of surgical procedures requiring anesthesia, including open lung biopsy, bronchoscopy, laparotomy, pyloroplasty, and procedures on the vocal cords. The primary considerations for the anesthesiologist are hemodynamic and concern the transplanted heart; these have been discussed previously. Because of unpredictable ventilatory patterns under anesthesia, controlled ventilation is advisable. At extubation, patients are able to cough only when alert enough to do so consciously.

Because the respiratory depressant effects of anesthetics and analgesics may produce prolonged alterations in ventilation, these patients should receive careful attention in the immediate postoperative period. Drug doses should be adjusted for probable renal insufficiency. Silent coronary artery disease must be anticipated. Signs of impending respiratory failure may be masked because of the denervation of pulmonary stretch receptors, which are thought to be responsible for the sensation of dyspnea accompanying early interstitial pulmonary edema. Continuous oxygen saturation monitoring and judicious use of fluids are helpful. Fluid therapy can be difficult; the transplanted heart functions optimally with a high preload during periods of hemodynamic stress such as anesthesia and surgery, but the transplanted lungs may become excessively edematous when preload is increased. Early extubation is of great importance because of the potential for pulmonary infection from nosocomial airway colonization. All patients require steroid supplementation because of chronic adrenal suppression from prednisone.

As with any immunosuppressed patient, careful attention must be given to sterile technique. Surgeons performing these noncardiac procedures are generally unfamiliar with the special requirements of the heart-lung transplant patient, and the responsibility for considering all aspects of the patient's care often rests with the anesthesiologist.

## SUMMARY AND CONCLUSIONS

In conclusion, accumulated clinical experience over the past 17 years has firmly established heart transplantation as a major therapeutic alternative in the management of end-stage heart disease. Although clinical heart-lung transplantation has only a five-year history, it remains the only potentially curative therapy for patients with end-stage cardiopulmonary disease. Advances in the field of organ transplantation have recently been profound; there are now substantial improvements in survival rates. The advancements in organ preservation research, the advent of the new immunosuppressive agent cyclosporine, improved protocols using various combinations of immunosuppressant therapy, and a better understanding of the immune response are primarily responsible for these improved results.

According to the Heart Transplant Registry (December 31, 1984) 44 centers had active heart transplant programs. In 1984, 440 heart transplants were performed world wide.[129] It is accepted that this number will increase as the survival of recipients improves. The overall survival of patients as reported from the Heart Transplant Registry were 80 per cent at one year and 47 per cent at six years in transplantations performed after 1978. The success rates being reported are the result of extensive experience, years of research, improved intensive postoperative management, and support from other services such as cardiology, pathology, anesthesiology, infectious diseases, nephrology, and nursing.

A major limitation on the wider application of heart and heart-lung transplantation as a treatment method is the overall cost associated with the procedure. Currently the estimated cost for the first year of care for a cardiac recipient is $100,000. The total first-year cost of a national heart transplant program is estimated to be $200 million if 2000 procedures are performed annually. This cost figure is lower than previously reported.[50,130] Rehabilitation following heart transplantation is excellent, returning over 80 per cent of the survivors to their previous activities; the long-term economic and social consequences favor this therapeutic approach.[131] The long-range outlook for heart-lung transplant recipients must remain closely guarded at this point, and therapy cannot be justified on the basis of economic potential of the recipients.

A further restriction to the expansion of heart and heart-lung transplantation is the availability of donors. It has been estimated that 20,000 Americans die from brain injury, brain tumor, or stroke each year that could permit removal of viable organs for transplantation.[132] The number of heart transplants needed annually in the United States has been estimated to be between 1000 and 5000.[50] Approximately only 20 per cent of potential heart donors are acceptable lung donors as well.[92] Another area of potential growth in cardiopulmonary transplantation involves pediatric patients. Now that continued growth of donor organs in children appears well established, more attention will undoubtedly be directed toward the many patients with congenital heart defects currently amenable only to palliative surgery.

Prolonged survival of heart transplant recipients has increased the importance of the complications resulting from immunosuppressive therapy.[133] Long-term steroid therapy increases the incidence of infections, diabetes mellitus, compression fractures, and cataracts. The introduction of cyclosporine resulted in a reduction in steroid dosages, but it soon became apparent that cyclosporine has its own adverse effects. Therefore, continuing research is now being directed toward the further refinement of immunosuppressive regimens. The degeneration in pulmonary function seen in late survivors of heart-lung transplantation may also be a problem of suboptimal immunosuppression. Research and experience will continue to add to the understanding of optimal anesthetic management for cardiopulmonary transplant patients, and the anesthesiologist must frequently refine techniques in view of this rapidly growing body of knowledge.

## REFERENCES

1. Carrel A, Guthrie CC: The transplantation of veins and organs. Am J Med 10:1101, 1905.

2. Mann FC, Priestly JR, Markowitz J, et al: Transplantation of the intact mammalian heart. Arch Surg 26:219, 1933.

3. Shumway NE: The experimental basis for heart transplantation. Bull Amer Coll Surg 66:6, 1981.

4. Demikhov VP: Experimental transplantation of vital organs (translated by B Haigh), New York, Consultants Bureau, 126, 1962.

5. Barnard CN, Barnard MS, Cooper DKC, et al: The present status of heterotopic cardiac transplantation. J Thorac Cardiovasc Surg 81:433, 1981.

6. Goldberg M, Berman EF, Akman CL: Homologous transplantation of the canine heart. J Int Coll Surgeons 30:575, 1958.

7. Lower RR, Shumway NE: Studies on orthotopic transplantation of the canine heart. Surg Forum 2:18, 1960.

8. Lower RR, Dong E Jr, Shumway NE: Suppression of rejection crises in the cardiac homografts. Ann Thorac Surg 1:645, 1965.

9. Lower RR, Dong E Jr, Glazener FS: Electrocardiograms of dogs with heart homografts. Circulation 33:455, 1966.

10. Hardy JD, Chavez CM, Kurrus FD, et al: Heart transplantation in man: Developmental studies and report of a case. JAMA 188:1132, 1964.

11. Barnard CN: A human cardiac transplant: An interim report of a successful operation performed at Groote Schuur Hospital. S Afr Med J 41:1257, 1967.

12. Jamieson SW, Stinson EB: Coronary heart disease. In Conner WE, Bristow JD (eds): Cardiac Transplantation for End-Stage Ischemic Heart Diseases. 25:437, 1985.

13. DeVries WC, Anderson JL, Joyce LD, et al: Clinical use of the total artificial heart. N Engl J Med 310:273, 1984.

14. Rose DM, Colvin SB, Culliford AT, et al: Late functional and hemodynamic status of surviving patients following insertion of the left heart assist device. J Thorac Cardiovasc Surg 86:639, 1983.

15. Baumgartner WA, Reitz BA, Bieber CP, et al: Current expectations in cardiac transplantation. J Thorac Cardiovasc Surg 75:525, 1978.

16. Baumgartner WA, Reitz BA, Oyer PE, et al: Cardiac homotransplantation. Curr Probl Surg 16(9):1, 1979.

17. Copeland JG, Stinson EB: Human heart transplantation. Curr Probl Cardiol 3:4, 1980.

18. Bieber CP, Griep RB, Oyer PE, et al: Use of rabbit antithymocyte globulin in cardiac transplantation. Relationship of serum clearance rate to clinical outcome. Transplantation 22:478, 1976.

19. Bieber CP, Lydick E, Griep RB, et al: Relationship of rabbit ATG serum clearance rates to circulating T-cell levels, rejection onset and survival in cardiac transplantation. Transplant Proc 9:1031, 1977.

20. Caves PK, Stinson EB, Billingham ME: Percutaneous transvenous endomyocardial biopsy in human heart recipients. Ann Thorac Surg 16:325, 1973.

21. Griepp RB, Stinson EB, Bieber CP: Control of graft atherosclerosis in human heart transplant recipients. Surgery 81:262, 1977.

22. Jamieson SW, Burton NA, Bieber CP: Cardiac

allograft survival in rats treated with cyclosporin-A. Surg Forum 30:289, 1979.

23. Jamieson SW, Burton NA, Oyer PE: Cardiac allograft survival in primates treated with cyclosporin A. Lancet 1:548, 1979.

24. Oyer PE, Stinson EB, Jamieson SW: Cyclosporin A in cardiac allografting: A preliminary experience. Transplant Proc 15:1247, 1983.

25. Lough ME, Lindsey AD, Shinn JA, et al: Life satisfaction following heart transplantation. Heart Transplant 4:446, 1985.

26. Goodman DJ, Rossen RM, Rider AK, et al: The effect of cycle length on cardiac refractory periods in the denervated human heart. Am Heart J 91:332, 1976.

27. Cannom DS, Graham AF, Harrison DC: Electrophysiological studies in the denervated transplanted human heart. Circ Res 32:268, 1973.

28. Mason JW, Winkle RA, Rider AK, et al: The electrophysiologic effects of quinidine in the transplanted human heart. J Clin Invest 59:481, 1977.

29. Stinson EB, Griepp RB, Schroeder JS, et al: Hemodynamic observations one and two years after cardiac transplantation in man. Circulation 45:1183, 1972.

30. Dong E Jr, Hurley EJ, Lower RR, et al: Performance of the heart two years after autotransplantation. Surgery 56:270, 1964.

31. Pope SE, Stinson EB, Daughters GT, et al: Exercise response of the denervated heart in longterm cardiac transplant recipients. Am J Cardiol 46:312, 1980.

32. Cannom DS, Rider AK, Stinson EB, et al: Electrophysiologic studies in the denervated transplanted human heart: II. Response to norepinephrine, isoproterenol and propranolol. Am J Cardiol 36:859, 1975.

33. Lurie KG, Bristow MR, Reitz BA: Increased β adrenergic receptor density in an experimental model of cardiac transplantation. J Thorac Cardiovasc Surg 86:195, 1983.

34. Homcy CJ: The ligand binding assay and its role in understanding adrenergic receptor function. J Thorac Cardiovasc Surg 86:193, 1983.

35. Goodman DJ, Rossen RM, Cannom DS, et al: Effect of digoxin on atrioventricular conduction; studies in patients with and without cardiac autonomic innervation. Circulation 51:251, 1975.

36. Schroeder JS, Berke DK, Graham AF, et al: Arrhythmias after cardiac transplantation. Am J Cardiol 33:604, 1974.

37. Romhilt DW, Doyle M, Sagar KB, et al: Prevalence and significance of arrhythmias in longterm survivors of cardiac transplantation. Circulation Suppl I, p 219, 1982.

38. Orlick AE, Ricci DR, Alderman EL: Effects of alpha adrenergic blockade on coronary hemodynamics. J Clin Invest 62:459, 1978.

39. Lower RR, Szentpetery S, Quinn J, et al: Selection of patients for cardiac transplantation. Transplant Proc 11:293, 1979.

40. Beecher HK, Adams RD, Barger C, et al: Report of the Harvard Medical School to examine the definition of brain death: A definition of irreversible coma. JAMA 205:337, 1968.

41. Mohandas A, Chou SN: Brain death: A clinical and pathological study. J Neurosurg 35:211, 1971.

42. Griepp RB, Stinson EB, Clark DA, et al: The cardiac donor. Surg Gynecol Obstet 133:792, 1971.

43. Bieber CP, Hunt SA, Schwinn DA, et al: Complications in long-term survivors of cardiac transplantation. Transplant Proc 13:207, 1981.

44. Thomas FT, Szentpetery SS, Mammana RE, et al: Long distance transportation of human hearts for transplantation. Ann Thorac Surg 26:344, 1978.

45. Watson DC, Reitz RA, Baumgartner WA, et al: Distant heart procurement for transplantation. Surgery 86:56, 1979.

46. Billingham ME, Baumgartner WA, Watson DC: Distant heart procurement for human transplantation. Circulation 62 (Suppl I):11, 1980.

47. Lurie KG, Billingham ME, Masek MA, et al: Ultrastructural and functional studies on prolonged myocardial preservation in an experimental heart transplant model. J Thorac Cardiovasc Surg 84:122, 1982.

48. Ceppelini R, Curtoni ES, Mattiuz PL, et al: Survival of test skin grafts in man: Effect of genetic relationship and of blood groups in compatibility. Ann NY Acad Sci 129:421, 1966.

49. Coulson AS, MacMillan F, Griepp RB, et al: Lymphocyte tissue culture studies on human heart transplant recipients: II. Screening the lymphocyte reactivity of the recipients in vitro. Transplantation 18:409, 1974.

50. Pennock JL, Oyer PE, Reitz BA, et al: Cardiac transplantation in perspective for the future. J Thorac Cardiovasc Surg 83:168, 1982.

51. Ozinsky J: Cardiac transplantation—the anesthetist's view: A case report. S Afr Med J 41:1268, 1967.

52. Keats AS, Strong MJ, Girgis KZ, et al: Observations during anesthesia for cardiac homotransplantation in ten patients. Anesthesiology 30:192, 1969.

53. Paiement B, Wielhorski WA, Grondin P, et al: Anesthetic management in nine heart transplantations. Laval Medical 41:186, 1970.

54. Fernando SA, Keenan RL, Boyan CP: Anesthetic experience with cardiac transplantation. J Thorac Cardiovasc Surg 75:531, 1978.

55. Grebenik C, Robinson PN: Cardiac transplantation at Harefield. A review from the anaesthetist's standpoint. Anaesthesia 40:131, 1985.

56. Garman JK: Anesthesia for cardiac transplantation. Cleve Clin Q 48:142, 1981.

57. Wetzel RC, Setzer N, Stiff JL, et al: Hemodynamic responses in brain dead organ donor patients. Anesth Analg 64:125, 1985.

58. Johnson B, Thomason R, Pallares V: Autonomic hyperreflexia: A review. Milit Med 140:345, 1975.

59. Naftchi NE, Wooten GF, Lowman EW, et al: Relationship between serum dopamine-B-hydroxylase activity, catecholamine metabolism, and hemodynamic changes during paroxysmal hypertension in quadriplegia. Circ Res 35:850, 1974.

60. Ducker TB: Increased intracranial pressure and pulmonary edema. Clinical study of 11 patients. J Neurosurg 28:112, 1968.

61. English TAH, Spratt P, Wallwork J, et al: Selection and procurement of hearts for transplantation. Br Med J 288:1889, 1984.

62. Mazze RI, Shue GL, Jackson SH: Renal dysfunction associated with methoxyflurane anesthesia. A randomized prospective clinical evaluation. JAMA 216:278, 1971.

63. Lowenstein E, Hallowell D, Levine LH: Cardiovascular response to large doses of intravenous morphine in man. N Engl J Med 281:1389, 1969.

64. Stanley TH, Webster LR: Anesthetic requirements and cardiovascular effects of fentanyl-oxygen and fentanyl-diazepam-oxygen anesthesia in man. Anesth Analg 57:411, 1978.

65. Moffitt EA, Sethna DH, Bussel JA, et al: Myocardial metabolism and hemodynamic response to halothane and morphine anesthesia for coronary artery surgery. Anesth Analg 61:979, 1982.

66. Conahan TJ, Ominsky AJ, Wollman H, et al: A prospective random comparison of halothane and morphine for open heart anesthesia. Anesthesiology 38:528, 1973.

67. Eisele JH, Reitan JA, Massumi RA: Myocardial performance and $N_2O$ analgesia in coronary artery diseases. Anesthesiology 44:16, 1976.

68. Schulte-Sasse U, Hess W, Tarnow J: Pulmonary vascular responses to nitrous oxide in patients with normal and high pulmonary vascular resistance. Anesthesiology 57:9, 1982.

69. Bieber CP, Stinson EB, Shumway NE, et al: Cardiac transplantation in man: VII. Cardiac allograft pathology. Circulation 41:753, 1970.

70. Kondo Y, Grogan JB, Cockrell JV, et al: Comparison of the efficacy of immuno-suppressive regimens on orthotopic heart allografts. J Thorac Cardiovasc Surg 67:612, 1974.

71. Bainhart GR, Goldman MH, Haastillo A: Comparison of immunosuppression therapy following heart transplantation: Pretransfusion azathioprine/ATG/prednisone versus cyclosporine/prednisone. Heart Transplant 4:381, 1985.

72. Bentwich Z, Douglas SD, Skultelsky E, et al: Sheep red cell binding to human lymphocytes treated with neuromanidase; enhancement of T-cell binding and identification of a subpopulation of B cells. J Exp Med 137:1532, 1973.

73. Billingham ME: Diagnosis of cardiac rejection by endomyocardial biopsy. Heart Transplant 1:25, 1981.

74. Billingham ME, Masek MA, Khanna K: Long-term cardiac allograft pathology in humans. Lab Invest 42:103, 1980.

75. Oyer PE, Stinson EB, Reitz BA, et al: Cardiac transplantation: 1980. Transplant Proc 13:199, 1981.

76. Haverich A, Scott WL, Dawkins KD, et al: Asymmetric pattern of rejection following orthotopic cardiac transplantation in primates. Heart Transplant 3:280, 1984.

77. Schroeder JS, Popp RL, Stinson EB, et al: Acute rejection following cardiac transplantation; phonocardiographic and ultrasound observations. Circulation 15:155, 1969.

78. Nowygrod R, Spotnitz HM, Dubroff JM: Organ mass: An indicator of heart transplant rejection. Transplant Proc 15:1225, 1983.

79. Dawkins KD, Oldershaw PJ, Billingham ME, et al: Noninvasive assessment of cardiac allograft rejection. Transplant Proc 17:215, 1985.

80. Mason JW, Stinson EB, Hunt SA: Infections after cardiac transplantation: Relation to rejection therapy. Ann Intern Med 85:69, 1976.

81. Krikorian JG, Anderson JL, Bieber CP: Malignant neoplasms following cardiac transplantation. JAMA 240:639, 1978.

82. Weintraub J, Warnke RA: Lymphoma in cardiac allotransplant recipients: Clinical and histological features and immunological phenotype. Transplantation 33:347, 1982.

83. Jamieson SW, Oyer PE, Bieber CP, et al: Transplantation for cardiomyopathy: A review of the results. Heart Transplant 2:28, 1982.

84. Hanto DW, Frizzera G, Gajl-Peczalska KJ: Epstein-Barr virus induced B-cell lymphoma after renal transplantation. N Engl J Med 306:913, 1982.

85. Myers BD, Ross J, Newton L, et al: Cyclosporine associated chronic nephropathy. N Engl J Med 311:699, 1984.

86. Isono SS, Woolson ST, Schurman DJ: Total joint replacement for steroid-induced osteonecrosis in cardiac transplant patients. Clin Orthop. (In press).

87. Kanter SF, Samuel SI: Anesthesia for major operations on patients who have transplanted hearts. A review of 29 cases. Anesthesiology 46:65, 1977.

88. Bricker SRW, Sugden JC: Anesthesia for surgery in a patient with a transplanted heart. Br J Anaesth 57:634, 1985.

89. Moore FD: Metabolic Care of the Surgical Patient. Philadelphia, WB Saunders Company, 1966.

90. Vetten KB: Immunosuppressive therapy and anesthesia. S Afr Med J 47:767, 1973.

91. Adu D, Turney J, Michael J, et al: Hyperkalemia in cyclosporine treated renal allograft recipients. Lancet 2:370, 1983.

92. Jamieson SW, Baldwin J, Stinson EB, Reitz BA, Oyer PE, Hunt S, Billingham M, Theodore J, Modsy D, Bieber CP, Shumway NE: Clinical heart-lung transplantation. Transplantation 37:81, 1984.

93. Cooley DA, Bloodwell RD, Hallman GL, Nova JJ, Harrison GM, Leachman RD: Organ transplantation for advanced cardiopulmonary disease. Ann Thorac Surg 8:30, 1969.

94. Lillehei CW, in discussion, Wildevuur C.R.H., Benfield, JR: A review of 23 human lung transplantations by 20 surgeons. Ann Thorac Surg 9:489, 1970.

95. Barnard CN, Cooper DKC: Clinical transplantation of the heart. A review of 13 years' personal experience. J R Soc Med 74:670, 1981.

96. Nakae S, Webb WR, Theodorides T, Gregg WL: Respiratory function following cardiopulmonary denervation in dog, cat and monkey. Surg Gyncol Obstet 125:1285, 1967.

97. Lower, RR, Stofer RC, Hurley EV, Shumway NE: Complete homograft replacement of the heart and both lungs. Surgery 50:842, 1961.

98. Reitz BA, Burton NA, Jamieson SW, et al: Heart and lung retransplantation in primates with extended survival. J Thorac Cardiovasc Surg 80:360, 1980.

99. Dawkins KD, Jamieson SW, Hunt SA, Baldwin JC, et al: Long-term results, hemodynamics, and complications after combined heart and lung transplantation. Circulation 71:919, 1985.

100. Jamieson SW: Personal communication, January 1986.
101. Jamieson SW, Dawkins KD, Burke C, Baldwin JW, et al: Late results of combined heart-lung transplantation. Transplant Proc 17:212, 1985.
102. Guz A, Noble MIM, Widdicombe JG, et al: The role of vagal and glossopharyngeal afferent nerves in respiratory sensation, control of breathing and arterial pressure regulation in conscious man. Clin Sci 30:161, 1966.
103. Comroe JH: Physiology of Respiration. Chicago, Year Book Medical Publishers, 1974.
104. Popovich B, Mihm FG, Hilberman M, et al: Reinnervation of the lungs after transplantation. Anesthesiology 57:A491, 1982.
105. Phillipson EA, Hickey RF, Bainton CR, et al: Effect of vagal blockade on regulation of breathing in conscious dogs. J Appl Physiol 29:475, 1970.
106. Theodore J, Robin ED, Burke CM, et al: Impact of profound reductions of $Pa_{O_2}$ on $O_2$ transport and utilization in congenital heart disease. Chest 87:293, 1985.
107. Nadel JA: Autonomic regulation of airway smooth muscle. In Nadel JA (ed): Physiology and Pharmacology of the Airways. New York, Marcel Dekker, 1980.
108. Nadel JA: Adoration of the vagi? N Engl J Med 311:463, 1984.
109. Dawkins KD, Jamieson SW, Hunt SA, et al: Long-term results, hemodynamics, and complications after combined heart and lung transplantation. Circulation 71:919, 1985.
110. Edmunds LH Jr, Graf PD, Nadel JA: Reinnervation of the reimplanted canine lung. J Appl Physiol 31:722, 1971.
111. Jamieson SW: Recent developments in heart and heart-lung transplantation. Transplant Proc 17:199, 1985.
112. Granger DN, Rutili G, McCord JM: Superoxide radicals in feline intestinal ischemia. Gastroenterology 81:22, 1981.
113. McCord JM: Organ radicals and lung injury. The state of the art. Chest 83:355, 1983.
114. Bieber CP, Stinson EB, Shumway NE, Payne R, Kosek J: Cardiac transplantation in man: VII. Cardiac allograft pathology. Circulation 31:753, 1970.
115. Theodore J, Jamieson SW, Burke C, et al: Physiologic aspects of human heart-lung transplantation: Pulmonary function status of the post-transplanted lung. Chest 85:349, 1984.
116. Burke CM, Morris AJR, Hawkins CGA, et al: Late airflow obstruction in heart-lung transplantation recipients. Heart Transplant 4:437, 1985.

117. Burke CM, Theodore J, Dawkins KD, et al: Post-transplant obliterative bronchiolitis and other late sequelae of human heart-lung transplantation. Chest 86:824, 1984.
118. Haworth SG: Primary pulmonary hypertension. Br Heart J 49:517, 1983.
119. Horn M, Ries A, Neveu C, et al: Restrictive ventilatory pattern in precapillary pulmonary hypertension. Am Rev Resp Dis 128:163, 1983.
120. James TN: On the cause of syncope and sudden death in primary pulmonary hypertension. Ann Intern Med 56:2523, 1962.
121. Ladowski JS, Hardesty RL, Griffith BP: Protection of the heart-lung allograft during procurement. Heart Transplant 3:351, 1984.
122. Jamieson SW, Stinson B, Oyer PE, Baldwin JC, Shumway NE: Operative technique for heart-lung transplantation. J Thorac Cardiovasc Surg 87:930, 1984.
123. Wagner RL, White PF, Kan PLB, et al: Inhibition of adrenal steroidogenesis by the anesthetic etomidate. N Engl J Med 310:1415, 1984.
124. Davidson JR, Chinyanga HM: Cardiovascular collapse associated with nitrous oxide anesthetic: A case report. Can Anaesth Soc J 29:484, 1982.
125. Jamieson SW, Stinson EB, Oyer PE, et al: Heart and lung transplantation for pulmonary hypertension. Am J Surg 147:740, 1984.
126. Scott WC, Haverich A, Billingham ME, Dawkins KD, Jamieson SW: Lethal lung rejection without significant cardiac rejection in primate heart-lung allotransplants. Heart Transplant 4:33, 1984.
127. Gryzan S, Paradis IL, Hardesty RL, Griffith BP, Dauber JH: Bronchoalveolar lavage in Heart-Lung Transplantation. Heart Transplant 4:414, 1985.
128. Aziz S, Bergdahl L, Baldwin JC, et al: Pancreatitis after cardiac and cardiopulmonary transplantation. Surgery 97:653, 1985.
129. Kaye MP: The International Heart Transplantation Registry—1984 Report. Heart Transplant 4:290, 1985.
130. Austen WG, Cosimi AB: Editorial retrospective. Heart transplantation after 16 years. N Engl J Med 311:1436, 1984.
131. Evans RW: Economic and social costs of heart transplantation. Heart Transplant 1:243, 1982.
132. Stuart FP, Veith FJ, Crawford RE: Brain death laws and patterns of consent to remove organs for transplantation from cadavers in the United States and 28 other countries. Transplantation 31:238, 1981.
133. Gamberg P: Clinical results: Cardiac transplantation. Transplant Proc 15:3135, 1983.

# 8

# *Liver Transplantation*

YOO GOO KANG
SIMON GELMAN

## ANATOMY AND PHYSIOLOGY OF THE LIVER

The liver is located in the right upper quadrant of the abdominal cavity, attached to the diaphragm. It weighs approximately 1500 gm in the adult and is divided into four lobes. The left and right lobes are divided at the line of attachment of the falciform ligament. The larger right lobe includes two smaller lobes, the quadrate and caudate lobes. A thin connective tissue capsule (Glisson's capsule) composed of regularly arranged collagen fibers covers the entire liver and the majority of vessels and nerves. Glisson's capsule also subdivides the parenchyma into lobules and provides an internal supporting framework for the hepatic parenchyma.

Structural concepts of liver lobulation have been developing since the middle of the seventeenth century. Detailed descriptions of liver anatomy and histology, including the review of structural concepts of liver lobulation, can be found in textbooks of histology.[1] The classic lobules are polyhedral prisms of liver tissue about 0.7 by 2 mm in size, separated one from another by connective tissue septa, biliary channels, and blood vessels. The approximate boundaries of the classic lobule can be visualized by locating the central vein (terminal hepatic venule) and the regularly displaced portal triads that encircle the periphery of the lobule. The hepatic arterioles, portal venules, and bile ductules originate from each portal triad and encircle the lobule supplying liver cells.

More than 30 years ago Rappaport defined the liver unit as an acinus.[2] According to his concept, hepatocytes are grouped into three zones surrounding the terminal afferent vessels (Fig. 8–1). Zone 1 cells are located close to the terminal vessels and are the first to receive blood, the first to regenerate, and the last to develop necrosis. Zones 2 and 3 receive blood with lesser amounts of oxygen and nutritives and therefore are less resistant to hepatotoxins, oxygen deprivation, and other damaging factors. Patterns obtained by scanning electron microscopy are in accordance with Rappaport's theory (Fig. 8–2). The concept of the lobule does not conflict with Rappaport's theory, but rather they complement each other and provide a basis for interpretation of the hepatic structure and function from different aspects.

### Liver Cells

The sinusoids form a rich intralobular vascular network and are larger and more variable in caliber than typical capillaries. The walls of sinusoids are lined with two distinct cell types: endothelial cells and Kupffer cells

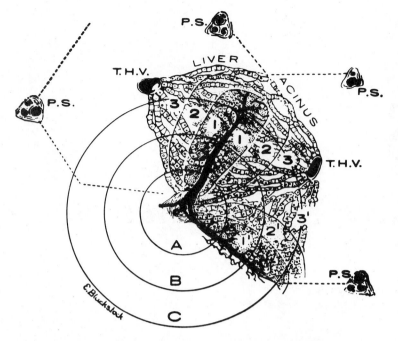

**Figure 8–1.** The blood supply of the hepatic structural unit: The structural unit occupies adjacent sectors of neighboring hexagonal fields. Zones 1, 2, and 3 represent areas supplied with blood of first, second, and third quality, respectively, with regard to oxygen and nutrients. These zones cluster about the terminal afferent vascular twigs and extend into the periportal field from which these twigs originate. Zones 1′, 2′, and 3′ designate corresponding areas in a portion of an adjacent structural unit. In zones 1 and 1′, the afferent vascular twigs empty into the sinusoids. The circles A, B, and C delimit concentric bands of the hepatic parenchyma arranged around a small portal field. (From Rappaport AM, Borowy ZJ, Lougheed WM, Lotto WN: Subdivision of hexagonal liver lobules into a structural and functional unit. Anat Rec 119:16, 1954, with permission of the authors and publisher.)

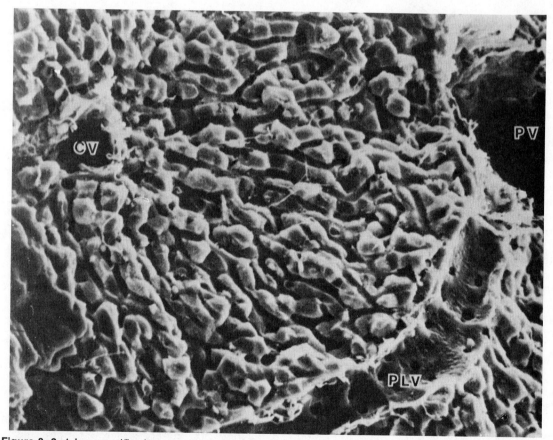

**Figure 8–2.** A low-magnification scanning electron micrograph depicting a portion of a liver lobule from a rat liver. Images such as this lend credence to the acinus lobule concept described by Rappaport. CV = central vein; PV = portal vein; PLV = perilobular venules ($\simeq \times 1{,}000$). (From Jones AL: Anatomy of the normal liver. In Zakim D, Boyer TD (eds): Hepatology: A Textbook of Liver Disease. Philadelphia, WB Saunders Company, 1982, p 3.)

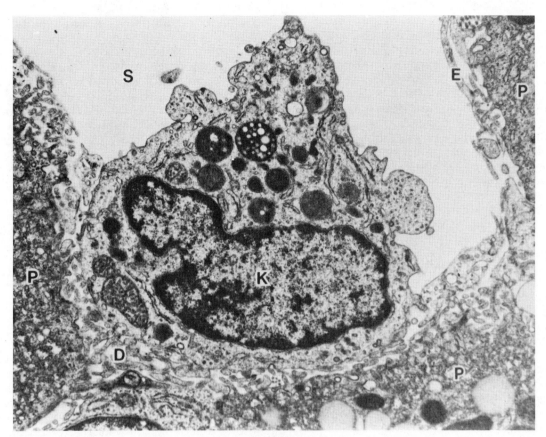

**Figure 8–3.** A transmission electron micrograph of a rat Kupffer cell (K). These large cells make up about a third of the sinusoidal (S) lining and have an extraordinary capacity for phagocytosis. Notice the numerous electron-dense lysosomes within the cytoplasm. D = space of Disse; E = endothelial cell with fenestrae; P = parenchymal cell ($\approx$ $\times$ 12,000). (From Jones AL: Anatomy of the normal liver. In Zakim D, Boyer TD (eds): Hepatology: A Textbook of Liver Disease. Philadelphia, WB Saunders Company, 1982, p 3.)

(Fig. 8–3). The volume of liver tissue occupied by sinusoids is much greater in the zone 3 area than in zone 1. The surface-to-volume ratio of zone 1 sinusoids is larger than that of zone 3 sinusoids. These observations support the idea of a greater probability for solute-membrane interaction in zone 1 than in zone 3. It has been estimated that hepatocytes constitute 78 per cent of the tissue volume.[3] Extracellular space accounts for approximately 16 per cent. The remaining 6 per cent of nonhepatocyte tissue consists of endothelial cells (2.8 per cent), Kupffer cells (2.1 per cent), and fat-storing cells (1.4 per cent).[3]

Endothelial cells are characterized by numerous pinocytotic vesicles, small mitochondria, and a few short profiles of endoplasmic reticulum. The space of Disse, or perisinusoidal space, is different in size and protrudes from the parenchymal cell surfaces.

Kupffer cells are the largest group of fixed macrophages in the organism. These cells have irregular surfaces and can be very large. They are active phagocytes, and their cytoplasm often contains phagocytic vacuoles with cellular debris and lysosomes. Kupffer cells endocytose bacteria, endotoxins, and effete erythrocytes from the blood stream, play a role in iron metabolism, and are probably also active in the clearance of circulating tumor cells and cellular debris after trauma.

Hepatic parenchymal cells, or hepatocytes, are large polyhedral cells approximately 20 by 30 $\mu$m in size. Each cell is in direct contact with other parenchymal cells, the biliary space, and the space of Disse. The cells have extraordinary regenerative ability and the capacity to tolerate increased metabolic demands. They secrete bile salts into the intestines, facilitating emulsification and absorption of dietary fats. They absorb digested material from the blood; store carbohydrates, proteins, vitamins, and lipids; and release these compounds into the blood. The hepatocytes synthesize glucose, fatty acids, cholesterol, phospholipids, albumin, and other proteins. These cells metabolize, detoxify, and inactivate many exogenous and endogenous compounds, including many drugs, steroids, and other hormones. They also convert some substances into more active forms, e.g., $T_4$ to $T_3$. Hepatocytes play an extremely important role in the immune system. To perform all of these functions, there is a well-developed system of organelles within the liver cells.

Mitochondria occupy approximately 18 per cent of the liver cell volume and are mainly responsible for oxidative phosphorylation and the oxidation of fatty acids. Lysosomes are also common in hepatocytes. Their function is to digest and catabolize certain substances, including effete organelles within the liver, and certain polypeptides. The rough and smooth endoplasmic reticulum (microsomes) is involved to certain degrees, directly or indirectly, in almost every function of liver cells. The rather sophisticated Golgi complex is mainly responsible for protein metabolism.

Cellular inclusions such as glycogen deposits first appear at the periphery of the classic liver lobule (or in zone 1 of Rappaport's acinus) during feeding and first disappear from centrilobular cells (zone 3) during starvation. However, other cellular inclusions are usually randomly distributed.

## Liver Blood Supply

The liver has a dual blood supply (Fig. 8–4). Hepatic blood flow equals approximately 100 ml·min$^{-1}$·100 gm$^{-1}$, which represents about 25 per cent of cardiac output; 65 to 80 per cent of total hepatic blood flow is supplied by the portal veins, and the remaining 20 to 35 per cent is supplied by the hepatic artery. Hepatic arterial blood contains more oxygen than portal blood and therefore provides about 50 per cent of the total oxygen delivered and consumed. The liver contains approximately 20 to 30 ml of blood per 100 gm of liver tissue, representing about 15 per cent of total blood volume. Half of this volume can be mobilized in conditions of increased tone of the sympathetic nervous system. Such data demonstrate that the liver is a major blood reservoir.

Portal venous blood flow is mainly controlled by the arterioles in the preportal splanchnic organs. This flow, combined with resistance to the flow in the portal vasculature within the liver, determines portal pressure (7 to 10 mm Hg). Presinusoidal (precapillary) sphincters determine the relatively uniform distribution of flow through the liver and play a role in the regulation of portal blood flow; however, it appears that the major site of venous resistance within the liver is postsinusoidal. The sinusoidal pressure is determined by the tone of presinusoidal and postsinusoidal sphincters and blood flow. Smooth muscle in the wall of the venules regulates venous compliance and blood volume. Both resistance and compliance in the portal venous vasculature are predominantly controlled by the sympathetic innervation mediated through alpha receptors. Pressure in the lobar hepatic veins approaches portal pressure, suggesting that the major site of resistance in the portal circuit is in the lobar hepatic veins. Changes in he-

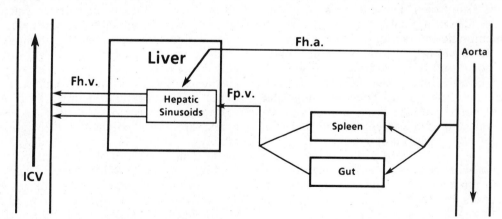

**Figure 8–4.** Schematic representation of liver blood supply. ICV = inferior caval vein; Fh.v. = hepatic venous flow; Fh.a. = hepatic arterial flow; Fp.v. = portal venous flow.

patic venous compliance play a major role in the overall control of cardiac output. Hepatic venous resistance is important in regulating both portal pressure and trans-sinusoidal fluid movements. Myogenic and metabolic intrinsic regulation play a very little role, if any, in controlling the hepatic venous resistance. The major regulating mechanism there appears to be sympathetic innervation mediated through alpha receptors. The sinusoids are relatively permeable to protein. As sinusoidal pressure increases, filtration of fluid increases, and protein passes more readily into the lymph vessels.

The major site of resistance in the hepatic arterial vasculature is the arterioles. The force of smooth muscles of these vessels is affected predominantly by local and intrinsic mechanisms that adjust hepatic arterial flow to compensate for changes in portal blood flow (the so-called arterial buffer response). A decrease in portal blood flow is usually accompanied by an increase in arterial hepatic blood flow.[4,5] From the teleological point of view, this increase (demonstrating hepatic arterial blood flow autoregulation) can be considered an attempt to maintain hepatic oxygen supply and/or total hepatic blood flow, which is essential for clearance of endogenic and exogenic compounds with a high hepatic extraction. The mechanism by which hepatic arterial blood flow increases when portal blood flow decreases involves neural, myogenic, and metabolic controls, quality of the portal blood, and washout effect.[4,5] The washout theory suggests that a substance (probably adenosine) is generated within the liver tissue. When portal blood flow decreases, this vasodilating substance is not washed out, and therefore it accumulates, leading to hepatic arterial vasodilation. Increased portal blood flow is associated with an effective washout of the substance and a reduction in the vasodilating effect on the arterial vasculature. Occlusion of the hepatic artery reduces portal pressure by 2 to 3 mm Hg and total hepatic blood flow by 20 to 33 per cent without any noticeable increase in portal blood flow. Thus, venous resistance remains unchanged.[6]

## Biliary System

A rich plexus of capillaries surrounds the bile duct within the portal canals. Blood subsequently flows into the sinusoids through intralobular branches of the portal vein. The location of the arterial peribiliary plexus is upstream to the sinusoids, and the bile vessels resemble the arrangement in another excretory organ, the kidney, providing the mechanism for countercurrent exchange. Blood enters the peribiliary plexus while the afferent arterioles and the efferent capillaries enter the straight sinusoids that are located along the wall of the excretory bile canaliculi. Efferent arterioles also enter into the portal venous system. The mixed arteriovenous blood enters the sinusoids and then drains into terminal hepatic venules (central veins). It appears that the peribiliary plexus supplies arterial blood to the stroma within the portal tracts and also provides a mechanism facilitating reabsorption of certain compounds from the bile via bile duct cells. These compounds can subsequently enter the circulation and be returned to the liver cells. Substances in arterial blood also can be removed by the bile duct epithelium and secreted into the bile lumen, bypassing the actual liver cells. The peribiliary plexus may also provide an intrahepatic feedback control mechanism for bile secretion. The passage of arterial blood into a capillary plexus before reaching the sinusoids represents a type of portal circulation. How much arterial blood actually reaches the sinusoids directly, bypassing the peribiliary plexus, remains to be determined.

Bile is produced by liver cells and proceeds down the bile canaliculi, traveling from zone 3 (the area surrounding the central vein or terminal hepatic venules) to zone 1 (the part of the acinus located near the portal triads). The bile then enters the small terminal bile ductules, then larger perilobular ductules and/or interlobular bile ducts, which then form a continuous passageway with progressively increasing size.

## Liver Function Tests

Different liver functions deteriorate to different degrees during the course of liver disease, making the evaluation of liver function sometimes very difficult. Tests characterizing liver function can be divided roughly into three groups. The first group evaluates liver excretory function and mainly characterizes the organic anion transport. This group includes sulfobromophthalein (Bromsulphalein, BSP) and indocyanine green (ICG) tests. Serum bilirubin concentration also reflects this function. The second group of tests determines hepatic metabolizing capacity. Drug metabolism, urea synthesis, and galactose elimination from the blood reflect this function. And, finally, serum concentrations of proteins of hepatic origin (albumin, globulins, lipoproteins, and specific clotting factors) evaluate the synthesizing ability of the liver.

It should be kept in mind that there are certain serum markers of hepatobiliary diseases. For example, an increase in the blood concentration of enzymes, specifically aspartate aminotransferase (AST) or serum glutamic-oxaloacetic transaminase (SGOT), alanine aminotransferase (ALT) or serum glutamic-pyruvic transaminase (SGPT), glutamate dehydrogenase, lactate dehydrogenase, and others, reflect liver cell damage and hepatocellular necrosis. Obstruction of the biliary tract and cholestasis are reflected in an increase in alkaline phosphatase, 5'-nucleotidase, lucine aminopeptidase, and gamma glutamyl transpeptidase. These tests sometimes lack specificity; however, there are disease-specific markers such as antibodies IgM and IgG for hepatitis A, antigens $HB_sAg$ and $HB_eAg$ for hepatitis B, and others. Detailed information concerning the evaluation of liver function can be found in a comprehensive review by Kaplowitz et al.[7]

## PATHOPHYSIOLOGY OF LIVER DISEASE

Obstructive jaundice is accompanied by an increase in portal venous pressure, a reduction in portal venous blood flow, an increase in portal-systemic shunting, and a decrease in peripheral vascular resistance and arterial pressure with a subsequent increase in cardiac output.[8] Similar alterations, although to a much greater degree, develop in patients with hepatic cirrhosis. It is interesting to note that biliary decompression may be accompanied by severe vasodilation and cardiovascular collapse.[9] The vasoconstricting ability in biliary obstruction is tremendously decreased. Experiments in rats have shown that equal blood loss is accompanied by substantially lower blood pressure in animals with biliary obstruction than in normal animals.[10] This hypotension was apparently due to an impaired reservoir function of the splanchnic system in animals with occluded common bile duct: splanchnic blood volume did not decrease at all in response to the blood loss in the experimental rats, while it did decrease by 15 per cent in control animals.[10]

Many liver diseases are accompanied by portal hypertension. Alcoholic liver disease, fatty liver, hepatitis, primary biliary cirrhosis, Wilson's disease, congenital hepatic fibrosis, sarcoidosis, schistosomiasis, carcinoma, veno-occlusive disease, hepatic vein thrombosis, certain cardiac diseases (cardiomyopathy, valvular heart disease with cardiac failure, constrictive pericarditis), increased portal vein blood flow due to arteriovenous fistula or idiopathic splenomegaly, and thrombosis or occlusion of portal or splenic veins may be complicated by portal hypertension.

The pathogenesis of portal hypertension is rather complex. The classic "backward theory" considers portal hypertension to be a result of liver cirrhosis (fibrosis) with subsequent increase in resistance to portal flow. However, experimentally induced restriction to portal flow is not always accompanied by an increase in portal pressure and is very rarely associated with bleeding from esophageal varices. More importantly, contrary to the pattern found in cirrhotic patients, experimentally induced restriction to portal flow is often accompanied by a decrease in mesenteric flow, an increase in mesenteric vascular resistance, an immediate decrease in oxygen content in portal blood, and an increase in arteriovenous oxygen content difference. The so-called "forward theory" of portal hypertension suggests that some factors lead to vasodilation and the formation of arteriovenous fistulas in the gut and spleen with increased splanchnic flow and development of a hyperdynamic state.[11,12] Interestingly, probably the first study suggesting the forward theory was published at the beginning of this century. Kretz, in 1904, demonstrated arteriovenous communications with "arterial mixture in the portal vein" in portal hypertension.[13] It appears that both an increase in splanchnic flow and an increase in resistance to portal flow are responsible for the well-known clinical picture of portal hypertension.[14]

What are the factors leading to splanchnic vasodilation? Glucagon concentrations are increased in patients with liver cirrhosis. Moreover, the increase in glucagon levels correlates very well with the increase in blood ammonia concentrations.[15] In rats with experimentally induced portal hypertension, glucagon concentrations are increased and are responsible for 40 per cent of the decrease in mesenteric vascular resistance and the increase in mesenteric flow.[16] The remaining 60 per cent of the observed decrease in mesenteric vascular resistance may be attributed to other vasodilating substances such as vasoactive intestinal polypeptide[17] or ferritin.[18]

The concentrations of many vasoconstricting substances are increased in patients with liver cirrhosis and portal hypertension. Levels of norepinephrine and epinephrine were found to be 314 and 280 per cent of controls respectively.[19] An increase in the norepinephrine concentrations correlated positively with the occluded hepatic venous pressure (which reflects well portal venous pressure) and inversely correlated with plasma volume. It is interesting to note that in portal hypertension the sensitivity to norepinephrine is substantially diminished.[20] Increased glucagon concentrations can be responsible for this decreased sensitivity to norepinephrine, since glucagon antagonizes the vasoconstricting effects of hepatic nerve stimulation and norepinephrine infusion.[21] A positive correlation was also found between occluded hepatic venous pressure and plasma renin activity in patients with liver cirrhosis and portal hypertension.[22]

It is clear that the complex pathogenesis of portal hypertension results in certain dysfunctions of practically all organs and systems (Fig. 8–5).

## Cardiopulmonary Sequelae of Liver Disease

Patients with liver cirrhosis and portal hypertension are usually in a hyperdynamic state with decreased vascular resistance and arterial blood pressure and increased cardiac output. If arterial hypotension results from hypovolemia due to hemorrhage and/or increased capillary permeability, calculated peripheral vascular resistance would increase. The low peripheral vascular resistance in liver disease, especially associated with liver cirrhosis and portal hypertension, is due mainly to an increased level of circulating vasoactive substances such as glucagon, vasoactive intestinal polypeptide, ferritin, and others. The increase in arteriovenous shunting, the decrease in sensitivity to catecholamines, and an abnormal plasma level of prostaglandins play an important role in the pathogenesis of the reduced vascular resistance. Venous oxygen saturation is increased and arteriovenous oxygen content difference is decreased in these patients. Despite the increased cardiac output, hepatic blood flow is reduced in liver cirrhosis as a result of the drastic reduction in portal blood flow. Hepatic arterial blood flow is maintained or even increased. Low peripheral vascular resistance with subsequent increases in stroke volume makes it possible to maintain a high cardiac output despite cardiomyopathy with impaired myocardial contractility, which very often develops in patients who have cirrhosis. An increase in heart rate, without other associated medical problems such as bleeding or pulmonary dysfunction, can often be interpreted as an early predictor of cardiac decompensation in these patients. Ascites *per*

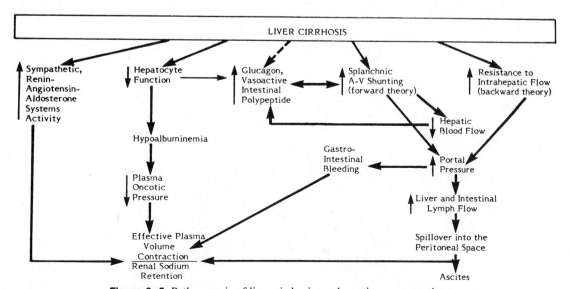

**Figure 8–5.** Pathogenesis of liver cirrhosis—schematic representation.

*se* can compromise the cardiovascular system by an increase in intra-abdominal and intrathoracic pressures with a subsequent decrease in venous return and cardiac output.

The majority of patients with liver cirrhosis and portal hypertension are hypoxemic. A reduction in arterial oxygen content may result from the following: intrapulmonary shunt, ventilation-perfusion abnormalities, alveolar hypoventilation (resulting from ascites), decreased pulmonary diffusing capacity, and a shift in the oxygen-hemoglobin dissociation curve to the right (decreased affinity of oxygen to hemoglobin).

Intrapulmonary shunt (venous admixture) in patients with portal hypertension is due to shunting of venous blood through arteriovenous fistulas similar to spider angiomas seen on the skin. Also, there are certain vascular communications between portal vein and pulmonary veins through azygos, mediastinal, and periesophageal veins. Additionally, during breathing of a low oxygen mixture, patients with cirrhosis do not increase their pulmonary vascular resistance. These and some other data strongly suggest that hypoxic pulmonary vasoconstriction is impaired in these patients, resulting in a ventilation-perfusion mismatch with a subsequent decrease in arterial oxygen content. Intrapulmonary vasodilation is also related to increased glucagon and vasoactive intestinal polypeptide concentrations in patients with liver disease.

Alveolar hypoventilation, which can be due to ascites and an increase in intra-abdominal pressure with a subsequent decrease in pulmonary functional residual capacity, can also be one of the reasons for hypoxemia. Impaired pulmonary diffusing capacity can result from an increase in extracellular fluid. Any kind of metabolic acidosis, which sometimes develops in patients with liver disease, reduces the affinity of hemoglobin for oxygen, leading to different degrees of arterial oxygen desaturation. The pathogenesis of hypoxemia in patients with liver cirrhosis is schematically represented in Figure 8–6.

Cardiopulmonary dysfunction in patients with liver disease often does not require special, vigorous measures. However, sometimes, especially in terminal stages of liver disease, pharmacological and ventilatory support is required.

## Renal Dysfunction and Hepatorenal Syndrome

The pathogenesis of renal dysfunction in patients with liver failure is not completely understood. The primary (partially due to increased levels of aldosterone) or secondary (due to reduced "effective" plasma volume) renal tubular retention/reabsorption of sodium is one of the most important features of renal dysfunction in patients with advanced liver disease. The decrease in effective plasma volume (due mainly to the redistribution of fluid from the intravascular space to interstitial fluid and ascites) is unavoidably accompanied by the activation of volume receptors with subsequent increase in sympathetic nervous activity and angiotensin concentrations, renin release, aldosterone secretion, and intrarenal blood flow redistribution. The elevated plasma concentration of aldosterone is attributed to increased adrenal secretion as well as to decreased metabolic degradation of the hormone. The rate of hepatic degradation of aldosterone is mainly related to hepatic blood flow, which is consid-

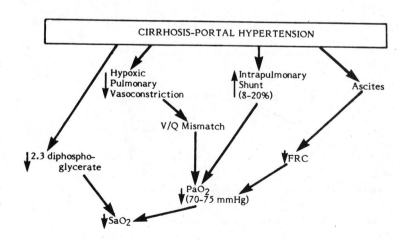

**Figure 8–6.** Hypoxemia in liver cirrhosis and portal hypertension—schematic representation of pathogenesis.

erably reduced in the majority of patients with severe liver disease, particularly cirrhosis.

Water diuresis in patients with liver disease might also be impaired. Water retention is mainly due to enhanced antidiuretic hormone (ADH) activity, as well as to decreased delivery of filtrate to the diluting segments of the nephron. An increased ADH concentration results in enhanced back-diffusion of free water in the collecting tubules. Most likely, increased ADH concentration in patients with liver disease is mediated through nonosmotic stimuli, including a decrease in peripheral vascular resistance and arterial pressure. Impaired metabolic clearance of ADH-vasopressin also contributes to the increased ADH activity. Dehydration and absorption of large amounts of nitrogenous substances from the gut following gastrointestinal bleeding and hypotension also contribute to renal dysfunction. Even severe renal dysfunction is often reversible, but sometimes renal lesions can be very serious, including acute tubular necrosis. Features of reversible renal dysfunction in patients with hepatic disease include normal urinary sediment and urinary sodium concentrations of less than 20 mM$^{-1}$. In patients who have hepatic disease the serum creatinine concentration is a much better index of the extent of renal dysfunction than the blood urea concentration, since hepatic failure sometimes is associated with a decrease in the rate of urea synthesis in the liver.

It appears that the renal failure in the hepatorenal syndrome is functional in nature. Despite the severe renal dysfunction, pathological abnormalities are minimal and inconsistent. Tubular functional integrity is manifested by relatively unimpaired concentrating ability. It has been demonstrated that kidneys transplanted from patients with hepatorenal syndrome are capable of resuming normal function in the recipients. The pathogenesis of hepatorenal syndrome remains unknown. Renal hemodynamic disorders with a particular reduction in cortical perfusion and the development of intrarenal shunts[23] play an important, if not a crucial, role in the development of hepatorenal syndrome. Activation of the renin-angiotensin system, an increase in sympathetic nervous activity, alterations in the endogenous release of renal prostaglandins, changes in the kallikrein-kinin system, increased levels of vasoactive intestinal polypeptide, and other vasoactive compounds play significant roles in the pathogenesis of hepatorenal syndrome.

The renin activity, aldosterone, and norepinephrine concentrations have been substantially increased—two- to five-fold—in patients with liver cirrhosis without renal failure when compared to healthy controls. These concentrations doubled or tripled when renal failure developed. The concentrations of some prostaglandins (PGE$_2$) and kallikreins in urine were two times higher in patients with liver cirrhosis without renal failure than in healthy controls. However, these values decreased to 50 to 25 per cent of controls when renal failure developed.[24] Obviously the renal plasma flow and glomerular filtration rate were much less in cirrhotic patients with renal failure than in patients without renal failure. The data strongly suggest that deterioration of renal function in patients with liver cirrhosis is directly related to an increase in renin activity, aldosterone, and norepinephrine concentrations in blood, while prostaglandins (PGE$_2$) and kallikreins play a compensatory protective role. When these protective mechanisms are exhausted, renal decompensation develops.

Clinically, patients with hepatorenal syndrome will usually have ascites, signs of increased sodium and water retention (hypernatremia or hyponatremia), and increased renin and aldosterone activity without signs of kidney damage (no salt waste, no hyposthenuria). The treatment of hepatorenal syndrome should include proper fluid load (preferably monitored by measurements of filling pressures), consisting of albumin, fresh frozen plasma (in cases with accompanying documented coagulopathy and bleeding), and crystalloids, with an appropriate concentration of sodium (usually hyponatremic or sodium-free solutions). Diuretic therapy is also important and includes furosemide, mannitol, and spironolactone. Small doses of dopamine, 0.5 to 3 $\mu$g·kg$^{-1}$·min$^{-1}$, appear to be useful. The beneficial effect of dopamine might be due to its antialdosterone effect,[25] as well as to the effect of dopamine on the renal circulation. Antialdosterone effect results in improved tubular solute transport (sodium and water excretion), while hemodynamic effects are presented by vasodilation within the kidneys and, to a certain extent, to an increase in cardiac output. The most effective treatment of hepatorenal syndrome is a surgically formed peritoneojugular shunt. The pathogenesis and treatment of renal dysfunction in patients with liver disease have been reviewed recently.[23]

## Electrolyte Disorders

Both hyponatremia and hypernatremia can occur in patients with hepatic dysfunction. Hypernatremia usually results from improper fluid therapy and renal retention of sodium. Hyponatremia can be due to excessive infusions of solutions with low sodium concentrations and excessive antidiuretic hormone activity, but is usually related to hemodilution resulting from retention of free water, as well as to failure of the sodium pump.[26,27]

Often-observed hypokalemia usually results from sodium retention, inadequate potassium intake, vomiting, diuretic therapy, and secondary aldosteronism. Hypocalcemia and hypomagnesemia can also develop in patients with hepatic disease.

## Acid-Base Imbalance

Both alkalosis and acidosis can develop in patients with severe liver dysfunction. Alkalosis is often due to hyperventilation and/or hypokalemia. Extensive hepatic necrosis with concomitant hemodynamic disorders may result in severe metabolic acidosis with accumulation of lactic acid, free fatty acids, citrate, succinate, acetoacetate, and other acidic compounds.

## Hypoglycemia

Hypoglycemia is common in patients with fulminant hepatic failure, owing to the depletion of glycogen stored in the liver, decreased gluconeogenesis, and interactions of the hormones regulating glucose metabolism. Profound hypoglycemia may lead to hypoglycemic coma. Glucose intolerance and high levels of circulating insulin are seen frequently in patients with chronic liver disease. Hypersecretion of insulin by the pancreas or inadequate hepatic clearance contributes to the high level of insulin. Insulin resistance is known to occur in patients with liver disease, before, at, or beyond the receptor level.[28] The blood glucagon level is usually high from hypersecretion and from the effects of portasystemic shunting.[29]

## Hepatic Encephalopathy

Central nervous system dysfunction is a common feature of severe liver disease. Clinically, hepatic encephalopathy is characterized by mental confusion, obtundation, asterixis (flapping tremor), and some other symptoms. A specific smell to the breath (fetor hepaticus) is easily recognized. Physical examination would reveal neuropsychiatric disorders (speech abnormalities, tremors), icterus, spider angiomas, characteristic liver palms, nail changes, alterations in the distribution of body hair, ascites, and hepatosplenomegaly. Laboratory investigation might reveal a decrease in albumin, an increase in globulins, diuretic-induced hypokalemic alkalosis, hypernatremia, and a decrease in hematocrit due to gastrointestinal bleeding. An increase in blood ammonia is probably one of the most specific determinants of hepatic encephalopathy. However, there is no close correlation between the blood ammonia concentrations and the severity of encephalopathy. Often present, electroencephalographic abnormalities are nonspecific and usually consist of predominance of theta activity (4 to 7 cycles per second) of various amplitude.

The pathogenesis of hepatic encephalopathy is rather complex. Apparently the syndrome results from inadequate hepatic removal of certain substances, predominantly nitrogenous compounds that are ingested and formed in the gastrointestinal tract. The inadequate removal of these compounds is due to hepatocyte dysfunction as well as to a decrease in hepatic blood flow. These compounds enter the central nervous system and interact reversibly with certain processes within the neural tissue. Recent data indicate that compounds other than ammonia (i.e., mercaptans, short-chain fatty acids, false neurotransmitters, and GABA) are also responsible for the development of hepatic encephalopathy.

The management of hepatic encephalopathy is based on general supportive measures, including aspiration of blood from the gastrointestinal tract in case of gastrointestinal bleeding, that reduce ammonia generation. Ammonia absorption from the gastrointestinal tract can be substantially reduced by oral administration of neomycin, which suppresses intestinal bacteria. This therapy is accompanied by reduction of bacteria-catalyzed hydrolysis of intraluminal nitrogen-containing compounds and reduction in ammonia formation.

Lactulose is also used to facilitate excretion of ammonia from the body: ammonia is trapped in the acidified fecal masses and becomes unavailable for absorption. There are some data suggesting that dopamine agonists (L-dopa) can decrease the symptoms of hepatic encephalopathy without significant alterations in the blood ammonia levels. It has been suggested that L-dopa influences hepatic encephalopathy by displacement of false neurotransmitters in the central nervous system by the physiological neurotransmitter substance. It is also possible that L-dopa influences hepatic encephalopathy by facilitating renal ammonia excretion. Branched-chain amino acids and other nutrient mixtures have also been used in the treatment of hepatic encephalopathy. Antibacterial therapy, proper diuretic therapy, correction of electrolyte disorders, and dietary treatment (a decrease in protein intake and an increase in carbohydrate intake) are also of great value.

Hepatic failure may be associated with cerebral edema due to disruption of the blood-brain barrier, failure of cellular osmoregulation, and/or expansion of the extracellular space.

## Coagulopathy

Hepatic failure is unavoidably associated with coagulopathy, which predisposes to hemorrhage. The coagulopathy results from thrombocytopenia and the reduced plasma concentrations of liver-produced clotting factors. Thrombocytopenia is due to bone marrow depression, hypersplenism (especially in viral hepatitis), and disseminated intravascular coagulation.[30]

The liver synthesizes the following clotting factors: I (fibrinogen), II (prothrombin), V, VII, IX, and X. Hepatic failure is associated with a decrease in the synthesis of these factors, resulting in prolongation of prothrombin time (PT) and partial thromboplastin time (PTT). Changes in prothrombin time usually reflect well the extent of liver dysfunction. Factors II, VII, IX, and X are vitamin K dependent, while Factors I and V are not. Factor VIII, which is not synthesized in the liver, can be increased during liver failure. Because of the relatively short half-life of Factor VII, it decreases earlier, probably to a greater extent than other liver-produced clotting factors.[31] Fibrinogen (Factor I) synthesis deteriorates the least. Some data indicate that the rate of fibrinogen degradation and consumption may be enhanced in hepatic failure. The abnormal metabolism of fibrinogen can be corrected, at least partially, by the administration of heparin.[32] These data suggest the

possible development of disseminated intravascular coagulation with secondary fibrinolysis in hepatic failure. Coagulopathy in hepatic failure has been recently reviewed.[33,34]

## Pathophysiological Effect of Treatment Methods

Surgical and pharmacological treatment of portal hypertension can produce certain pathophysiological alterations in functions of many systems and organs.

**Portacaval shunt** (direct portacaval or one of the peripheral shunts involving renal, splenic, or mesenteric veins) is usually accompanied by a decrease in portal pressure, an increase of flow through the portal vein to the caval vein, and a decrease in hepatic blood flow due to a decrease in portal blood flow to the liver. Hepatic arterial blood flow usually increases. These changes can sometimes be very dramatic. For example, one study demonstrated that portal flow to the caval vein, as well as hepatic arterial blood flow, doubled after portacaval shunt formation.[35] Hepatic arterial blood flow is usually increased after portacaval shunt formation in patients rated class A, according to Child's classification. However, in class B and C patients, hepatic arterial blood flow usually does not increase.[36] Generally speaking, after portacaval shunt formation, patients with increased hepatic arterial blood flow have a better prognosis than patients with no increase in hepatic arterial blood flow.

Total hepatic blood flow usually decreases in this situation, leading to an increase in concentration in the blood of many vasoactive substances that would bypass the liver to a greater extent than before formation of the portacaval shunt. Such substances include vasoactive intestinal polypeptide, glucagon, ferritin, and probably some others. In addition, the decrease in portal pressure is accompanied by a decrease in arterial resistance in the gut and spleen, with a subsequent increase in blood flow through the preportal tissues. An increase in the levels of vasodilating substances and a decrease in vascular resistance in the preportal area lead to a considerable decrease in total peripheral vascular resistance with a subsequent increase in venous return and cardiac output.[37] The chain of events developing after portacaval shunt formation is depicted on Figure 8–7.

**Vasopressin** is a common drug used in an attempt to stop bleeding from esophageal

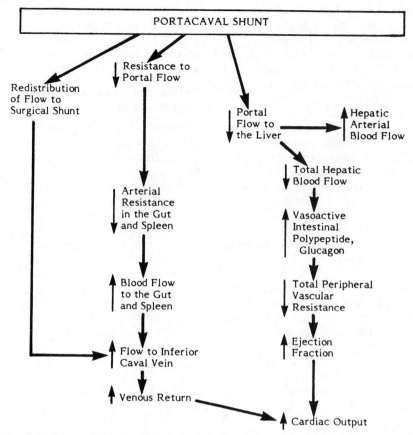

**Figure 8–7.** Schematic representation of cardiovascular consequences of portacaval shunt.

varices in patients with liver cirrhosis and portal hypertension. The beneficial effect of vasopressin in this case is due to preportal vasoconstriction with a subsequent decrease in portal blood flow and portal pressure. Hepatic arterial blood flow during vasopressin infusion is reduced at the very beginning of treatment, but then restores to and usually exceeds baseline values.[38] Vasopressin, however, has some undesirable effects, including coronary vasoconstriction that can sometimes be detrimental. The combination of vasopressin with a vasodilating drug, namely, sodium nitroprusside or nitroglycerin, was demonstrated to be beneficial, producing a slight, further decrease in portal pressure and an increase in hepatic arterial blood flow.[38–40]

**Somatostatin** has not gained as much recognition as vasopressin in the treatment of bleeding from esophageal varices. However, some data clearly demonstrate that somatostatin can be as effective as vasopressin in controlling bleeding.[41] It seems that soma-

tostatin decreases portal blood flow and portal pressure by a substantial reduction in intestinal motility and glucagon activity that results in a decrease in mesenteric blood flow.[42]

**Propranolol** has gained tremendous popularity during recent years as a treatment for the prevention of gastrointestinal bleeding in patients with portal hypertension.[43] Experimental data suggest that propranolol decreases portal pressure by both $beta_1$ and $beta_2$ adrenergic blockade. $Beta_1$ adrenergic blockade leads to a decrease in cardiac output with a subsequent decrease in portal blood flow, while $beta_2$ adrenergic blockade results in splanchnic vasoconstriction.[44] A decrease in azygos blood flow during propranolol treatment was much greater than the decrease in cardiac output, hepatic vein–portal vein pressure gradient, or hepatic blood flow.[45] The specific antirenin activity of propranolol probably plays a certain role in the effectiveness of the drug. The beneficial effect of propranolol can also be attributed partially to a decrease in anxiety, resulting in a decreased level of alcohol abuse. Adverse effects of propranolol treatment include a decrease in the efficacy of diuretic therapy, an increase in ammonia concentration in blood with signs of encephalopathy, sometimes observed hypoglycemia, and decreased clearance of other drugs. If propranolol treatment is terminated, a severe withdrawal syndrome may develop, resulting in gastrointestinal bleeding. As Conn stated, "Once treatment with propranolol is begun, it is a lifetime sentence."[46]

## Pharmacokinetic Implications of Liver Disease

The pharmacokinetics of many drugs are altered in patients with liver disease. There are three primary factors that may be involved in these alterations. First, reduction in hepatic blood flow considerably decreases clearance and prolongs the half-life of drugs and compounds with a high hepatic extraction ratio. Second, reduction in hepatic intrinsic clearance due to a decrease in hepatocyte enzyme activity also decreases clearance and increases the half-life of drugs with a relatively low extraction ratio. Finally, altered plasma protein binding and changes in volume of distribution often play a substantial role in the pharmacokinetics of many drugs.

The volume of distribution, clearance, and elimination half-life of sodium thiopental are not significantly changed in patients with liver cirrhosis; since thiopental has a low extraction ratio, its clearance is independent of hepatic blood flow.[47] The results of this study indicate that, despite its hepatic-dependent elimination, the risk of prolonged action of thiopental in cirrhotic patients is unlikely. However, the doubled free fraction of thiopental (due to a decrease in albumin concentration in the blood) may enhance the effect of a single dose.[47]

The volume of distribution of morphine is not changed significantly, but clearance is decreased and the elimination half-life is prolonged considerably: Elimination half-life is seven times longer in cirrhotic patients than in healthy controls.[48] The volume of distribution, elimination half-life, and clearance of fentanyl are approximately similar in patients with and without liver cirrhosis.[49] The pharmacokinetic differences between morphine and fentanyl can be attributed to the extrahepatic ways of fentanyl elimination.[49] Al-

fentanil, however, may exert a prolonged and pronounced effect in patients with liver cirrhosis because of low clearance and a large free fraction of the drug.[50]

A decreased plasma level of pseudocholinesterase has been observed in patients receiving liver transplants.[51] The level increased toward normal values after transfusion of blood and was normalized when the graft liver became functional. Although the duration of action of succinylcholine and the plasma level of pseudocholinesterase are inversely related,[52] the increased duration of muscle relaxation is not significant during liver transplantation. Decreased response to nondepolarizing relaxants, atracurium, and d-tubocurarine, has been demonstrated in patients with severe hepatic disease.[53,54] It appears that this effect is related to increased binding of the relaxant to globulin. In chronic liver disease, hypoalbuminemia is usually accompanied by hyperglobulinemia. Volume of distribution and elimination half-life of pancuronium are increased, while clearance is reduced in patients with liver cirrhosis.[55]

Detailed information regarding pharmacokinetics of different drugs in patients with liver disease can be found in comprehensive reviews.[56,57]

## Surgical Intervention and Anesthesia in Patients with Liver Disease

Surgical intervention induces certain splanchnic circulatory disturbances. Available data strongly suggest that laparotomy *per se* reduces blood flow through the gut.[58] A study devoted specifically to the role played by anesthesia and surgical intervention separately on the liver circulation has shown that anesthesia alone can be accompanied by different degrees of reduction of liver blood flow. When a surgical procedure is superimposed with anesthesia, liver blood flow is further decreased. The degree of this decrease depends on the specific type of surgical intervention. Minor peripheral procedures are accompanied by a small degree of blood flow reduction, while major procedures, such as upper laparotomy, are associated with a much larger decrease in liver blood flow.[59] Moreover, when standard surgical stress, i.e., laparotomy, was applied under different types of anesthesia, the degree of reduction in splanchnic blood flow varied greatly. The data demonstrate that, first, surgical intervention, rather than anesthesia, is the main determinant of alterations in the splanchnic circulation, and second, that anesthesia can play a modifying role for developing circulatory disturbances during surgical stress. The results of this study were confirmed indirectly by other investigators.[60-63]

Phenobarbital pretreated (liver enzyme–induced) rats anesthetized with halothane developed liver necrosis after laparotomy alone or after laparotomy with ligation of the hepatic artery. Under similar conditions, halothane anesthesia without laparotomy did not lead to liver necrosis.[61] This suggests that laparotomy *per se* was accompanied by a reduction in the liver oxygen supply severe enough to cause liver necrosis.

It has been demonstrated that laparotomy was accompanied by a decrease in portal venous and therefore total liver blood flow, while hepatic arterial blood flow was increased.[60] Apparently unavoidable traction and manipulation on the splanchnic organs play a certain role in the mechanisms of splanchnic circulatory disturbances developing during surgical stress. However, a general biological response to surgical stress seems to be important. It has been shown that laparotomy *per se* causes marked mesenteric vasoconstriction and reduction in gastrointestinal blood flow, which could be abolished by hypophysectomy.[64] The results of this study indicate that both the renin-angiotensin system and antidiuretic hormone play important roles in the control of the mesenteric vascular resistance during laparotomy. Catecholamine release, which almost always accompanies surgery, also plays a notable role in decreasing splanchnic blood volume and flow.[65,66] It is important to realize that splanchnic circulatory disturbances can affect systemic hemodynamics and reduce clearance of drugs and hormones with high hepatic extraction ratios.[56]

Liver function apparently is compromised when splanchnic blood flow is reduced; it has been shown that major surgery was associated with a significant increase in the concentration of liver enzymes. The degree of increase was similar, regardless of the anesthesia provided. This increase was not observed when the same kind of anesthesia was provided during minor surgery.[62,63] Other studies have also demonstrated that postoperative liver dysfunction is mainly due to

the operation *per se* rather than to a chosen anesthetic technique.[62,67-69]

Thus, as we have seen, laparotomy does induce certain changes in liver circulation and function, but usually without detrimental consequences. However, in patients with severe liver disease, laparotomy *per se* might be extremely risky. In the 1960's the mortality from laparotomy alone in patients with acute hepatitis was approaching 10 per cent.[70] During the last 20 years the situation has not improved significantly: Powell-Jackson et al.[71] reported 31 per cent mortality within one month after laparotomy in 36 patients with hepatitis.

In conclusion, it appears that hepatic injury resulting from a combination of surgery and anesthesia has various reasons and degrees (Table 8–1). Hepatic oxygen deprivation due to respiratory and/or circulatory depression, including a decrease in cardiac output, blood pressure, and hepatic blood flow, is one of the most frequent causes of postoperative liver dysfunction. The possibility of accumulation of free radicals and other toxic intermediates, as a result of the reductive metabolism of halothane in hypoxic conditions, also cannot be excluded.[72,73] Often the degree of these alterations is relatively mild, but sometimes it can lead to liver necrosis with subsequent hepatic failure. Some patients can have surgery dur-

### TABLE 8–1. Postoperative Liver Dysfunction

A. Hepatic $O_2$ deprivation
   1. hypoxia
   2. ↓ BP and ↓ CO
   3. ↓ HBF
B. Viral hepatitis, acute
C. Aggravated chronic hepatitis
   1. Immunity depression by anesthesia and/or surgery
   2. Respiratory/circulatory depression resulting in liver hypoxia
   3. Deteriorated hepatic artery blood flow autoregulation
   4. Relative overdose (altered pharmacokinetics)
D. Fulminant hepatitis with specific halothane-related antibodies
E. Free radicals produced by reductive metabolism of halothane
F. Specific drug therapy
G. Blood transfusion
H. Infection

ing the incubation period for acute viral hepatitis.[74–76] Surgery and anesthesia can aggravate chronic hepatitis. There is a very rare possibility for fulminant hepatitis with specific halothane-related antibodies to occur.[77,78]

## HISTORY OF LIVER TRANSPLANTATION

The first hepatic transplantation was a form of heterotopic (auxiliary) transplantation performed in dogs by Welch and associates in 1955; they reported that the donor liver was functional.[79,80] Studies by Moore and associates[81] and Starzl and colleagues[82] followed. In these early years of liver transplantation, heterotopic liver transplantation seemed attractive. The first such procedure in a human was reported by Absolon et al. in 1965.[83] The removal of the native liver was thought unnecessary. It was thought the graft liver placed in the paravetebral gutter or in the pelvis would provide extra hepatic function, and the surgical procedure would be easier than orthotopic liver transplantation. However, the auxiliary liver graft frequently did not receive portal venous blood and had less than optimal biliary drainage and hepatic

blood inflow and outflow, so it atrophied rapidly. Heterotopic liver transplantation was successfully performed in patients by Fortner et al. in 1973;[84] they supplied splanchnic blood to the homograft (Fig. 8–8) Although favorable results were obtained, auxiliary liver transplantation would be beneficial only for patients with potentially reversible liver disease when the objective is temporary life support during which the native liver can recover.[85] It may be theoretically advantageous in certain patients in whom orthotopic liver transplantation would pose a great surgical risk, in patients with thrombosis of the portal vein in the hepatic hilum, or in patients with previous extensive surgery in the right upper quadrant.[86]

The first successful orthotopic homotransplantation of the liver in a human was performed in 1963 by Starzl and colleagues,[87] followed by Moore et al. in Boston[88] and Demirleau and associates in Paris.[89] Most clinical experience since then has been obtained by Starzl's group in Pittsburgh and by Calne's group in Cambridge. Despite wide experience in centers in Denver and then in Pittsburgh and Cambridge, liver transplantation was considered experimental until recently. Major obstacles in liver transplanta-

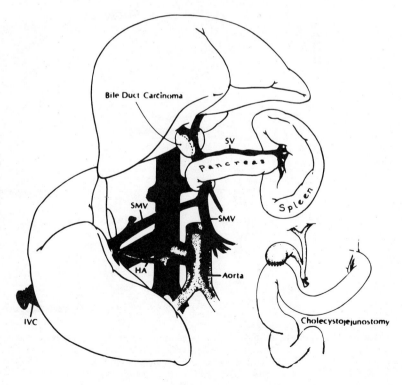

**Figure 8–8.** Heterotopic (auxiliary) hepatic transplantation. HA = hepatic artery; IVC = inferior vena cava; SMV = superior mesenteric vein; SV = splenic vein. (From Fortner JG, et al: Clinical liver heterotopic (auxiliary) transplantation. Surgery 74:740, 1973, with permission.)

tion were difficulty in the surgical technique and poor outcome. Although orthotopic liver transplantation seems simple in principle, its execution has been extremely complicated by the poor physical condition of recipients and massive bleeding caused by the abnormal vascularization and defects in the coagulation system. Also, patients have often had previous intra-abdominal surgery, which further complicates liver transplantation. Other factors include difficulty in preserving the graft organ, low survival and high morbidity rates, and the enormous economic burden of the procedure.[86] Initially, hepatectomy required cross-clamping of the portal vein, inferior vena cava, and hepatic artery, following revascularization of the graft liver. However, the procedure was complicated by cardiovascular instability due to decreased venous return and surgical bleeding associated with the persistent portal hypertension. Calne and associates introduced a partial cardiopulmonary bypass to improve venous return during cross-clamping of the major vessels.[90] They used a femorofemoral bypass with a pump-oxygenator, which collected blood from the inferior vena cava through the femoral vein and returned it to the femoral artery (Fig. 8–9). The aortic pressure could be maintained, preserving vital organ perfusion and reducing the strain on the myocardium, while acidosis and hypothermia could be reduced. In addition, the bypass could autotransfuse blood by recirculating blood aspirated from the hepatic fossa during the vascularization of the graft liver. However, the necessary systemic heparinization impaired the coagulation system, and uncontrollable bleeding occurred. Starzl and associates in Pittsburgh introduced a venous bypass system (the femoral and portal veins to the axillary vein) using a cardiopulmonary bypass apparatus with a roller head pump and cardiotomy reservoir after systemic heparinization. This technique was also complicated by coagulopathy and had to be abandoned.[91] In 1983, Griffith and associates introduced a venovenous bypass system that uses a centrifugal force pump and heparin-bound Gott aneurysm shunt without systemic

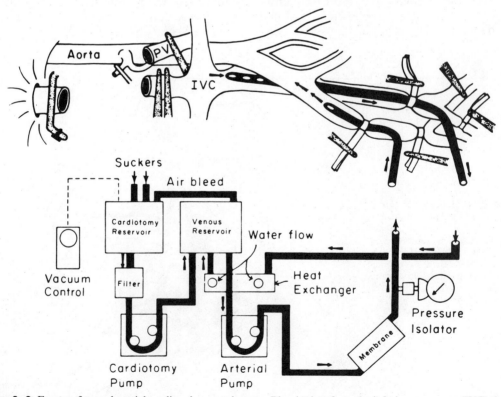

**Figure 8–9.** Femoro-femoral partial cardiopulmonary bypass. Blood taken from the inferior vena cava (IVC) through the right common femoral vein is oxygenated, warmed, and pumped into the right common femoral artery. PV = portal vein. (From Wheeldon DR, et al: Liver Transplantation: The Cambridge–King's College Hospital Experience. New York, Grune & Stratton, 1983, p 145, with permission.)

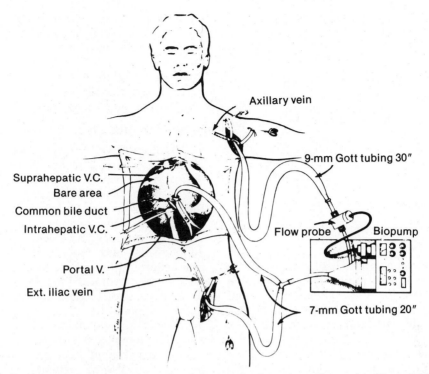

**Figure 8–10.** Veno-venous bypass (the femoral and the portal vein to the axillary vein). (From Griffith BP, et al: Veno-venous bypass without systemic anticoagulation for transplantation of the human liver. Surg Gynecol Obstet 160:270, 1985, by permission of Surgery, Gynecology & Obstetrics.)

heparinization[92] Fig. 8–10. The system decreased surgical blood loss, minimized physiological insult in the recipient, and simplified surgery.[91] Their bypass technique is now the most commonly used for adult and for some pediatric patients in the United States.

In addition to advances in surgical technique, improvements in understanding of rejection phenomena, immunosuppression therapy, intraoperative and postoperative medical management, understanding and control of the coagulation system, and management of infection have made the procedure manageable. Many centers have developed liver transplantation programs, and experience world wide has accumulated to more than 1000 recipients with a five-year survival rate, as high as 62.8 per cent in a Pittsburgh series.[93]

## PROCUREMENT AND SURGICAL PROCEDURE

### Procurement

Preparation of the donor organ begins with the identification of a possible donor, legally supported by The Uniform Anatomical Gift Act. The potential organ donor should be pronounced dead before the procurement process begins, according to the criteria of the individual hospital. Once a donor has been identified, information regarding availability of the donor organ, blood type, weight, age, and gender is reported to the 24-ALERT computer system of the North American Transplant Coordinators Organization (NATCO), and the most suitable recipient is located, while attempts are made to coordinate ethical and medicolegal requirements.[94] Recently, the number of organ donors has increased to 2500 per year,[95] although 0.7 to 3.5 per cent of the in-hospital deaths occurring could yield 7000 to 35,000 potential donor organs for transplantation each year.[96] The identified donor is assessed according to the general criteria listed in Table 8–2.

### Donor Hepatectomy

The surgical procedure for the donor liver has been described by Starzl and associates.[85] A midline incision is made from the suprasternal notch to the pubis, and the sternum is split. The aorta is dissected for cross-

**TABLE 8–2. Criteria for an Acceptable Liver Donor**

Age between 2 months and 40 years
No untreated systemic infection
No history of malignant neoplasms other than primary
 brain tumors
No prolonged ischemia or hypothermia
No history of hepatobiliary disease or severe trauma
Acceptable laboratory test results:
  SGPT, SGOT, total and direct bilirubin
  Prothrombin time, activated partial thromboplastin
   time
  Platelet count
Compatible size and ABO blood type with available
 recipient

clamping at a level that will allow intra-aortic infusion of cold solution into the organ to be removed. The liver is skeletonized and flushed with 1 to 2 L of cold lactated Ringer's solution via the aorta and the portal vein. The liver is then removed, and the liver's vascular tree is flushed with either cold electrolyte solution of intracellular composition (Euro-Collins' solution)[97] or hypothermic plasma solution.[98] Both solutions yield similar results. The liver is then placed in a plastic bag, which is suspended in slushed ice for transportation. A continuous perfusion technique using different perfusates was attempted, but the complexity of the technique and its failure to improve results have made a simple hypothermic storage technique the most popular for preservation. If the cardiovascular system of the donor is unstable or if the donor has suffered cardiac arrest, the organ can be removed swiftly by cross-clamping the aorta near the diaphragm and infusing the cold solution via the celiac axis and the portal vein. The liver is very sensitive to warm ischemia and has a relatively large tissue mass with double blood supply. Therefore, rapid cooling of the donor liver is essential to minimize ischemic injury. The limit of safe cold ischemia time for a donor liver is arbitrarily set at 10 hours, although efforts are made to keep the ischemia time as low as possible. The surgical technique for multiorgan procurement has been well described by Starzl et al.[99]

### Recipient Matching

Many patients awaiting orthotopic liver transplantation are viable candidates for only a brief period, and highly discriminative selection of donors is not practical. Fortunately the hyperacute rejection seen in renal trans-

plantation is not seen in liver transplantation.[86] Transplantation of livers to recipients whose serum contained cytotoxic antigraft antibodies did not cause serious rejection of the grafts. Therefore, transplantation is often performed across the ABO blood group barriers without significant ill effects.[100]

### Indications for Liver Transplantation

Orthotopic liver transplantation can benefit all patients with irreversible liver disease, although the benefit is doubtful for patients with primary hepatic malignant disease or in the terminal phase of advanced liver failure. Liver transplant recipients undergo very stressful surgery and chronic immunosuppression, and patients should meet certain criteria, although none of the contraindications is absolute.[85] Pre-existing systemic or local infections would not allow long-term immunosuppression. Patients older than 50 years may not withstand the surgical stress and the intensive immunosuppression; postoperative complications are more frequent and severe in older patients. However, recent improvements in the transplantation program have allowed successful surgery in patients older than 60, and chronological age may no longer be a barrier to liver transplantation. Patients with coexisting disease in organs other than the liver, such as severe cardiac disease, pulmonary disease, or renal disease, or patients with a history of sociopathic behavior may not be suitable candidates. Although organ dysfunction secondary to liver disease may not be a contraindication to surgery, it is difficult to differentiate whether the disease is primary or secondary to the liver disease in origin. Shaw and colleagues assessed risk factors in a series of 160 patients who underwent orthotopic liver transplantation, using a scoring system designed to distinguish high-risk from low-risk patients.[101] Primary indications for orthotopic liver transplantation are summarized in Table 8–3.

### Surgical Procedure for Recipients

The patient is placed on a padded operating table with arms abducted, and prepared for operation with antiseptic solution from the clavicle to upper thigh, including both axillary areas. The abdominal cavity is entered, the liver is isolated, and adhesions caused by previous surgery are dissected. The hilum is located and the liver is dearterialized. During the hilar dissection, the bile duct is tran-

**TABLE 8–3.    Indications for Primary Liver Transplantation Performed
Between March 1963 and December 1984**

| | Number of Patients | | |
|---|---|---|---|
| **Liver Disease** | Mar. 1963–Feb. 1980 | Mar. 1980–Dec. 1984 | Total |
| Biliary atresia | 50 | 72 | 122 |
| Cirrhosis | 61 | 70 | 131 |
| Inborn errors of metabolism* | 17 | 43 | 60 |
| Primary biliary cirrhosis | 6 | 39 | 45 |
| Sclerosing cholangitis | 7 | 30 | 37 |
| Primary liver tumor | 20 | 10 | 30 |
| Secondary biliary cirrhosis | 4 | 8 | 12 |
| Familial cholestasis | 0 | 9 | 9 |
| Budd-Chiari syndrome | 1 | 6 | 7 |
| Acute liver necrosis | 1 | 5 | 6 |
| Neonatal hepatitis | 1 | 4 | 5 |
| Hepatic fibrosis | 2 | 1 | 3 |
| Hepatic adenoma | 0 | 2 | 2 |
| Polycystic disease | 0 | 1 | 1 |
| Miscellaneous | 0 | 7 | 7 |
| Total | 170 | 307 | 477 |

* Inborn errors of metabolism include alpha$_1$-antitrypsin deficiency, Wilson's disease, tyrosinemia, glycogen storage disease, hemochromatosis, and hypercholesterolemia. Adapted from Gordon R, et al: Indications for liver transplantation in the cyclosporine era. Surg Clin North Am. In press.

sected as high as possible. The infrahepatic inferior vena cava is encircled, and the left triangular and falciform ligaments are incised until the suprahepatic inferior vena cava has been identified and encircled. The portal vein is isolated and encircled. Hepatectomy can be performed after occlusion of the suprahepatic and infrahepatic inferior vena cava, the portal vein, and the hepatic artery. When unheparinized venovenous bypass is used, the axillary vein is identified and cannulated. Cannulas are inserted in the femoral vein and the portal vein. These cannulas are connected to the centrifugal bypass system, and the blood drained from the two vessels is diverted to the axillary vein. Once the bypass system has been established the diseased liver is removed.[92]

The first vascular anastomosis is made in the suprahepatic vena cava. As the infrahepatic vena caval anastomosis is constructed, a slow infusion of electrolyte solution is continued through the portal vein. The infusion flushes preservative solution of intracellular composition and air bubbles out of the vascular tree of the donor liver. The completed portal venous anastomosis is followed by the reperfusion of the graft liver by unclamping of the suprahepatic and infrahepatic inferior vena cava and the portal vein to minimize the

warm ischemia time. Once major vascular hemostasis has been obtained, the hepatic artery is anastomosed by a microvascular surgical technique. When the surgery is performed with venovenous bypass, the portal venous cannula is removed during the portal anastomosis. Bypass is discontinued after reperfusion of the graft liver but before anastomosis of the hepatic artery. Upon completion of the hepatic arterial anastomosis, the patient is allowed to recover from hypothermia, coagulopathy, and the altered physiological condition. The biliary reconstruction is performed mainly by duct-to-duct reconstruction (choledochocholedochostomy), although choledochojejunostomy to a Roux-en-Y limb is used for patients whose biliary anatomy is altered (Fig. 8–11). Patency of the biliary tree is confirmed by intraoperative cholangiography before the completion of surgery.

## ANESTHETIC CARE OF THE ORGAN DONOR

Once a potential organ donor has been identified, it must be established that criteria for brain death are met. If the donor must be transported to another hospital for procurement of the organ, it is mandatory that the

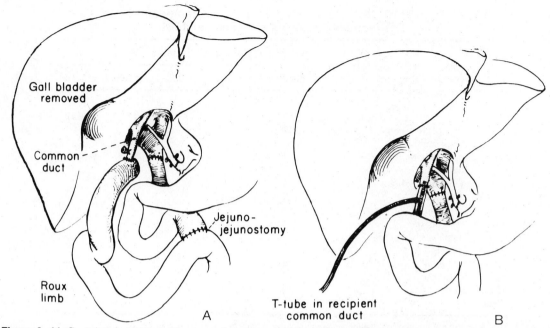

**Figure 8–11.** Completed orthotopic liver transplantation. *A*, Biliary tract reconstruction with choledochojejunostomy, using Roux limb. *B*, Biliary reconstruction with choledochocholedochostomy. (From Starzl TE, et al: Orthotopic liver transplantation in ninety-three patients. Surg Gynecol Obstet 142:491, 1976, by permission of Surgery, Gynecology & Obstetrics.)

criteria for brain death of the second hospital are met. Maintaining optimal oxygenation and organ perfusion is the major goal in donor management. The monitoring and medications required for donor anesthesia are listed in Table 8–4. ECG, arterial blood pressure, and central venous pressure are monitored throughout the procurement procedure. Because donors are already mechanically ventilated, anesthetic care is primarily to provide optimal conditions for the surgeons and to

### TABLE 8–4. Preparation for Donor Anesthesia

1. Proper medical and legal documentation for procurement of organ
2. Monitoring
   ECG, arterial blood pressure, central venous pressure, urine volume, body temperature
4. Laboratory tests
   Arterial blood gas tensions and acid-base state, hematocrit, serum electrolytes
5. Others
   Warming blanket, steroids, antibiotics, vasodilators, vasopressors, diuretics, mannitol, Pitressin, heparin, solutions (crystalloid and colloid), blood

maintain physiological conditions to avoid ischemia and acidosis of the donor organ. Therefore, muscle relaxants may be used to facilitate surgery. Although donors are brain dead, a pressor response to nociceptive stimuli occurs frequently,[102] and inhalation anesthetics can be added to correct the increased sympathetic response.

Victims of brain death have complete loss of brain stem function and are dependent on mechanical ventilation. Pulmonary function may be impaired by pulmonary complications secondary to prolonged ventilatory support, trauma, aspiration of gastric contents, and/or cardiovascular instability. Optimal ventilatory support often necessitates the use of a high $F_{IO_2}$ to maintain adequate arterial oxygenation. Arterial blood gas tensions and acid-base state are monitored frequently and corrected to normal levels. Intravascular volume is often decreased by decreased secretion of antidiuretic hormone, hemorrhage, diuretic therapy, inadequate hydration, or loss of vasomotor tone. To maintain perfusion of the donor organ, arterial blood pressure is kept above the critical level (systolic pressure greater than 100 mm Hg and mean arterial blood pressure greater than 70 mm Hg) by expanding blood volume with crystalloid or colloid solution to maintain central venous pressure at 6 to 10 cm $H_2O$. Blood transfusion is often required to keep hematocrit greater than 30 per cent. Only when volume expansion does not stabilize the cardiovascular system are vasopressors administered. Alpha vasopressors are discouraged to avoid vasoconstriction of the splanchnic vessels. Infusion of dopamine (less than 15 $\mu g \cdot kg^{-1} \cdot min^{-1}$) maintains perfusion pressure with minimal impairment of organ perfusion. Urine volume and serum electrolyte levels are monitored. Excessive urine output (more than 1 $L \cdot hr^{-1}$) resulting from decreased secretion of the antidiuretic hormone may be controlled by intravenous infusion of vasopressin (Pitressin—50 units in 500 ml). The body temperature should be kept above 34°C to maintain cardiac stability.

## ANESTHETIC MANAGEMENT OF THE RECIPIENT

### Preoperative Assessment of the Recipients

Patients for liver transplantation present a wide spectrum of pathophysiological changes. The patient with a primary hepatoma may be fairly healthy with well-preserved hepatic function, whereas the patient with postnecrotic cirrhosis may have multiple organ disease and very poor hepatic function. The characteristic multiple organ involvement of end-stage liver disease mandates thorough preoperative assessment of the transplant recipient, which can be done ideally in two phases. First, patients are assessed when they are admitted for their initial screening as a transplantation candidate. A thorough examination of all organ systems is routine at this time, and the urgency of surgery may preclude a lengthy assessment immediately prior to surgery. If the patient has correctable disease, attempts can be made to optimize his or her condition. Patients with severely abnormal cardiopulmonary function should be discouraged from undergoing surgery, because this condition greatly increases surgical morbidity and mortality. Nevertheless, liver transplantation may be the only chance the patient has to survive.

The decision for candidacy should be made after all physicians involved in the patient's care, including anesthesiologists, have weighed the benefits and risks of surgery.

The patient and family should be informed of anesthetic care, postoperative care, and the risk of anesthesia and surgery at this time. A second visit may be made before surgery when a donor organ has been located for the patient. The information obtained from the previous visit is compared with the current physical status. All consent forms should be reviewed, and frequently the consent of both the recipient and the family is required because of the questionable mental status of the recipient.

Generally, light premedication is recommended because of poor physical status and encephalopathy. Since gastric emptying time is frequently prolonged, an antacid may be included in the premedication, especially when the recipient has had recent oral intake. Pathophysiological changes that frequently occur in recipients are described below.

**Cardiopulmonary System.** The pathophysiological consequences of advanced liver disease are discussed earlier in this chapter. The evaluation of the degrees of cardiopulmonary, hepatic, renal, and other dysfunctions is mandatory. For example, the preoperative physiological variables measured in 12 liver transplant candidates are shown in Table 8–5.

Minimally, the preoperative evaluation of the cardiopulmonary system should include

**TABLE 8–5. Cardiopulmonary Variables Measured in 12 Patients with Chronic End-Stage Liver Disease**

| Variable | Value (Mean ± SE) |
| --- | --- |
| Cardiac index | 4.9 ± 0.3 L/min/sq m |
| Mean arterial pressure | 78 ± 5 mm Hg |
| Central venous pressure | 6 ± 1 mm Hg |
| Mean pulmonary arterial pressure | 14 ± 2 mm Hg |
| Left ventricular stroke work | 51 ± 3 gm/sq m |
| Systemic vascular resistance index | 408 ± 32 dynes/sec/ cm$^{-5}$/sq m |
| Pulmonary vascular resistance index | 28 ± 6 dynes/sec/ cm$^{-5}$/sq m |
| Pa$_{CO_2}$ | 32 ± 1 mm Hg |
| pH | 7.44 ± 0.2 |
| A–a gradient | 24 ± 5 mm Hg |
| Oxygen transport | 1080 ± 74 ml/min |
| Oxygen consumption | 122 ml/min |
| Hemoglobin | 10.0 ± 0.5 gm/dl |

From Martin DJ, et al: Unpublished data. By permission of Dr. DJ Martin.

history, physical examination, ECG, chest roentgenogram, and arterial blood gas analysis. Further investigation is required to rule out any suspected serious cardiac dysfunction. If the cardiac output is less than normal, cardiovascular instability during surgery can be anticipated. Pulmonary function tests are helpful in patients with questionable pulmonary function.

**Renal System.** Renal dysfunction is common in patients with end-stage liver disease. Poor renal function of hepatic origin can be improved by successful liver transplantation and is not a contraindication to surgery. Laboratory measurements for differential diagnosis of impaired renal function in patients with liver disease are listed in Table 8–6. The preoperative evaluation should include urine output, urinalysis, creatinine clearance test, and determination of blood urea nitrogen, creatinine, and serum electrolyte levels.

**Fluid and Electrolyte Balance.** Hyponatremia often observed in patients scheduled for liver transplantation is usually not corrected in the immediate preoperative period. Intraoperative transfusion of fresh frozen plasma, sodium bicarbonate, and crystalloid solutions would provide needed sodium load.

A serum potassium level of less than 3 $mEq \cdot L^{-1}$ is not uncommon in patients with liver disease. In most patients, total body potassium is reduced even in the absence of hypokalemia, and the magnitude of the decrease is related to the severity of hepatic dysfunction.[103] Patients have been anesthetized for hepatic transplantation without immediate preoperative correction of hypokalemia because of the urgency of surgery and lack of response to supplementation therapy. In addition, intraoperative ill effects of hypokalemia have not occurred, while lethal

levels of hyperkalemia have occurred on reperfusion of the graft liver.[104] Hyperkalemia is seen in patients with moderate to severe renal disease, and every effort should be made preoperatively to reduce the serum potassium by dialysis or by administration of cation-exchange resins.

Preoperative reduction in the level of ionized calcium is sometimes seen, especially after transfusion of multiple units of blood products, and it is correctable by administration of calcium chloride. Although hyperphosphatemia and hypomagnesemia are seen in these patients, the clinical effects of these abnormalities are relatively minor.

**Central Nervous System.** Hepatic encephalopathy is common in patients with severe liver disease. The pathophysiology is discussed earlier. The severity of hepatic encephalopathy ranges from altered mental state to deep coma and generalized convulsions (Table 8–7). When the degree of central nervous system dysfunction is being evaluated, it is important to remember that close to 50 per cent of autopsied patients after fulminant hepatic failure showed signs of cerebral edema,[105] which necessitates precautions not to increase intracranial pressure. Unsuspected chronic subdural hemorrhage was also seen,[106] suggesting that recent changes in neurological signs or mental status should not be automatically assumed to be hepatic in origin.

**Blood Coagulation System.** It is not surprising that prothrombin time and activated partial thromboplastin time are prolonged, and levels of all coagulation factors except fibrinogen and factor VIII are decreased preoperatively in patients who receive liver transplants (Table 8–8). Although the fibrinogen level is generally high in patients with

**TABLE 8–6.    Differential Diagnosis of Impaired Renal Function in Patients with Liver Disease**

|  | Prerenal | Hepatorenal | Acute Renal Failure |
|---|---|---|---|
| Urine sodium concentration | $<10 \ mEq \cdot L^{-1}$ | $<10 \ mEq \cdot L^{-1}$ | $> 30 \ mEq \cdot L^{-1}$ |
| Urine-to-plasma–creatinine ratio | $>30:1$ | $>30:1$ | $<20:1$ |
| Urine osmolality | At least 100 mOsm > plasma Osm | At least 100 mOsm > plasma Osm | Equal to plasma osmolality |
| Urinary sediment | Normal | Unremarkable | Casts, cell debris |

From Epstein M: Renal functional abnormalities in cirrhosis: Pathophysiology and management. In Zakim D, Boyer TD (eds): Hepatology. Philadelphia, WB Saunders Company, 1982, p 460.

**TABLE 8–7. Staging of Neurological Signs of Hepatic Encephalopathy**

| Clinical Signs | Asterixis |
| --- | --- |
| Stage 1 | |
| Exaggerated behavior pattern, changes in personality, euphoria, agitation, subtle confusion, slowing of intellect, poor computation, sleep rhythm reversal, impaired handwriting | Uncommon |
| Stage 2 | |
| Inappropriate behavior, gross mental confusion, slow responses, drowsiness, speech disorder, poor memory, lethargy | Usually present |
| Stage 3 | |
| Increasing obtundation, sleeping most of the time, obvious confusion, somnolence, stupor, delirium | Present |
| Stage 4 | |
| Comatose, may respond to pain, decerebrate posture | Inability to elicit |

liver disease, dysfibrinogenemia is known to occur, evidenced by moderately prolonged thrombin time and reptilase time. The clinical significance of the acquired dysfibrinogenemia in patients receiving liver transplants is not known. Factor VIII level increases from increased production related to a stress response, release from damaged cells, or impaired catabolism of Factor VIII.[107] Platelet count is generally low owing to sequestration secondary to hypersplenism. In addition, abnormal platelet function may be related to a preponderance of small, hypofunctional platelets.[108] Fibrinolytic activity is increased, presumably because of defective synthesis of fibrinolytic inhibitors or delayed removal of plasminogen activators. Fibrin degradation products are positive in one third of recipients and euglobulin lysis time is not infrequently less than one hour. The role of disseminated intravascular coagulation is controversial. A patient with chronic liver disease may have a defective vascular phase of hemostasis, although it is not well understood. In addition, frequent upper gastrointestinal tract bleeding from esophageal varices requires multiple preoperative transfusions, and dilutional coagulopathy may occur. The preoperative coagulation profile is scored by disease group and the score compared with the blood products used during liver transplantation.[109] More blood

products were transfused in patients with postnecrotic cirrhosis, sclerosing cholangitis, and acute fulminant hepatitis, and the degree of hepatocellular damage appeared to be associated with the blood transfusion volume.

Thus a complete preoperative coagulation profile is very useful for assessing the coagulation system and anticipating the magnitude of intraoperative blood transfusion. Preoperative correction of the coagulation system may seem to be beneficial for intraoperative management, but it is not practical. Candidates for transplantation are given vitamin K, but this does not always improve coagulation. Patients may be given blood products preoperatively. However, the transfused blood products may be destroyed or may not function in the presence of the diseased liver. The urgency of surgery may not allow preparation time, and exchange transfusion in the absence of hemodynamic monitoring may interfere with cardiopulmonary performance. Therefore, correction of the coagulation system is best accomplished intraoperatively.

Anemia (hematocrit less than 30 per cent) is seen frequently. It may be microcytic hypochromic anemia due to gastrointestinal bleeding or macrocytic anemia from folic acid deficiency.

Blood glucose concentration should be determined preoperatively and hypoglycemia or hyperglycemia appropriately corrected.

The preoperative evaluation of hepatic function *per se* should include the possibility of transmission of hepatitis. Screening should be done for the hepatitis antigen and antibody to protect other surgical patients and health care personnel. Precautions should be taken not to be contaminated by hepatitis (see Appendix A), and all patients with a history of hepatitis are regarded infective unless the absence of antigenemia is proven.

## Monitoring and Preparation

**Monitoring.** Aggressive monitoring and proper interpretation of the monitored variables are essential for the successful conclusion of surgery and uneventful recovery. The cardiovascular system is monitored by ECG, radial arterial pressure, central venous pressure, pulmonary arterial pressure, and cardiac output determination by thermodilution technique. On-line constant monitoring of mixed-venous oxygen saturation of hemoglo-

**TABLE 8–8. Preoperative Coagulation Profile of 63 Liver Transplantation Patients (Mean ± SD)**

| Variables | Normal Range | Neoplasm | Primary Biliary Cirrhosis | Postnecrotic Cirrhosis | Sclerosing Cholangitis | Miscellaneous Disease | Retransplant | All patients |
|---|---|---|---|---|---|---|---|---|
| Number of patients | | 9 | 13 | 11 | 6 | 9 | 15 | 63 |
| PT (sec) | 10.8–13.0 | 13.3 ± 4.0 | 13.9 ± 1.7 | 15.7 ± 1.4 | 13.3 ± 3.6 | 18.9 ± 5.4 | 13.2 ± 1.5 | 14.8 ± 3.7 |
| aPTT (sec) | 26–34 | 34.1 ± 6.3 | 41.0 ± 8.7 | 40.2 ± 4.1 | 42.4 ± 10.1 | 46.7 ± 10.6 | 41.7 ± 14.2 | 41.5 ± 13.9 |
| Platelets (1000/mm$^3$) | 150–450 | 245 ± 151 | 181 ± 199 | 162 ± 178 | 86 ± 19 | 82 ± 64 | 116 ± 115 | 147 ± 144 |
| Fibrinogen (mg %) | 150–450 | 323 ± 166 | 382 ± 116 | 247 ± 134 | 238 ± 44 | 167 ± 86 | 301 ± 149 | 292 ± 138 |
| Factor V (U/ml) | 0.5–1.5 | 0.82 ± 0.41 | 0.54 ± 0.27 | 0.35 ± 0.12 | 0.47 ± 0.20 | 0.28 ± 0.23 | 0.66 ± 0.29 | 0.53 ± 0.32 |
| Factor VII (U/ml) | 0.5–1.5 | 0.56 ± 0.25 | 0.83 ± 0.35 | 0.35 ± 0.25 | 0.71 ± 0.49 | 0.28 ± 0.24 | 0.53 ± 0.26 | 0.57 ± 0.39 |
| Factor VIII (U/ml) | 0.5–1.5 | 1.42 ± 0.33 | 2.03 ± 0.73 | 1.82 ± 0.93 | 2.53 ± 1.30 | 2.30 ± 0.70 | 1.92 ± 1.35 | 2.00 ± 0.90 |
| ELT (min) | >300 | 218 ± 48 | 215 ± 77 | 163 ± 87 | 218 ± 67 | 132 ± 68 | 247 ± 86 | 202 ± 81 |

From Kang YG, Martin DJ, Marquez J, et al: Intraoperative changes in blood coagulation and thromboelastographic monitoring in liver transplantation. Anesth Analg 64:892, 1985, with permission of the publisher.

bin has been extremely helpful in determining cardiovascular performance. Monitoring also includes serial measurements of arterial blood gas tensions and end-tidal $CO_2$ tension. Hourly measurement of urine output and urine specific gravity aids in assessing renal function. Body temperature is monitored by measuring rectal, esophageal, and blood temperatures. The laboratory determinations needed during surgery are arterial blood gas tensions and acid-base state, hemoglobin, hematocrit, and serum levels of sodium, potassium, ionized calcium, and glucose. These are measured hourly or more frequently, when needed. Finally, the blood coagulation system is evaluated by means of the prothrombin time, activated partial thromboplastin time and platelet count; determination of thrombin time, reptilase time, plasma clot lysis time, levels of Factors I, II, and VIII, fibrin split products, results of the ethanol gel test, and euglobulin lysis time are also helpful. Thromboelastography has been very helpful in assessing the function of the blood coagulation system at the bedside.[110,111]

**Preoperative Preparation.** The equipment and medications found necessary in anesthesia for liver transplantation are shown in Tables 8–9 and 8–10. The anesthesia gas machine is prepared with a compressed air supply to provide an $F_{IO_2}$ of less than 70 per cent during surgery. A volume ventilator is preferable to overcome the high airway pressure that may occur during surgery. To prevent hypovolemia and hypothermia, a rapid-infusion system with a delivery capacity of

**TABLE 8–9.    Equipment Required for Anesthesia and Intraoperative Management of Liver Transplantation**

1. Anesthesia gas machine with compressed air supply
2. Ventilator
3. Inspired-gas humidifier
4. Multiple-channel vital sign monitor and recorder
5. Cardiac output computer (thermodilution)
6. On-line mixed-venous oximetry
7. Mass spectrometer
8. Thromboelastograph
9. Rapid-infusion system
10. Blood pump with blood warmer
11. Autotransfusion system
12. Cardiac defibrillator
13. Warming blanket
14. Liver transplantation supply cart

**TABLE 8–10.    Medications Immediately Accessible for Liver Transplantation**

| Agent* | Amount | |
| --- | --- | --- |
| Thiopental | 1000 mg | (25 mg/ml) |
| Ketamine | 200 mg | (10 mg/ml) |
| Succinylcholine | 200 mg | (20 mg/ml) |
| d-Tubocurarine | 9 mg | (3 mg/ml) |
| Pancuronium | 20 mg | (2 mg/ml) |
| Fentanyl | 500 μg | (50 μg/ml) |
| Lorazepam | 8 mg | (2 mg/ml) |
| Atropine | 1.2 mg | (0.4 mg/ml) |
| Ephedrine | 50 mg | (5 mg/ml) |
| Epinephrine | 100 μg | (10 μg/ml) |
| Dopamine infusion set | 200 mg in 250 ml of saline | |
| Lidocaine | 100 mg | (10 mg/ml) |
| Calcium chloride | 3000 mg | (100 mg/ml) |
| Sodium bicarbonate | 2 ampules | (80 mEq) |
| Insulin (regular) | (in refrigerator) | |
| Dextrose 50% | 50 ml | |
| Cefotaxime | 1 gm | q 4 h |
| Ampicillin | 1 gm | q 4 h |
| Cyclosporine A | 2.5 mg/kg | q 12 h |
| Solu-Medrol | 1 gm | |
| Neosporin ointment | 1 oz | |

* Other necessary medications are available on the liver transplantation anesthesia supply cart.

2 to 3 L/min of prewarmed blood is essential[111,112] (Fig. 8–12). A warming blanket and blood warmers are needed, and the ambient temperature of the operating room should be controllable. A multiple-channel monitor for ECG and pressures monitoring is required, and a recorder helps to follow trends in the hemodynamic status. An autotransfusion system is useful to decrease the complications related to multiple transfusion and the burden on the blood bank. A cardiac defibrillator should be easily accessible.

The blood bank should be notified before surgery and an adequate amount of blood and blood components secured. Ten units of packed red blood cells (RBC) and 10 units of fresh frozen plasma (FFP) inside the operating room at the beginning of surgery is sufficient in most cases. More blood products should be ready in the blood bank for use on demand: RBC, 20 units; FFP, 20 units; platelets, 10 to 20 units; and cryoprecipitate, 12 units. The blood products needed for a specific recipient cannot be predicted, and the blood bank should be prepared to provide 200 units of RBC and FFP within a 12 to 24 hour period. A laboratory facility must be available to process "stat" laboratory tests during

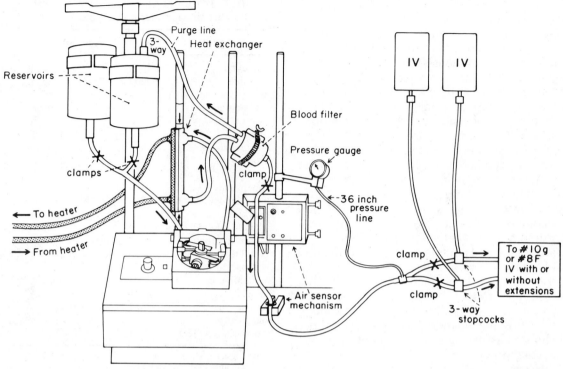

**Figure 8–12.** A rapid infusion system, developed by JJ Sassano, M.D., of the University of Pittsburgh School of Medicine. (From Kang YG, et al: Intraoperative changes in blood coagulation and thromboelastographic monitoring in liver transplantation. Anesth Analg 64:889, 1985.)

surgery. A telephone system inside the operating room is essential for communication with personnel in the blood bank, laboratory, and intensive care unit. Last, but most important, the anesthesiologist should discuss the anesthesia plan with well-prepared residents or nurse anesthetists to achieve well-coordinated, optimal anesthetic care.

**Preparation of the Patient.** The patient is placed on the operating table in the supine position with the arms abducted and the elbows flexed. The patient is positioned properly to prevent stretch injury of the brachial plexus and is well padded, especially at pressure points such as the elbows, heels, and sacrum. ECG electrodes are placed and secured by tape. Since the patient is lightly premedicated, anesthesia can be induced with minimal preparation if the physical status of the patient is acceptable: One radial arterial catheter and one peripheral intravenous catheter are inserted. Generally, two indwelling catheters (20-gauge) are placed in the radial arteries after Allen's test—one for blood pressure monitoring and the other for drawing blood samples and back-up pressure mon-

itoring. Surgery lasts up to 24 hours, and occasionally an intra-arterial catheter fails to monitor blood pressure. A second catheter is very helpful on those occasions, and it is removed at the end of surgery. Unless a normal or hypercoagulable state is demonstrated by thromboelastography, the catheters may be continuously flushed with normal saline without heparin (4 ml/hr) via a flush device to eliminate a heparin effect without untoward effect(s). Patients should be prepared to receive a fluid volume of up to 40 times their blood volume in a period of 12 hours with a rate reaching 1000 to 3000 ml/min. Insertion of two large-bore peripheral intravenous catheters (larger than 12-gauge) is recommended. Generally, two 8.5 French indwelling catheters (introducers for pulmonary arterial catheter) are inserted using the Seldinger technique—one in the antecubital vein contralateral to the axillary vein to be used for venous bypass and the other in the left external jugular or the left internal jugular vein. A flow-directed pulmonary arterial catheter capable of on-line mixed venous oximetry is inserted via the right internal jugular vein and is floated into the pulmonary artery. The subclavian vein is used when the jugular veins are not accessible. A Foley indwelling urinary catheter and esophageal and rectal thermistors are inserted. A precordial stethoscope is replaced with an esophageal stethoscope after the induction of anesthesia. Precaution should be taken not to traumatize esophageal varices while inserting the esophageal stethoscope and nasogastric tube. A Doppler device may be helpful in detecting air emboli, but its application may interfere with surgery. The patient's airway is attached to a mass spectrometer to monitor end-tidal gas tensions. A peripheral nerve stimulator is used to assess the degree of muscle relaxation.

## Intraoperative Anesthetic Management

### Induction and Maintenance of Anesthesia

Most relatively young patients without serious cardiac disease tolerate induction of anesthesia fairly well. All patients are considered to have a full stomach because gastric emptying time is frequently prolonged, urgency of surgery does not allow ample time for gastric emptying, and nausea and vomiting are common side effects of cyclosporine A. Preoxygenation followed by rapid-sequence induction with cricoid pressure, or awake intubation in a patient with a compromised airway, is used in all patients. Ketamine (1 to 2 mg·kg$^{-1}$) is the common induction agent, and thiopental (4 mg·kg$^{-1}$) is used in patients whose cardiovascular system is relatively stable. Succinylcholine is used to facilitate intratracheal intubation and atracurium is used when hyperkalemia is present. The patient is ventilated with a tidal volume of 10 to 15 ml·kg$^{-1}$, and the respiratory rate is adjusted to maintain end-tidal $CO_2$ at 4 to 4.5 per cent, or $Pa_{CO_2}$ of 35 to 40 mm Hg. PEEP (5 cm $H_2O$) is added to the ventilatory circuit and $F_{IO_2}$ is controlled between 50 and 70 per cent.

Nitrous oxide is not recommended for maintenance of anesthesia. Prolonged exposure to nitrous oxide excessively distends bowel loops, making surgical closure of the abdomen difficult. It also depresses cardiovascular function and increases the size of air emboli.[113]

Although all potent inhalation anesthetics have been used to maintain anesthesia,[114] isoflurane is used most frequently. It depresses the cardiovascular system less than other inhalation agents, it is biologically stable compared with other agents, and it has not demonstrated hepatotoxicity in animals or in humans.[115] Halothane undergoes a reductive pathway in the hypoxic condition, producing reactive intermediary metabolites that may be hepatotoxic. Since cold and warm hepatic ischemia is unavoidable, halothane is better avoided. Enflurane may increase inorganic fluoride to a high level during long surgery,[116,117] and it may not be suitable for patients who are likely to develop renal complications. A relatively low concentration of an inhalation anesthetic appears to be sufficient in these patients,[118] although this requires further investigation.

A narcotic is frequently used as a primary agent or as an adjunct to an inhalation agent, along with sedatives such as lorazepam. A short-acting narcotic, fentanyl, is preferred to allow early postoperative neurological assessment. Narcotics are reported to cause choledochoduodenal sphincter spasm occasionally, but it may not be clinically significant.[119] Scopolamine is avoided because it may cause prolonged pupillary dilation. Pancuronium, metacurine, and atracurium have been used safely for muscle relaxation without complication. Maintaining desired levels of drug at the receptors and in plasma may be difficult during surgery with massive blood transfusion. However, the loss of intravenous agents may not be significant if they are highly lipophilic.[120]

### Maintenance of the Physiological State

Maintaining a close to normal physiological state is a major determinant of successful outcome. The primary difficulties encountered during anesthesia for liver transplantation are cardiovascular instability, hypotension, arrhythmias, massive fluid shift, electrolyte imbalance, and coagulopathy. The operation can be divided into three distinct stages, based on the characteristic physiological changes and for the convenience of discussion. Stage 1, the preanhepatic phase, extends from induction of anesthesia to complete dissection of the hepatic vasculature. Stage 2, the anhepatic phase, begins when hepatic circulation is interrupted or when the native liver is removed and ends when the donor liver is reperfused. Stage 3, the postanhepatic phase, is the period between reperfusion of the graft liver and the end of surgery.

**Cardiovascular System.** Cardiac output stays high during the early part of surgery. The major cardiovascular change seen in stage 1 stems from intravascular volume depletion caused by surgical bleeding and by the drainage of large amounts of ascitic fluid. Numerous collateral channels and fragile vessels make surgical hemostasis very difficult. The degree of blood loss depends largely on the severity of hepatic hilar scarring, portal hypertension, and coagulopathy. A blood mixture high in coagulation factors is administered. During the rapid blood loss, cardiac output decreases and hypotension develops. Hypotension is treated initially by volume expansion, followed by administration of calcium chloride when reduction in the level of ionized calcium is observed. Surgical manipulation of the hilum of the liver may compress major vessels, reducing venous return, and unexpected or prolonged hypotension should be reported to the surgical team. If hypotension and decreased cardiac output persist, a vasopressor may be administered. Since peripheral vascular resistance is remarkably low in these patients, phenylephrine would be an appropriate drug, except that it may constrict nutrient vessels and increase the shunt fraction. Dopamine (3 to 10 $\mu g \cdot kg^{-1} \cdot min^{-1}$) is the preferred agent. During the hepatic hilar dissection, compression of the thoracic cavity and irritation of the diaphragm may result in hypotension and arrhythmia. Occasionally, low cardiac output and hypotension in conjunction with increased ventricular filling pressure are seen in the early stage of surgery. A large pleural effusion or pericardial effusion should be sought and drained via thoracentesis or pericardial window. Communication with the surgical team is essential to prevent and treat severe hypovolemia, reactive hypervolemia, arryhthmia, and cardiac tamponade.

The second stage of surgery has been carried out in two different ways. Hepatectomy may be performed after simple occlusion of the inferior vena cava, hepatic artery, and portal vein. With this technique, venous return decreases to as low as 50 per cent, and hypotension develops.[121] The preload can be increased by transfusion before and during cross-clamping of the vessels; calcium chloride or a small dose of vasopressor also may be used at that time, if needed. Cross-clamping of the portal vein aggravates the pre-existing portal hypertension, increasing surgical bleeding. Obstruction of the inferior vena cava decreases perfusion of the kidney, and oliguria and hematuria can be noted. These physiological changes that occur with the occlusion of the major vessels can be eased by using the venovenous bypass system described earlier. Cardiopulmonary profiles of patients who received venovenous bypass are shown in Table 8–11. The bypass did not change heart rate or cardiac filling pressure, although cardiac index decreased and sys-

**TABLE 8–11.  Cardiopulmonary Profiles of 28 Patients Who Received Venovenous Bypass Liver Transplantation (Mean ± SD)**

| Variable | Prebypass | Bypass |
|---|---|---|
| Temperature (°C) | 34.9 ± 0.98 | 33.8 ± 1.16* |
| Heart rate (bpm) | 85.6 ± 14.3 | 84.1 ± 14.2 |
| MAP (mm Hg) | 75.0 ± 17.1 | 83.0 ± 17.6 |
| PAO (mm Hg) | 12.0 ± 4.2 | 10.5 ± 3.3 |
| CVP (mm Hg) | 9.9 ± 4.4 | 9.2 ± 4.9 |
| Cardiac index ($L \cdot min^{-1} \cdot m^{-2}$) | 4.37 ± 1.44 | 3.44 ± 1.09* |
| Systemic vascular resistance index ($dynes \cdot sec \cdot cm^{-5} \cdot m^{-2}$) | 443.7 ± 233 | 660 ± 366* |
| Pulmonary vascular resistance index ($dynes \cdot sec \cdot cm^{-5} \cdot m^{-2}$) | 34.3 ± 23.9 | 44.1 ± 39.1 |
| pH | 7.42 ± 0.07 | 7.40 ± 0.08 |
| Pa$_{O_2}$ (mm Hg) | 380 ± 92.4 | 398 ± 91.6 |
| Pa$_{CO_2}$ (mm Hg) | 33.3 ± 5.2 | 29.9 ± 4.8* |

* $p < 0.05$
Adapted from Shaw BW Jr, Martin DJ, Marquez JM, et al: Venous bypass in clinical liver transplantation. Ann Surg 200:526, 1984.

temic vascular resistance increased. The authors attributed the decrease in cardiac index to the decrease in oxygen demand from low body temperature and hepatectomy.[121] The centrifugal bypass system uses the patient's intravascular volume as a reservoir. The bypass blood flow is influenced mainly by the availability of blood at the inflow site and the resistance of the bypass circuit. When the bypass blood flow is significantly reduced or when it is less than 20 per cent of the cardiac output, the surgeon should be warned to clear obstruction in the circuit. The bypass system appears to activate the coagulation system when bypass flow is less than 800 ml/min.[122] It is customary to discontinue bypass when the flow is less than 1 L/min to avoid thromboembolism,[123] although the safe limit of flow rate may be still lower (Kam I, et al., unpublished data). The anesthesiologist should monitor bypass flow and be prepared for a sudden decrease in venous return. Once a satisfactory bypass system with adequate flow is established, the physiological changes are minimal and a very smooth second stage is maintained. During the lower caval anastomosis formation, the hepatic vascular tree is irrigated with 300 to 500 ml of cold lactated Ringer's solution via the portal vein. This maneuver flushes the preservation solution and metabolites out of the donor liver and evacuates air from the inferior vena cava. At the end of the second stage, serum electrolyte levels, arterial blood gas tensions, and acid-base state are measured and corrected to minimize the hemodynamic changes associated with reperfusion of the graft liver.

The third stage of surgery begins with reperfusion of the graft liver. Partial hepatic circulation is reinstituted by unclamping the inferior vena cava and the portal vein to decrease the warm ischemia time of the donor liver. Anastomosis of the hepatic artery follows. The most dramatic changes in the cardiovascular system are seen on reperfusion of the graft liver: severe hypotension, bradycardia, supraventricular and ventricular arrhythmias, electromechanical dissociation, and occasionally cardiac arrest (Fig. 8–13). The changes in hemodynamic variables and electrolyte levels after reperfusion of the graft liver are shown in Table 8–12.[124] The hemodynamic changes include a significant decrease in heart rate, mean arterial pressure, cardiac index, and mixed-venous oxygen saturation of hemoglobin and are associated with a significant increase in potassium, decrease in ionized calcium and in pH, and an increase in base deficit. Pulmonary arterial and central venous pressures increase, although a transient decrease in the cardiac filling pressure may develop when hemostasis is not adequate. These alterations are due to a sudden influx of a large quantity

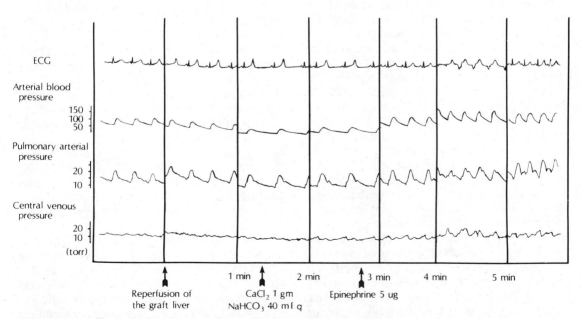

**Figure 8–13.** Electrocardiographic changes seen on reperfusion of the graft liver.

**TABLE 8–12. Hemodynamic Changes on Reperfusion of the Graft Liver in 12 Patients (Mean ± SD)**

| Variable | Before Reperfusion | After Reperfusion |
| --- | --- | --- |
| Heart rate (bpm) | 82 ± 21 | 73 ± 13* |
| Mean arterial pressure (mm Hg) | 80 ± 21 | 69 ± 15* |
| Cardiac index (L·min$^{-1}$·m$^{-2}$) | 3.7 ± 1.4 | 2.9 ± 1.4* |
| Potassium (mEq·L$^{-1}$) | 3.7 ± 0.6 | 5.1 ± 1.0* |
| Calcium (ionized) (mM·L$^{-1}$) | 0.84 ± 0.08 | 0.77 ± 0.12* |
| pH | 7.42 ± 0.10 | 7.37 ± 0.11* |

* $p < 0.05$ vs before reperfusion.
From Martin DJ, Marquez JM, Kang YG, et al: Liver transplantation: Hemodynamic and electrolyte changes seen immediately following revascularization. Anesth Analg 63:246, 1984, with permission of the publisher.

**TABLE 8–13. Physiological Changes Before and After Reperfusion of the Graft Liver with Calcium Chloride (1 gm) Pretreatment in 11 Patients (Mean ± SD)**

| Variables | Before Reperfusion | After Reperfusion |
| --- | --- | --- |
| Heart rate (bpm) | 83 ± 15 | 68 ± 21* |
| Mean arterial pressure (mm Hg) | 82 ± 11 | 63 ± 13* |
| Cardiac index (L·min$^{-1}$·m$^{-2}$) | 3.2 ± 1.2 | 3.6 ± 1.3 |
| Potassium (mEq·L$^{-1}$) | 3.9 ± 0.95 | 5.1 ± 1.5* |
| Calcium (ionized) (mM·L$^{-1}$) | 0.66 ± 0.26 | 0.96 ± 0.32* |
| pH | 7.40 ± 0.04 | 7.30 ± 0.09* |

* $p < 0.05$ vs before reperfusion.
From Martin DJ, Marquez JM, Kang YG, et al: Liver transplantation: Hemodynamic and electrolyte changes seen immediately following revascularization. Anesth Analg 63:246, 1984, with permission of the publisher.

of potassium originating from ischemic hepatocytes and from the organ preservation solution, changes in conduction of electrical activity, and depression of the myocardium and vascular tone. Acidic substances from the graft liver and congested viscera and large amounts of cold blood or unknown toxic substances from the graft liver may also play a role in decreased cardiac contractility and peripheral vascular resistance. This short-lived impairment of cardiovascular function can be abated partially by infusion of calcium chloride and sodium bicarbonate to treat hyperkalemia and to normalize the ionized calcium level and acid-base state. The cardiovascular profile and serum electrolyte levels of a group of patients who received calcium chloride (1 gm) immediately before reperfusion of the graft liver are shown in Table 8–13.[124] The calcium chloride pretreatment prevented the cardiac index from falling, but hypotension and bradycardia persisted. The bradycardia is most likely associated with hyperkalemia, and it returns toward normal heart rate without the use of a chronotropic agent in most patients. In some patients, glucose and insulin have been administered to reduce the serum potassium level, but this long-acting therapeutic regimen is seldom necessary. A small dose of inotropic agent (epinephrine, 5 to 10 µg bolus) has been very effective in overcoming the transient cardiovascular depression. The preload can be increased to treat hypotension. However, an overzealous increase in preload may aggravate the already increased filling pressures, resulting in an additional burden on the heart, increased impedance to hepatic blood outflow, and subsequent impairment in hepatic blood flow and oxygen supply. Although the dramatic hemodynamic changes may subside within 10 to 15 minutes after reperfusion of the graft liver, pulmonary hypertension, high central venous pressure, and a moderate degree of hypotension may persist. The origin of the pulmonary hypertension is not clear. It may be caused by embolization or pulmonary vasoactive substances released by the graft liver.

Thromboembolism or air embolism in pulmonary or cerebral circulation is one of the major complications during surgery.[125] It may happen at any time, but most commonly occurs at the beginning of the anhepatic stage if venovenous bypass is used or on reperfusion of the graft liver. When portal thrombosis exists in the recipient, the thrombus may embolize via the bypass system at the onset of bypass. If massive pulmonary emboli significantly obstruct pulmonary flow, early diagnosis is essential for surgical correction.

Once acute hemodynamic changes are under control, the rest of the third stage is relatively calm. However, when the hepatic arterial anastomosis must be made between the aorta of the recipient and the hepatic artery of the donor liver, continuous bleeding may occur during the dissection of the retroperitoneal area. Irritation of the diaphragm and compression of the thoracic cavity continue during surgical hemostasis. Enough blood and blood products should be always on hand to treat massive bleeding, which can occur at any time.

**Pulmonary System.** Pulmonary gas exchange can be maintained relatively easily in most patients. $F_{IO_2}$ is kept below 70 per cent, whenever possible, to prevent absorption atelectasis[126] and oxygen toxicity.[127] In patients who show signs of pleural effusion on preoperative assessment, chest tubes to drain fluid are inserted during the first stage of surgery. This improves gas exchange and decreases ventricular filling pressure. Frequent measurements of blood gas tensions and continuous monitoring of end-tidal gas tensions by mass spectrometer ensure adequate ventilation and oxygenation. In patients with pre-existing cardiopulmonary disease, pulmonary edema may occur, mostly after reperfusion of the graft liver. Treatment of intraoperative pulmonary edema can be very difficult. Increasing PEEP and maintaining minute ventilation by using a volume ventilator may prevent hypoxemia. Diuretics are rarely effective in patients with marginal renal function. Blood transfusion is withheld to decrease intravascular volume. The intraoperative mortality associated with pulmonary edema is high, and every effort should be made to prevent it.

**Blood Transfusion and Blood Coagulation** (see also Chapter 11). Massive intraoperative bleeding is a characteristic feature of liver transplantation, and transfusion of a large quantity of warmed blood is necessary to prevent cardiovascular instability. This is possible by using a rapid infusion system that can deliver blood warmed to 30 to 34°C. An autotransfusion system has been used[128] and is effective in salvaging up to 20 to 30 per cent of the blood loss during liver transplantation. Because of possible ill effects of heparin, citrate phosphate and dextrose with adenine (CPDA-1) is preferred for anticoagulation during the collection cycle. However, possible contaminations by ascites, infectious organisms, and gastrointestinal tract contents require further investigation. The volume of blood transfused varies, ranging, according to reports from different centers, from less than 10 units to more than 200 units of RBC. The observations at the University of Pittsburgh are shown in Table 8–14; the number of used units of RBC has been re-

**TABLE 8–14. Number of Units of Red Blood Cells (RBC) Transfused for Patients Who Received Liver Transplants in 1983 at the University of Pittsburgh**

| Units of RBC | No. of Patients |
|:---:|:---:|
| 0–10 | 21 |
| 11–20 | 20 |
| 21–30 | 11 |
| 31–50 | 4 |
| 51–70 | 2 |
| >100 | 5 |

duced further in a recent series of patients. Although some patients have required less than 10 units of RBC, the anesthesiologist and blood bank personnel must be prepared for the transfusion of more than 200 units of RBC.

Maintaining a close-to-normal quantity of coagulation factors may not be possible or even desirable in a patient undergoing major vascular surgery without systemic or local heparinization. Maintaining normal blood coagulability without increasing the danger of thromboembolism is paramount. Intraoperative changes in the coagulation profile are seen in Table 8–15.[110] During stage 1 of surgery, prothrombin time (PT) and activated partial thromboplastin time (aPTT) remain prolonged, and levels of all coagulation factors, including platelet count, decrease progressively. In stage 2, the coagulation profile does not change significantly except that aPTT is prolonged and euglobulin lysis time (ELT) shortened. The most dramatic changes are seen on reperfusion of the graft liver. PT and aPTT are remarkably prolonged, and concentrations of all coagulation factors are decreased. The coagulation profile improves slowly and returns toward clinically acceptable values, except for Factor V level. The fall and rise of concentration of the coagulation factors appear to be related to a dilutional effect and poor or absent hepatic synthetic function. However, the decreases in factors VIII:C and V seem to involve destruction during active fibrinolysis,[129] demonstrated by a sudden decrease in factor VIII:C concentration associated with the short ELT on reperfusion of the graft liver. Plasmin produced by plasminogen activator may cleave factor VIII:C and factor V. Severe fibrinolytic activity can develop any time during surgery, but it is most likely

**TABLE 8–15.  Intraoperative Changes in Coagulation in 11 Patients with Primary Biliary Cirrhosis (Mean ± SD)**

| | Before Operation | Stage 1 | Stage 2 | | Stage 3 | | | |
| --- | --- | --- | --- | --- | --- | --- | --- | --- |
| | | 120 MIN | 5 MIN | 30 MIN | 5 MIN | 30 MIN | 120 MIN | END |
| PT (sec) | 13.9 ± 1.7 | 13.7 ± 1.0 | 14.0 ± 1.3 | 13.8 ± 1.2 | 15.4 ± 1.6[a] | 15.7 ± 1.5[a] | 15.0 ± 1.4 | 14.6 ± 1.4 |
| aPTT (sec) | 41.0 ± 8.7 | 40.2 ± 7.7 | 46.0 ± 12.9 | 51.2 ± 16.0 | 75.2 ± 39.2[a] | 61.5 ± 23.6[a] | 46.0 ± 9.7 | 38.4 ± 3.8 |
| Platelets (1000/cu mm) | 181 ± 199 | 150 ± 122 | 149 ± 120 | 154 ± 122 | 124 ± 63[a] | 132 ± 61 | 134 ± 82 | 143 ± 74 |
| Fibrinogen (mg/dl) | 323 ± 166 | 288 ± 100 | 252 ± 113 | 235 ± 88 | 194 ± 93[a] | 195 ± 101[a] | 191 ± 90[a] | 210 ± 92 |
| Factor V (U/ml) | 0.54 ± 0.27 | 0.43 ± 0.22 | 0.35 ± 0.19 | 0.38 ± 0.19 | 0.26 ± 0.18[a] | 0.22 ± 0.13[a] | 0.21 ± 0.11[a] | 0.23 ± 0.13[a] |
| Factor VII (U/ml) | 0.83 ± 0.35 | 0.71 ± 0.37 | 0.62 ± 0.31 | 0.65 ± 0.27 | 0.52 ± 0.23[a] | 0.52 ± 0.18[a] | 0.53 ± 0.18 | 0.51 ± 0.17 |
| Factor VIII (U/ml) | 2.03 ± 0.73 | 1.81 ± 0.86 | 1.51 ± 0.88 | 1.49 ± 0.75 | 1.11 ± 0.70[a] | 0.82 ± 0.53[a] | 0.87 ± 0.44[a] | 0.93 ± 0.35[a] |
| ELT (min) | 215 ± 77 | 134 ± 93 | 140 ± 88 | 101 ± 77[a] | 68 ± 53[a] | 108 ± 45 | 155 ± 63 | 185 ± 70 |
| R (min) | 8.5 ± 2.4 | 8.2 ± 3.6 | 6.6 ± 3.4 | 7.5 ± 2.3 | 11.2 ± 5.0[a] | 9.7 ± 2.7 | 8.8 ± 3.0 | 8.0 ± 2.9 |
| R + k (min) | 12.0 ± 2.7 | 12.0 ± 6.3 | 9.5 ± 2.5 | 11.0 ± 2.2 | 23.5 ± 16.4[a] | 15.0 ± 6.1 | 12.5 ± 4.5 | 10.0 ± 2.6 |
| α (°) | 55.5 ± 8.5 | 53.8 ± 12.2 | 53.6 ± 10.4 | 53.1 ± 7.4 | 39.1 ± 17.5[a] | 48.6 ± 10.5 | 50.6 ± 12.0 | 55.1 ± 8.0 |
| MA (mm) | 54.6 ± 11.2 | 57.3 ± 9.4 | 52.3 ± 11.0 | 51.3 ± 9.4 | 38.2 ± 14.5[a] | 51.7 ± 8.9 | 51.5 ± 11.9 | 52.1 ± 10.8 |
| $A_{60}/MA \cdot 100$ (%) | 83.0 ± 7.8 | 76.4 ± 14.5 | 73.9 ± 27.0 | 65.5 ± 35.5 | 75.8 ± 34.4 | 79.8 ± 29.3 | 92.2 ± 8.6[a] | 91.7 ± 6.7[a] |

[a] Significantly different from the corresponding preoperative value ($p < 0.05$).

From Kang YG, Martin DJ, Marquez J, et al: Intraoperative changes in blood coagulation and thromboelastographic monitoring in liver transplantation. Anesth Analg 64:892, 1985, with permission of the publisher.

during the anhepatic stage and on reperfusion of the graft liver when ELT is less than one hour in more than 40 per cent of patients.[110] The fibrinolytic activity improves after reperfusion of the graft liver, and ELT becomes longer than two hours in most patients. Intraoperative changes in ELT, plasminogen, and antiplasmin are shown in Figure 8–14.[129] ELT decreases progressively, especially during the anhepatic stage; antiplasmin level follows a similar pattern, whereas plasminogen level remains relatively unchanged. Fibrinolysis during liver transplantation may be caused by multiple factors: release of tissue plasminogen activators, a decrease in hepatic clearance of plasmin, a decrease in antiplasmin level, and activation of protein C.[130,131]

Similar changes are observed during intraoperative monitoring by thromboelastography (Table 8–16): prolonged reaction time (r) and coagulation time (r + K), decreased maximum amplitude (MA), and decreased fibrinolytic index (A60/MA). The most abnormal thromboelastographic variables are seen on reperfusion of the graft liver. The changes in the coagulation system on reperfusion of the graft liver are caused by several factors. The influx of preservative solution may have a dilutional effect. The role of fibrinolysis is described above. Heparin from the donor liver or an endogenous heparin-like substance may play a role, but it is not thought to be significant.[110] Disseminated intravascular coagulation does not appear to play a major role, because most coagulation factors and platelet count are better maintained than Factor VIII, and fibrin degradation products and fibrin monomer are detected in only moderate quantities.[129] The metabolic effects of reperfusion on coagulation should be emphasized. Hypothermia, acidosis, hypocalcemia, and cardiovascular instability could adversely affect the coagulation system. Coagulation inhibitors released by the graft liver and changes in physiological homeostasis may impair coagulability even when coagulation factors are adequate. Lack of direct correlation between coagulability and concentrations of coagulation factors is well demonstrated by the improved blood coagulability on thromboelastography 30 minutes after reperfusion while levels of coagulation factors decrease or remain at the same level.[132]

Intraoperative management of the coagulation system consists of aggressive monitoring, proper replacement therapy, and selective pharmacological therapy. A coagulation profile can be obtained relatively quickly in experienced laboratories, but thromboelastography is essential for minute-to-minute monitoring of blood coagulability, as opposed to quantity of coagulation elements. Thromboelastography differentiates coagulopathy from surgical bleeding, and it identifies pathological coagulation processes.

Replacement therapy is instituted from the beginning of surgery. Blood components can be infused separately, according to the need of the patient. However, transfusion of premixed red blood cells with fresh frozen plasma makes replacement therapy easier, because of the complexity of component therapy during massive blood transfusion in patients whose coagulation factors are almost uniformly decreased. Transfusion of fresh whole blood may decrease the number of blood donors the patient is exposed to, but a large quantity of fresh whole blood may not be available. To accommodate the need for massive blood transfusion while blood coagulability is maintained, a blood mixture is prepared in the cardiotomy reservoir of the rapid infusion system, composed of 2 units (600 ml) of RBC, 2 units (400 ml) of fresh frozen plasma (FFP), and 500 ml of electrolyte solution (Plasmalyte A R, Travenol Laboratories, Deerfield, Ill.). The blood mixture delivers blood with a hematocrit of $27 \pm 2$ per cent, fibrinogen 130 mg·dl$^{-1}$, Factor V 0.21 units·ml$^{-1}$, and Factor VIII 0.57 units·ml$^{-1}$.[110] Electrolyte solution is added to replace third-space loss, to decrease the loss of RBC, and to decrease viscosity, thereby improving peripheral circulation in patients with inadvertent hypothermia. Transfusion of the premixed blood has demonstrated favorable results, but it requires further investigation. During surgery, non-glucose-containing electrolyte solution is used to avoid hyperglycemia, and all intravenous lines are kept open. Intravascular volume is replaced mainly by the blood mixture in the rapid infusion system. Dilutional coagulopathy and pathological coagulation processes are expected, and transfusion of additional FFP, platelets, and cryoprecipitate may be required, according to thromboelastographic measurements (Table 8–16). When thromboelastography is not available, platelets are transfused to maintain platelet count greater than 100,000/cu mm, and cry-

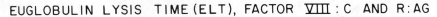

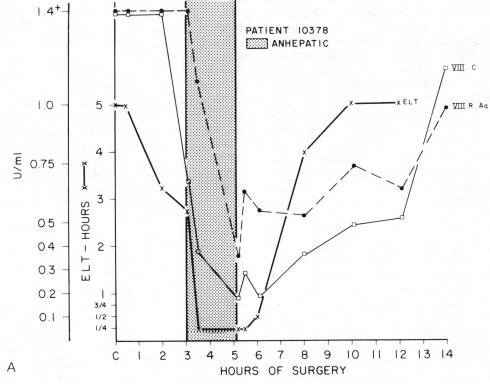

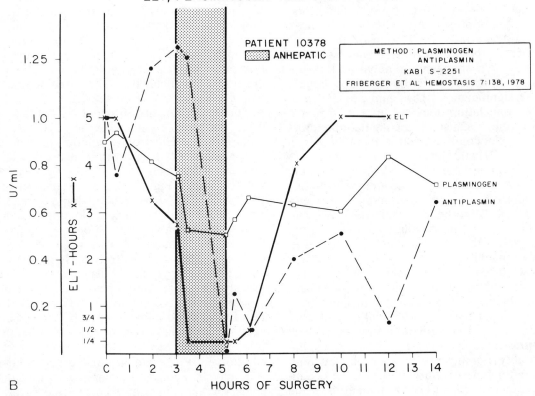

**Figure 8–14.** Intraoperative changes in euglobulin lysis time, plasminogen, and antiplasmin in a liver transplant recipient. (From Lewis JH, et al: Intraoperative coagulation changes in liver transplantation. In Winter PM, Kang YG (eds): Hepatic Transplantation: Anesthetic and Perioperative Management in Hepatic Transplantation. Philadelphia, Praeger, 1986.)

**TABLE 8–16. Intraoperative Management of Coagulation by Thromboelastographic Monitoring**

1. Maintenance of physiological homeostasis
2. Replacement therapy
   a. FFP for prolonged reaction time (r >15 min)
   b. Platelets for small MA (MA <40 mm)
   c. Cryoprecipitate for persistent coagulopathy and/or slow clot formation rate (α <40)
3. Pharmacological therapy
   a. Epsilon aminocaproic acid or protamine sulfate—after the effectiveness of the drug is confirmed by in vitro test
   b. Heparin: may be harmful

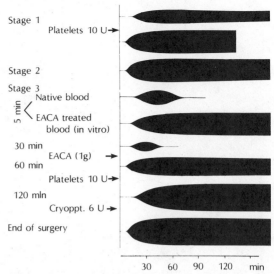

**Figure 8–15.** Thromboelastographic monitoring, replacement therapy, and pharmacologic therapy in a liver transplant recipient. See text for details.

oprecipitate is added when Factors I and VIII are less than 30 per cent of normal values. Clinical significance of PT and aPTT measurements is very limited because they are usually prolonged and may not respond to transfusion of FFP. Transfusion of platelets and cryoprecipitate is withheld during the second stage to avoid thromboembolism when the venovenous bypass without systemic heparinization is used. Once the graft liver is in the systemic circulation, the coagulation system is allowed to recover for 30 minutes. Thereafter, aggressive replacement therapy should be reinstituted. Persistent poor coagulability is expected in a patient who receives a poorly functioning graft liver, and continuous replacement therapy is required on those occasions.

Pharmacological therapy may include antifibrinolytic therapy and reversal of the heparin effect by protamine sulfate. Epsilon aminocaproic acid has been used for patients who demonstrated severe fibrinolytic activity, after the effectiveness of the drug was tested *in vitro* by comparing results of thromboelastography of blood treated with epsilon aminocaproic acid (0.1 per cent) and of untreated blood.[133] A small dose (1 gm) of epsilon aminocaproic acid has been effective in stopping very active fibrinolysis without thrombotic complications. However, antifibrinolytic therapy requires proper monitoring of coagulation before its use, because mild fibrinolysis subsides spontaneously, and indiscriminate use of epsilon aminocaproic acid may cause lethal thrombosis.[134] Protamine sulfate may be given when a heparin effect is seen on thromboelastography; it has been found to be effective in a selected but small number of patients (Kang YG, unpub-

lished data). The combination of replacement therapy, restoration of physiological variables, and pharmacological therapy improves blood coagulability within two hours after reperfusion of the graft liver, and surgery is concluded with normal or close-to-normal blood coagulability (Fig. 8–15).

**Fluid and Electrolyte Balance.** Deranged acid-base balance has been seen in many transplant recipients. Intraoperative metabolic acidosis is very common, especially during the second and third stages of surgery[135] (Fig. 8–16). The acidosis is caused by rapid transfusion of acidotic blood; release of lactic acid by the tissues after crossclamping of the major vessels; decreased metabolism of citrate, lactate, and other acids owing to absence of or poor hepatic function; and decreased tissue perfusion. Base deficit is corrected frequently by administration of sodium bicarbonate. However, overzealous correction may cause intraoperative hypernatremia, leading to postoperative metabolic alkalosis. Therefore, sodium bicarbonate is given only in a minimal dose and when base deficit exceeds 6 to 8 mM/L.[114,135] Nevertheless, these authors prefer aggressive correction of acidosis to minimize the cardiovascular instability on reperfusion of the graft liver. In addition, the degree of postoperative metabolic alkalosis does not correlate with the intraoperative dose of sodium bicarbonate.

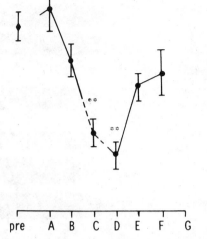

**Figure 8–16.** Changes in base deficit during liver transplantation. Mean + SEM of nine patients. A, After induction of anesthesia; B, dissection of the liver; C, beginning of the anhepatic stage; D, reperfusion of the graft liver; E, biliary reconstruction; F, skin closure; and G, end of surgery. $p < 0.01$ vs preoperative values. (From Carmichael FJ, et al: Anesthesia for hepatic transplantation. Cardiovascular and metabolic alterations and their management. Anesthes Analg 64:112, 1985.)

Serum ionized calcium concentration decreases progressively during surgery (Fig. 8–17), reaching the lowest levels during the anhepatic stage and on reperfusion of the graft liver.[136] Serum citrate level increases pro-

gressively and begins to decrease after reperfusion of the graft liver. The highest serum citrate level, similar to that contained in the transfused blood, is reached during the anhepatic stage. Citrate intoxication, which is noted as a decrease in serum ionized calcium concentration, elevation of serum citrate level, and myocardial depression, occurs very frequently. Citrate intoxication develops when massive blood transfusion is administered to a patient with decreased hepatic function and/or decreased hepatic blood flow in the presence of hypothermia or acidosis.[137] A decrease in serum ionized calcium concentration to 0.56 mM/L has been associated with a decrease in both left ventricular stroke index and right atrial pressure and unchanged systemic vascular resistance.[136] Administration of calcium chloride increases ionized calcium concentration and improves cardiovascular function. Thus, citrate intoxication is a serious intraoperative complication during liver transplantation, although it has not been clearly demonstrated in other surgical patients.[138] A prolonged QT interval on the ECG is a sign of hypocalcemia, and its relation to the degree of hypocalcemia requires further investigation. Frequent measurement of serum ionized calcium and aggressive correction of ionic hypocalcemia are mandatory; approximately 1 gm of calcium chloride may be required for

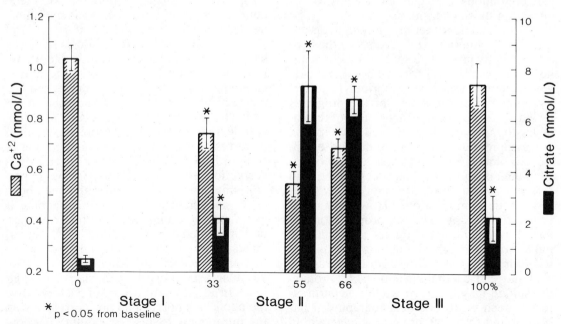

**Figure 8–17.** Serum ionized calcium and citrate levels during liver transplantation. (From Marquez JM: Citrate intoxication during hepatic transplantation. In Winter PM, Kang YG (eds): Hepatic Transplantation: Anesthetic and Perioperative Management in Hepatic Transplantation. Philadelphia, Praeger, 1986.)

every 6 units of citrated blood products. Hypercalcemia has been noted after overcorrection of hypocalcemia, but ill effects have not been observed.

Intraoperative potassium supplementation to treat sometimes-observed hypokalemia is not recommended as long as cardiovascular irritability is not encountered. Serum potassium concentration increases abruptly (to 7 to 10 mEq·L$^{-1}$) immediately after reperfusion of the graft liver starts. The concentration decreases rapidly within three to five minutes, presumably by redistribution. A tall T wave is seen on the ECG, and arrhythmia develops, although transiently. Changes in heart rhythm range from bradycardia to cardiac arrest. The effects of hyperkalemia on the cardiovascular system can be treated best by administration of calcium chloride and sodium bicarbonate. In most patients, cardiac arrest of hyperkalemic origin responds to resuscitation. It has been suggested that potassium is taken up by the graft liver and hypokalemia develops after reperfusion of the graft liver.[139] In our experience, however, plasma potassium concentration is maintained at an acceptable level (above 3.5 mEq·L$^{-1}$) and infrequently requires supplementation.

The diseased liver does not store a sufficient amount of glycogen, and gluconeogenesis may be impaired; therefore hypoglycemia is expected. However, blood glucose concentrations have been reported in the normal range during the anhepatic stage in patients who did not receive exogenous glucose other than blood transfusion.[140] Furthermore, hyperglycemia has been observed throughout surgery if a glucose-containing solution was administered.[135] In animals receiving liver transplants without exogenous glucose administration, including that contained in blood, normoglycemia was well maintained during the anhepatic stage, and hyperglycemia developed after reperfusion of the graft liver (DeWolf A, unpublished data). The normal to high glucose level in patients receiving liver transplants is reportedly related to the decrease in glucose utilization as well as to the administration of glucose contained in the transfused blood. A blood sugar level of less than 100 mg/dl is rarely seen during the anhepatic stage when blood transfusion is minimal. On those occasions glucose is administered as 5 per cent dextrose solution. During reperfusion of the graft liver a glucose level frequently exceeds 200 mg/dl. This hyperglycemia is probably due to the release of glucose from the ischemic hepatocytes of the newly transplanted liver and may last for several hours.

**Renal System.** Intraoperative oliguria is not uncommon. Pre-existing hepatorenal syndrome; reduction of renal perfusion, especially during the anhepatic stage without bypass; hypovolemia during massive fluid shifts; and the nephrotoxicity of cyclosporine A all contribute to renal dysfunction. Oliguria during this stage has been less problematic since the venovenous bypass system was introduced. The renal complications associated with intravascular hemolysis after massive blood transfusion are not clear. Maintaining adequate urine output may help prevent acute tubular necrosis and the pathological process associated with intravascular hemolysis. A low dose of dopamine (3 µg·kg$^{-1}$·min$^{-1}$) has been used, although its role in renal protection is controversial. Administration of mannitol has been suggested to prevent postoperative renal failure, but its effectiveness has not been clearly defined.

**Body Temperature.** A decrease in body temperature is unavoidable during major abdominal surgery of prolonged duration.[141] Body temperature falls steadily from the beginning of surgery, especially when massive blood transfusion is required. The decrease is more pronounced during the second (anhepatic) stage when the venovenous bypass system is used without a heat exchanger. A sudden fall in body temperature (as low as 31°C) is seen on reperfusion of the graft liver when cold preservation solution is flushed into the systemic circulation. At that time, central blood temperature falls 1 to 2°C within 3 minutes. It rises slowly afterward, reaching 34–35°C at the end of surgery. Therefore, at present, it is recommended that hypothermia be avoided by using a warming blanket, incorporating a heat exchanger in the blood delivery system and a humidifier in the respiratory circuit, irrigating the abdominal cavity with warm solution, and raising the temperature in the operating room. Inadvertent hypothermia may protect a graft liver suffering from ischemic injury. However, the effects of body temperature on the graft liver function and survival need investigation. On the other hand, hypothermia may interfere with the cardiovascular and coagulation functions.

## Conclusion of Surgery

Unless unusual surgical or medical complications occur, the patient's clinical condition becomes stable, most of the physiological variables are normalized, and the graft liver begins to produce bile within 2 to 4 hours of the graft liver reperfusion. At the conclusion of surgery patients are transported to the intensive care unit with ECG, arterial blood pressure, and precordial or esophageal heart tone monitoring. Action of muscle relaxants is not antagonized, and mechanical ventilation is provided while patients recover from hypothermia and the influence of anesthetics and other drugs.

### Pediatric Considerations

Anesthetic management for pediatric patients has been well described by Borland et al.[114] Biliary atresia is the most common indication for liver transplantation, followed by an inborn error of metabolism.[93] Patients are usually premedicated with intramuscular atropine, morphine sulfate, and pentobarbital. Multiple intravenous catheters are inserted for replacement of blood volume. Intra-arterial and central venous pressure catheters are commonly placed. A pulmonary arterial catheter is inserted when required. Intravenous thiopental or ketamine is frequently used to induce anesthesia. Maintenance of anesthesia is quite similar to that in adults. The surgical technique is also similar to that in adults. Previous intra-abdominal procedures, such as portoenterostomy (Kasai operation), make recipient hepatectomy very difficult. Intraoperative changes in the cardiopulmonary system are quite similar to those in adults. However, the vast majority of children tolerate the anhepatic stage with minimal change in hemodynamic status resulting from greater cardiac reserves and proportionally larger collateral vessels.[123] Therefore, the anhepatic stage is performed after simple cross-clamping of major vessels in most patients. Venovenous bypass may be used only in children with body weight greater than 20 kg because the cannula size and safe flow rate of the bypass limit its use in small patients.[123] Blood loss during surgery ranges between 0.5 and 25 blood volumes (mean, 3.95 blood volumes).[114] Intraoperative changes in the coagulation system are like those in adults, with less incidence of coagulopathy and fibrinolysis.

### Retransplantation of the Liver

Some patients receive second or third liver transplants when the first graft liver does not function properly because of rejection, primary nonfunction of the graft, or surgical complications. According to their physical status, these patients can be divided into two groups. One group has acute rejection or a nonfunctioning liver, and the search for another liver has been prolonged. The deteriorating graft liver has caused multiple systemic complications: coma, a very unstable cardiovascular system, adult respiratory distress syndrome, renal failure, coagulopathy, hypoglycemia, hyperkalemia, and hypocalcemia. Frequently these patients receive inotropic drugs, multiple blood transfusions, and ventilatory support. The anesthetic care is similar to that of patients with fulminant hepatitis. The other group of patients has some degree of hepatic function after chronic rejection, and their physical condition is relatively stable. Generally, hepatectomy is less complicated, and anesthetic management and surgery in these cases is simpler. However, intravenous and intra-arterial catheterization is often difficult. In patients who have had prolonged steroid therapy, vessels are fragile and their trauma might lead to massive bleeding.

### Postoperative Care

Postoperative care of recipients has been thoroughly described by Shapiro et al.[142] General supportive care is similar to that of other critically ill patients. Upon the patient's arrival at the surgical intensive care unit the following baseline studies are performed: chest radiograph; ECG; complete blood cell count with differential; serum concentrations of electrolytes (potassium, sodium), ionized calcium, magnesium and phosphate, creatinine, blood urea nitrogen, total and direct bilirubin, serum glutamic-oxaloacetic transaminase, serum glutamic-pyruvic transaminase, gamma glutamic-pyruvic transaminase, alkaline phosphatase, amylase, total protein, albumin; and coagulation profile (PT, aPTT, and platelet count). The tests are repeated every six hours or daily, according to the need of the individual patient.

Postoperative pain can be significant after liver transplantation. Narcotics may interfere with the neurological assessment of the patient, and altered drug metabolism may prolong the elimination of the drug; therefore, morphine sulfate is carefully titrated against effect, using minimal incremental doses (1 to 2 mg).

For immunosuppression therapy, methylprednisolone, cyclosporine A, and occasionally monoclonal antibody (OKT 3) are administered, as described in Chapter 4. Cyclosporine A (2 mg·kg$^{-1}$) is administered intravenously every 8 to 12 hours, and orally (17.5 mg·kg$^{-1}$·day$^{-1}$) when absorption of the drug in the gastrointestinal tract is satisfactory. The dose is adjusted according to the blood level of cyclosporine A and its side effects, which include reversible nephrotoxicity, hypertension, hyperkalemia, hepatotoxicity, hirsutism, tremor or seizures, vague abdominal pain, and lymphoproliferative syndrome. OKT 3, a T-cell-specific antilymphocyte globulin, is used to treat acute rejection. Its side effects consist of bronchospasm, fever, rigor, diarrhea, vomiting, chest tightness, possibly pulmonary edema, and even respiratory arrest.[143,144] Clinically significant postoperative extrahepatic complications in a large series of patients have been described[144] and are listed in Table 8–17.

The cardiovascular system is relatively stable in most patients, although some may have persistent arrhythmia or require cardiovascular support. Drugs such as dopamine, dobutamine, and epinephrine are titrated against the cardiovascular effects. Postoperative hypertension is not uncommon and may require an antihypertensive drug. Hydralazine (5 to 10 mg intravenously) is used frequently, and nitroprusside may be administered. Diuretics and beta blocking drugs may be added to treat sustained hypertension. Pulmonary edema is sometimes seen postoperatively, and diuretics are used liberally.

Pulmonary supportive care is critical for patients who receive immunosuppression therapy. In most patients the endotracheal tube is removed within 48 hours postoperatively after pulmonary function, clinical condition, and chest radiograph are evaluated. Atelectasis is common, and aggressive pulmonary toilet is required to improve gas exchange and to prevent pneumonia. Pleural effusion is also a common occurrence, and thoracentesis may become necessary. Adult respiratory distress syndrome is seen in patients with sepsis or acute rejection. This is treated by controlling infection or retransplanting the liver.

Many patients are confused in the early postoperative period. However, this mild mental disorder clears rapidly when the graft liver begins to function. The most common neurological complication consists of seizures, which occur within the first four days

**TABLE 8–17. Clinically Significant Postoperative Extrahepatic Complications in 225 Hepatic Transplant Recipients**

| Complication | No. of Patients |
|---|---|
| Cardiovascular system | |
| Arrhythmia | 6 |
| Acute myocardial infarction | 3 |
| Endocarditis | 3 |
| Pulmonary system | |
| Infection | 42 |
| Pleural effusion requiring thoracentesis | 40 |
| Atelectasis requiring bronchoscopy | 42 |
| Respiratory failure requiring tracheostomy | 25 |
| Aspiration pneumonia | 7 |
| Persistent pneumothorax | 3 |
| Renal system | |
| Renal failure | 70 |
| Central nervous system | |
| Seizure | 23 |
| Intracranial hemorrhage | 10 |
| Meningitis | 3 |
| Psychosis and depression | 5 |
| Digestive system | |
| Hemorrhage | 21 |
| Perforation of the bowels | 9 |
| Obstruction | 8 |
| Pancreatitis | 5 |
| Hematological system | |
| Lymphoma | 5 |
| Hodgkin's disease | 1 |
| Surgical complications | |
| Surgical bleeding | 5 |
| Medical bleeding | 14 |
| Biliary tract complications | 40 |
| Intra-abdominal infection | 57 |
| Wound complications | 25 |
| Others | |
| Thrombophlebitis | 6 |
| Decubitus ulcer | 7 |
| Multiple vertebral fracture | 4 |
| Infected seroma | 7 |
| Tooth abscess | 3 |
| Brachial plexus injury | 2 |
| Knotty pulmonary artery catheter | 1 |

Data based on Wood RP, Shaw BW Jr, Starzl TE: Extrahepatic complications of liver transplantation. Semin Liver Dis 5:384, 1985.

after operation. The cause is unknown, although cyclosporine A may precipitate the seizures. In most patients the seizures are controlled with phenobarbital. Intracranial hemorrhage or meningitis is seen occasionally.

A wide spectrum of renal dysfunction is seen postoperatively. Patients with a urine output of more than 20 ml·hr$^{-1}$ with adequate ventricular filling pressure do not require special treatment. Patients with less urine output with a low ventricular filling pressure are treated with fluid administration. Some patients develop renal failure, requiring hemodialysis, although persistent renal failure is uncommon. The immunosuppression therapy schedule and dose are adjusted to avoid the nephrotoxic effects of cyclosporine A.

Major postoperative bleeding that requires re-exploration is rare. The blood coagulability decreases in the immediate postoperative period, presumably because of inadequate hepatic synthetic function. Prolonged PT and aPTT and thrombocytopenia are observed, and the thromboelastographic pattern may also deteriorate. The coagulation function is supported by the transfusion of FFP, platelets, and cryoprecipitate. However, replacement therapy is guided by the combination of coagulation profile and clinical signs to avoid thrombotic complications.

Fluid therapy is determined by the clinical and laboratory assessment of the patient. FFP is used frequently to expand intravascular fluid volume and to supplement coagulation factors. RBC is transfused to maintain hematocrit greater than 30 per cent. Crystalloid solution is used when fluid shift to the interstitial space persists. A decrease in ionized calcium concentration is uncommon unless the patient requires massive blood transfusion. Mild hypokalemia is seen frequently and is treated with daily supplementation of potassium. Hyperkalemia occurs in patients with poor renal or hepatic function. Mild hyperglycemia is common, but rarely requires special treatment. Hypoglycemia can be seen in patients with poor hepatic function and is treated with glucose supplementation. Frequently observed metabolic alkalosis results from potassium depletion and diuretic therapy and is treated by potassium supplementation. Metabolic acidosis in the early postoperative period is a sign of poor hepatic function. Oral intake of liquid is encouraged as soon as motility of the gastrointestinal tract returns. Enteral feeding is required in some patients, and intravenous hyperalimentation is used for patients who develop prolonged gastrointestinal tract complications.

Patients often develop bacterial infection and/or infection by fungus or cytomegalovirus. Infectious complications of organ transplantation are presented in detail in Chapter 5. Forty per cent of the mortality is associated with infection, the primary site of which is the abdominal cavity. Therefore, preventing and controlling infection cannot be overemphasized. The prophylactic antibiotic therapy with cefotaxime and ampicillin begins intraoperatively and continues postoperatively. Fever is common in the early postoperative period; its source should be investigated and proper therapy initiated. The assessment includes physical examination and roentgenography of the chest and abdomen. Cultures and sensitivity tests are obtained on blood, respiratory secretions, drains, tubes, indwelling catheters, and urine. When the clinical assessment indicates, tests are performed for cytomegaloviral infection, tuberculosis, legionnaires' disease, and hepatitis. When pneumonia develops, the cause is identified by bronchoalveolar lavage. Few patients develop cytomegaloviral hepatitis, which may destroy the graft liver. Epstein-Barr viral infection may be associated with development of the lymphoma syndrome. Documented herpes viral infection is treated by daily administration of acyclovir (5 mg·kg$^{-1}$). Fungal infection is prone to develop in patients who receive immunosuppression and antibiotics. Mycostatin mouthwash is given for prophylaxis of oral and esophageal candidiasis. Aspergillus infection has been invariably associated with mortality.

The most common hepatic complication is rejection of the graft liver. Early postoperative fever, abdominal pain, fatigue, and failure to thrive are the early signs of rejection. Liver function tests are evaluated, and quantity and quality of bile are assessed to rule out infection. Acute rejection is treated with additional steroid administration. If signs of rejection do not improve, OKT 3 is administered. Sometimes hepatic dysfunction is associated with thin, watery bile. It is not clear whether this phenomenon is related to rejection or a nonfunctioning liver.

Hepatic dysfunction may continue and progress after the transplantation, indicating primary nonfunction of the graft. The patient's condition deteriorates eventually, resulting in coma, metabolic acidosis, hypoglycemia, coagulopathy, renal failure, adult respiratory distress syndrome, and cardiogenic shock. The main cause of primary nonfunction of the liver is believed to be prolonged cold or warm ischemia of the donor organ. Retransplantation of the liver is considered when the diagnosis is made.

Surgical complications include surgical bleeding, thrombosis of anastomosed vessels, and biliary obstruction or leakage. Thrombosis of the hepatic artery or the portal vein leads to rapid destruction of the graft liver and is more common in the pediatric population. Early postoperative anticoagulation therapy is instituted for patients with Budd-Chiari syndrome to prevent hepatic venous thrombosis. Biliary tract complications are diagnosed by T-tube cholangiography and endoscopic retrograde cholangiopancreatography and corrected surgically.

## RESULTS OF LIVER TRANSPLANTATION

The outcome of liver transplantation can be analyzed from the series of Calne et al. in Cambridge and Starzl et al. in Pittsburgh. In Calne's series, 118 patients received liver transplants between 1968 and 1982.[145,146] Ten patients died within 36 hours; eight from uncontrollable bleeding and two from cardiac arrest on reperfusion of the graft liver. In the first postoperative week, six more patients died from uncontrollable bleeding, and one died from chronic subdural hemorrhage that was unnoticed before surgery. Many recipients died in the early postoperative period; the three-month survival rate was 42 per cent. The authors reported a one-year survival rate of 23.7 per cent and a five-year survival rate of 4.2 per cent. In their recent series, one-year survival improved to greater than 50 per cent.[145]

In Starzl's group, 170 patients received liver transplants in Denver between 1963 and 1979.[146] The causes of early postoperative death in Starzl's patients were ischemic graft, intraoperative hemorrhage, thrombosis of graft vessels, cerebral air emboli, and portal thrombosis in the recipient.[86] The one-year survival in this group was 32.4 per cent and survival to June 1984 was 18.2 per cent with follow-up of 4.75 to 14.75 years. Cyclosporine A and steroids have been the main immunosuppression agents since 1980. Between July 1980 and June 1984, 244 patients received liver transplants in Denver and Pittsburgh, with a one-year survival of 68 per cent. Starzl and associates reported outcome

by calendar year: One-year survival was 78.6 per cent in 1980, 65.4 per cent in 1981, 50 per cent in 1982, and 70 to 80 per cent in 1983.[146] It is interesting that except for a decrease in 1982, the one-year survival has increased every year to a high of 80 per cent. Survival may be affected by several factors: age and physical condition of the patient, type and severity of liver disease, and surgical and medical technique. Analyzing the statistics from these two major transplantation centers, it is reasonable to project a continuous increase in both short- and long-term survival.

## SUMMARY AND CONCLUSIONS

Although liver transplantation has been performed for two decades, progress was initially slow and survival poor. Painstaking efforts at the two leading centers kept the program alive in the 1970's, and remarkable results have been achieved since 1981. The number of recipients and survival rates have increased dramatically, and the procedure has become manageable. Surgically, the biliary reconstruction technique has decreased postoperative complications; venovenous bypass has decreased intraoperative stress for recipients; and early consideration of retransplantation has decreased overall mortality. Obviously, better understanding of rejection phenomena and the introduction of cyclosporine A helped to improve long-term survival. The increased support by health insurance companies has lessened the economic burden of the procedure. An essential contribution has come from health care personnel behind the scene—an almost unlimited supply of blood products from blood banks, the continuous search for new techniques by supporting laboratory personnel, and dedicated preoperative and postoperative support by intensive care personnel and nurses.

Great progress has been made in anesthetic management. Liver transplantation anesthesia was pioneered by Aldrete and Farman and has been refined by teams in Pittsburgh and other centers. Clinical and basic research have contributed to decreasing intraoperative morbidity and mortality. Development of a rapid infusion system has tremendously reduced hypovolemia- and hemorrhage-related mortality; clinical thromboelastographic monitoring has helped control coagulopathies; and understanding of calcium and potassium homeostasis has practically eliminated the incidence of cardiac arrest.

Nevertheless, many topics require further studies. Candidates at high surgical risk should be better defined to reduce perioperative morbidity and mortality. Dramatic changes in the cardiopulmonary and coagulation systems developing on reperfusion of the graft liver presumably result from intermediary metabolites or other unknown substances originating from the graft liver. Isolation of those substances will help prevent intraoperative complications. Improved liver preservation technique will decrease the waste of donor organs and ultimately allow liver transplantation to become an elective procedure.

The joint efforts of dedicated teams of medical and nonmedical professionals will help patients enjoy survival with an excellent quality of life.

## REFERENCES

1. Jones AL, Spring-Mills E: The liver and gallbladder. In Weiss L, Greep RO (eds): Histology, 4th ed. New York, McGraw-Hill Book Company, 1977, p 701.
2. Rappaport AM, Borowy ZJ, Lougheed WM, Lotto WN: Subdivision of hexagonal liver lobules into a structural and functional unit. Anat Rec 119:16, 1954.
3. Blouin A, Bolender RP, Weibel ER: Distribution of organelles and membranes between hepatocytes and nonhepatocytes in rat liver parenchyma. J Cell Biol 72:441, 1977.
4. Gelman S, Ernst E: Role of pH, $Pco_2$ and $O_2$ content of portal blood in hepatic circulatory autoregulation. Am J Physiol 233:E255, 1977.
5. Lautt WW: Mechanism and role of intrinsic regulation of hepatic arterial blood flow: Hepatic arterial buffer response. Am J Physiol 249:G549, 1985.
6. Greenway CV: Physiology of blood circulation. In Abramson DI, Dobrin PB (eds): Blood Vessels and Lymphatics in Organ Systems. New York, Academic Press, 1984, p 477.
7. Kaplowitz N, Eberle D, Yamada T: Biochemical tests for liver disease. In Zakim D, Boyer TD (eds): Hepatology: A Textbook of Liver Disease. Philadelphia, WB Saunders Company, 1982, p 583.
8. Bosch J, Enriquez R, Groszmann RJ, Storer EH: Chronic bile duct ligation in the dog: Hemodynamic characterization of a portal hypertensive model. Hepatology 3:1002, 1983.
9. Tamakuma S, Wada N, Ishiyama M, et al: Relationship between hepatic hemodynamics and biliary pressure in dogs: Its significance in clinical shock following biliary decompression. Jap J Surg 5:255, 1975.
10. Aarseth S, Bergan A, Aarseth P: Circulatory homeostasis in rats after bile duct ligation. Scand J Clin Lab Invest 39:93, 1979.
11. Witte CL, Witte MH: Splanchnic circulatory and tissue fluid dynamics in portal hypertension. Fed Proc 42:1685, 1983.
12. Vorobioff J, Bredfeldt JE, Groszmann RJ: Increased blood flow through the portal system in cirrhotic rats. Gastroenterology 87:1120, 1984.
13. Kretz R: Lebercirrhose. Path Gesselsch 8:54, 1904.
14. Benoit JN, Womack WA, Hernandez L, Granger DN: "Forward" and "backward" flow mechanisms of portal hypertension. Gastroenterology 89:1092, 1985.
15. Sherwin R, Joshi P, Hendler R, Felig P, Conn HO: Hyperglucagonemia in Laennec's cirrhosis. The role of portal-systemic shunting. N Engl J Med 290:239, 1974.
16. Benoit JN, Barrowman JA, Harper SL, Kvietys PR, Granger DN: Role of humoral factors in the intestinal hyperemia associated with chronic portal hypertension. Am J Physiol 247:G486, 1984.
17. Kulik TJ, Johnson DE, Elde RP, Lock JE: Pulmonary vascular effects of vasoactive intestinal peptide in conscious newborn lambs. Am J Physiol 246:H716, 1984.
18. Keren G, Boichis H, Zwas TS, Frand M: Pulmonary arterio-venous fistulae in hepatic cirrhosis. Arch Dis Child 58:302, 1983.
19. Henriksen JH, Christensen NJ, Ring-Larsen H: Noradrenaline and adrenaline in various vascular beds in patients with cirrhosis—relation to haemodynamics. Clin Physiol 1:293, 1981.
20. Kiel JW, Pitts V, Benoit JN, Granger DN, Shepherd AP: Reduced vascular sensitivity to norepinephrine in portal-hypertensive rats. Am J Physiol 248:G192, 1985.
21. Richardson PDI, Withrington PG: Glucagon inhibition of hepatic arterial responses to hepatic nerve stimulation. Am J Physiol 233:H647, 1977.
22. Bosch J, Arroyo V, Betriu A, et al: Hepatic hemodynamics and the renin-angiotensin-aldosterone system in cirrhosis. Gastroenterology 78:92, 1980.
23. Epstein M: Renal functional abnormalities in cirrhosis: Pathophysiology and management. In Zakim D, Boyer TD (eds): Hepatology: A Textbook of Liver Disease. Philadelphia, WB Saunders Company, 1982, p 446.
24. Perez-Ayuso RM, Arroyo V, Camps J, et al: Renal kallikrein excretion in cirrhotics with ascites: Relationship to renal hemodynamics. Hepatology 4:247, 1984.
25. Racz K, Buu NT, Kuchel O, DeLean A: Dopamine 3-sulfate inhibits aldosterone secretion in cultured bovine adrenal cells. Am J Physiol 247:E431, 1984.
26. Alam AN, Wilkinson SP, Poston L, et al: Intracellular electrolyte abnormalities in fulminant hepatic failure. Gastroenterology 72:914, 1977.
27. Alam AN, Poston L, Wilkinson SP, et al: A study *in vitro* of the sodium pump in fulminant hepatic failure. Clin Sci Molec Med 55:355, 1978.
28. Flier JS, Kahn CR, Roth J: Receptors, antireceptor antibodies and mechanisms of insulin resistance. N Engl J Med 300:413, 1979.
29. Marco J, Diego J, Villanueba ML, et al: Elevated plasma glucagon levels in cirrhosis of the liver. N Engl J Med 28:1107, 1973.
30. Gazzard BG, Rake MO, Flute PT, et al: Bleeding in relation to the coagulation defect of fulminant

hepatic failure. In Williams R, Murray-Lyon IM (eds): Artificial Liver Support. Tunbridge Wells, England, Pitman Medical, 1975, p 63.

31. Dymock IW, Tucker JS, Woolf IL, et al: Coagulation studies as a prognostic index in acute liver failure. Br J Haematol 29:385, 1975.

32. Flute PT: Blood coagulation defects in FHF. Am J Gastroenterol 69:363, 1978.

33. Verstraete M, Vermylen J, Collen D: Intravascular coagulation in liver disease. Annu Rev Med 25:447, 1974.

34. B'oom AL: Intravascular coagulation and the liver. Br J Haematol 30:1, 1975.

35. Delin NA, Ekestrom S, Lindahl J, Nylander G, Sundblad R: Immediate changes in blood flow and oxygen metabolism of the cirrhotic liver following portacaval shunt operations. Surg Gynecol Obstet 144:499, 1977.

36. Steegmuller KW, Marklin HM, Hollis HW Jr: Intraoperative hemodynamic investigations during portacaval shunt. Arch Surg 119:269, 1984.

37. Gelman S, Aldrete JS, Halpern N: Hemodynamics during portacaval shunt operation in humans. Anesth Analg 61:185, 1982.

38. Gelman S, Ernst E: Nitroprusside prevents adverse hemodynamic effects of vasopressin. Arch Surg 113:1465, 1978.

39. Groszmann RJ, Kravetz D, Bosch J, et al: Nitroglycerin improves the hemodynamic response to vasopressin in portal hypertension. Hepatology 2:757, 1982.

40. Changler JG: Vasopressin and splanchnic shunting. Ann Surg 195:543, 1982.

41. Kravetz D, Bosch J, Teres J, Bruix J, Rimola A, Rodes J: Comparison of intravenous somatostatin and vasopressin infusions in treatment of acute variceal hemorrhage. Hepatology 4:442, 1984.

42. Price BA, Jaffe BM, Zinner MJ: Effect of exogenous somatostatin infusion on gastrointestinal blood flow and hormones in the conscious dog. Gastroenterology 88:80, 1985.

43. Benhamou JP, Lebrec D: Drug therapy of portal hypertension due to cirrhosis. Semin Liver Dis 2:231, 1982.

44. Koreger RJ, Groszmann RJ: The effect of the combination of nitroglycerin and propranolol on splanchnic and systemic hemodynamics in a portal hypertensive rat model. Hepatology 5:425, 1985.

45. Bosch J, Mastai R, Kravetz D, Bruix J, Rigau J, Rodes J: Measurement of azygos venous blood flow in the evaluation of portal hypertension in patients with cirrhosis. J Hepatol 1:125, 1985.

46. Conn HO: Propranolol in portal hypertension: Problems in paradise? Hepatology 4:560, 1984.

47. Pandele G, Chaux F, Salvadori C, Farinotti M, Duvaldestin P: Thiopental pharmacokinetics in patients with cirrhosis. Anesthesiology 59:123, 1983.

48. Mazoit JX, Sandouk P, Zetlaoui P, Schermann JM: Pharmacokinetics of morphine in normal and cirrhotic subjects. Anesthesiology 61:A244, 1984.

49. Haberer JP, Schoeffler P, Couderc E, Duvaldestin P: Fentanyl pharmacokinetics in anaesthetized patients with cirrhosis. Br J Anaesth 54:1267, 1982.

50. Ferrier C, Marty J, Bouffard Y, et al: Alfentanil pharmacokinetics in patients with cirrhosis. Anesthesiology 62:480, 1985.

51. Aldrete JA, O'Higgins JW, Holmes J: Changes of plasma cholinesterase activity during orthotopic liver transplantation in man. Transplantation 23:404, 1977.

52. Foldes FF, Swerdlow M, Lipschitz E, et al: Comparison of the respiratory effects of suxamethonium and suxethonium in man. Anesthesiology 17:559, 1956.

53. Gyasi HK, Naguib M: Atracurium and severe hepatic disease: A case report. Can Anaesth Soc J 32:161, 1985.

54. Baraka A, Bagali F: Correlation between tubocurarine requirements and plasma protein pattern. Br J Anaesth 40:89, 1968.

55. Duvaldestin P, Agoston S, Henzel D, Kersten UW, Desmonts JM: Pancuronium and pharmacokinetics in patients with liver cirrhosis. Br J Anaesth 50:1131, 1978.

56. Wilkinson GR, Schenker S: Drug disposition and liver disease. Drug Metabol Rev 4:139, 1975.

57. Williams RL, Benet LZ: Hepatic function and pharmacokinetics. In Zakim D, Boyer TD (eds): Hepatology: A Textbook of Liver Disease. Philadelphia, WB Saunders Company, 1982, p 230.

58. Gelman S: Effects of anesthetics on splanchnic circulation. In Altura BM, Halevy S (eds): Cardiovascular Action of Anesthetics and Drugs Used in Anesthesia. New York, Karger Publishing Company. In press.

59. Gelman S: Disturbances in hepatic blood flow during anesthesia and surgery. Arch Surg 111:881, 1976.

60. Bohrer SL, Rogers EL, Koehler RC, Traystman RJ: Effect of hypovolemic hypotension and laparotomy on splanchnic and hepatic arterial blood flow in dogs. Curr Surg, Sept-Oct 1981, p 325.

61. Harper MH, Collins P, Johnson BH, et al: Postanesthetic hepatic injury in rats: Influence of alterations in hepatic blood flow, surgery, and anesthesia time. Anesth Analg 61:79, 1982.

62. Clarke RSJ, Doggart JR, Lavery T: Changes in liver function after different types of surgery. Br J Anaesth 48:119, 1976.

63. Viegas O, Stoelting RK: LDH$_5$ changes after cholecystectomy or hysterectomy in patients receiving halothane, enflurane, or fentanyl. Anesthesiology 51:556, 1979.

64. McNeill JR, Pang CC: Effect of pentobarbital anesthesia and surgery on the control of arterial pressure and mesenteric resistance in cats: Role of vasopressin and angiotensin. Can J Physiol Pharmacol 60:363, 1982.

65. Donald DE: Splanchnic circulation. In Shepherd JT, Abboud FM, Geiger ST (eds): Handbook of Physiology, Volume 3. Bethesda, American Physiological Society, 1983, p 219.

66. Greenway CV: Role of splanchnic venous system in overall cardiovascular homeostasis. Fed Proc 42:1678, 1983.

67. Zinn SE, Fairley HB, Glenn JD: Liver function in patients with mild alcoholic hepatitis, after enflurane, nitrous oxide-narcotic, and spinal anesthesia. Anesth Analg 64:487, 1985.

68. Loft S, Boel J, Kyst A, Rasmussen B, Hansen SH, Dossing M: Increased hepatic microsomal enzyme activity after surgery under halothane or spinal anesthesia. Anesthesiology 62:11, 1985.

69. Oikkonen M, Rosenberg PH, Neuvonen PJ: Hepatic metabolic ability during anaesthesia. Anaesthesia 39:660, 1984.

70. Harville DD, Summerskill WHJ: Surgery in acute hepatitis. JAMA 184:257, 1963.

71. Powell-Jackson P, Greenway B, Williams R: Adverse effects of exploratory laparotomy in patients with unsuspected liver disease. Br J Surg 69:449, 1982.

72. Gandolfi AJ, Brown BR: Hypoxia and halothane hepatotoxicity. Anesth Analg 62:859, 1983.

73. Van Dyke RA: Halogenated anaesthetic hepatotoxicity—Is the answer close at hand? Clin Anaesth 1:485, 1983.

74. Wataneeyawech M, Kelly KA: Hepatic diseases. Unsuspected before surgery. NY State J Med 75:1278, 1975.

75. Schemel WH: Unsuspected hepatic dysfunction found by multiple laboratory screening. Anesth Analg 55:810, 1976.

76. Dykes MHM, Gilbert JP, Schur PH, Cohen EN: Halothane and the liver: A review of the epidemiologic, immunologic and metabolic aspects of the relationship. Can J Surg 15:217, 1972.

77. Satoh H, Fukuda Y, Anderson DK, et al: Immunological studies on the mechanism of halothane-induced hepatotoxicity: Immunohistochemical evidence of trifluoroacetylated hepatocytes. J Pharmacol Exp Ther 233:857, 1985.

78. Neuberger J, Gimson AES, Davis M, Williams R: Specific serological markers in the diagnosis of fulminant hepatic failure associated with halothane anaesthesia. Br J Anaesth 55:15, 1983.

79. Welch CS: A note on transplantation of the whole liver in dogs. Transplant Bull 2:54, 1955.

80. Goodrich EO, Welch HF, Nelson JA, et al: Homotransplantation of the canine liver. Surgery 39:244, 1956.

81. Moore FD, Smith LL, Burnap TK, et al: One-stage homotransplantation of the liver following total hepatectomy in dogs. Transplant Bull 6:103, 1959.

82. Starzl TE, Bernhard VM, Benvenuto R, et al: A new method for one-stage hepatectomy in dogs. Surgery 46:880, 1959.

83. Absolon KB, Hagihara PF, Griffen WO Jr, et al: Experimental and clinical heterotopic liver homotransplantation. Rev Int Hepatol 15:1481, 1965.

84. Fortner JG, Kinne DW, Shiu MH, et al: Clinical liver heterotopic (auxiliary) transplantation. Surgery 74:739, 1973.

85. Starzl TE, Iwatsuki S: Transplantation of the liver. In Disease of the Liver. Philadelphia, JB Lippincott Company. In press.

86. Starzl TE, Iwatsuki S, Van Thiel DH, et al: Evolution of liver transplantation. Hepatology 2:614, 1982.

87. Starzl TE, Marchioro TL, von Kaulla KN, et al: Homotransplantation of the liver in humans. Surg Gynecol Obstet 117:659, 1963.

88. Moore FD, Birtch AG, Dagher F, et al: Immunosuppression and vascular insufficiency in liver transplantation. Ann NY Acad Sci 102:729, 1964.

89. Demirleau J, Noureddine M, Vignes P, et al: Tentative d' homogreffe hepatique. Mem Acad Chir 90:177, 1964.

90. Calne RY, Smith DP, McMaster P, et al: Use of partial cardiopulmonary bypass during the anhepatic phase of orthotopic liver grafting. Lancet 1:612, 1979.

91. Shaw BW Jr, Martin DJ, Marquez JM, et al: Venous bypass in clinical liver transplantation. Ann Surg 200:524, 1984.

92. Griffith BP, Shaw BW Jr, Hardesty RL, et al: Veno-venous bypass without systemic anticoagulation for transplantation of the human liver. Surg Gynecol Obstet 160:270, 1985.

93. Gordon RD, Shaw BW Jr, Iwatsuki S, et al: Indications for liver transplantation in the cyclosporine era. Surg Clin North Am. In press.

94. Denny DW: Liver procurement for transplantation. In Winter PM, Kang YG (eds): Hepatic Transplantation: Anesthetic and Perioperative Management. New York, Praeger, 1986.

95. Denny D: Testimony on organ procurement and distribution for transplantation. Organ Transplants. US Government Printing Office, 1983, p 134.

96. Bart KJ, Macon EJ, Humphries AL Jr, et al: Cadaveric kidneys for transplantation: A paradox of shortage in the face of plenty. Transplantation 31:383, 1981.

97. Brettschneider L, Daloze PM, Porter KA, et al: The use of combined preservation techniques for extended storage of orthotopic liver homografts. Surg Gynecol Obstet 126:263, 1968.

98. Zimmermann FA, Calne RY, McMaster P, et al: Organ Preservation II. Edinburgh, Churchill Livingstone, 1979, p 267.

99. Starzl TE, Hakala TR, Shaw BW Jr, et al: A flexible procedure for multiple cadaveric organ procurement. Surg Gynecol Obstet 158:223, 1984.

100. Starzl TE: Introductory remarks about liver transplantation. In Winter PM, Kang YG (eds): Hepatic Transplantation: Anesthetic and Perioperative Management. New York, Praeger, 1986.

101. Shaw BW Jr, Wood RP, Gordon RD, et al: Influence of selected patient variables and operative blood loss on six-month survival following liver transplantation. Semin Liver Dis 5:385, 1985.

102. Wetzel RC, Setzer N, Stiff JL, et al: Hemodynamic responses in brain dead organ donor patients. Anesth Analg 64:125, 1985.

103. Casey TH, Summerskill WHJ, Orvis AL: Body and serum potassium in liver disease: I. Relationship to hepatic function and associated factors. Gastroenterology 48:198, 1965.

104. Farman JV, Lines JG, Williams RS, et al: Liver transplantation in man. Anesthetic and biochemical management. Anaesthesia 29:17, 1974.

105. Gazzard BG, Portmann B, Murray-Lyon IM, et al: Causes of death in fulminant hepatic failure and relationship to quantitative histological assessment of parenchymal damage. Q J Med 44:615, 1975.

106. Neuberger JM, MacDougall BRD, Williams R: Liver transplantation. In Calne RY (ed): The Cambridge-King's College Hospital Experience. New York, Grune & Stratton, 1983, p 343.

107. Green AJ, Ratnoff OD: Elevated antihemophilic factor (AHF, factor VIII) procoagulant activity and AHF-like antigen in alcoholic cirrhosis of the liver. J Lab Clin Med 83:189, 1974.

108. Karpatkin S, Freedman ML: Hypersplenic thrombocytopenia differentiated from increased peripheral destruction by platelet volume. Ann Intern Med 89:200, 1978.

109. Bontempo FA, Lewis JH, Ragni MV, et al: The

preoperative coagulation pattern in liver transplant patients. In Winter PM, Kang YG (eds): Hepatic Transplantation: Anesthetic and Perioperative Management. New York, Praeger, 1986.

110. Kang YG, Martin DJ, Marquez J, et al: Intraoperative changes in blood coagulation and thromboelastographic monitoring in liver transplantation. Anesth Analg 64:888, 1985.

111. Kang YG: Monitoring and treatment of coagulation. In Winter PM, Kang YG (eds): Hepatic Transplantation: Anesthetic and Perioperative Management. New York, Praeger, 1986.

112. Sassano JJ: The rapid infusion system. In Winter PM, Kang YG (eds): Hepatic Transplantation: Anesthetic and Perioperative Management. New York, Praeger, 1986.

113. Munson ES, Merrick HC: Effects of nitrous oxide on venous embolism. Anesthesiology 27:783, 1966.

114. Borland LM, Roule M, Cook, R: Anesthesia for pediatric orthotopic liver transplantation. Anesth Analg 64:117, 1985.

115. Eger EI II: The pharmacology of isoflurane. Br J Anaesth 56:71S, 1984.

116. Mazze RI, Calverly RK, Smith NT: Inorganic fluoride nephrotoxicity: Prolonged enflurane and halothane anesthesia in volunteers. Anesthesiology 46:265, 1977.

117. Ngai SH: Current concepts in anesthesiology. Effects of anesthetics and various organs. N Engl J Med 302:564, 1980.

118. Marquez J, Martin DJ: Anesthetic management in liver transplantation. In Winter PM, Kang YG (eds): Hepatic Transplantation: Anesthetic and Perioperative Management. New York, Praeger, 1986.

119. Jones RM, Detmer M, Hill AB, et al: Incidence of choledochoduodenal sphincter spasm during fentanyl-supplemented anesthesia. Anesth Analg 60:638, 1981.

120. Shanks CA, Avram MJ, Ronai AK, et al: Loss of tubocurarine with the washing of salvaged autologous blood. Anesthesiology 61:A316, 1984.

121. Papas G, Palmer WM, Martineau GL, et al: Hemodynamic alterations caused during orthotopic liver transplantation in humans. Surgery 70:872, 1971.

122. Denmark SW, Shaw BW Jr, Griffith BP, et al: Veno-venous bypass without systemic anticoagulation in canine and human liver transplantation. Surg Forum 34:380, 1983.

123. Shaw BW Jr: Venous bypass for clinical transplantation of the liver. In Winter PM, Kang YG (eds): Anesthetic and Perioperative Management. New York, Praeger, 1986.

124. Martin DJ, Marquez JM, Kang YG, et al: Liver transplantation: Hemodynamic and electrolyte changes seen immediately following revascularization (abstract). Anesth Analg 63:246, 1984.

125. Starzl TE, Schneck SA, Mazzoni G, et al: Acute neurological complications after liver transplantation with particular reference to intraoperative cerebral air embolus. Ann Surg 187:236, 1978.

126. Wagner PD, Laravuso RB, Uhl RR, et al: Continuous distributions of ventilation-perfusion ratios in normal subjects breathing air and 100% O$_2$. J Clin Invest 54:54, 1974.

127. Winter PM, Smith G: The toxicity of oxygen. Anesthesiology 37:210, 1972.

128. Lindrop MJ, Farman JV, Smith MF: Liver transplantation. In Calne RY (ed): The Cambridge-King's College Hospital Experience. New York, Grune & Stratton, 1983, p 128.

129. Lewis JH, Bontempo FA, Kang YG, et al: Intraoperative coagulation changes in liver transplantation. In Winter PM, Kang YG (eds): Hepatic Transplantation: Anesthetic and Perioperative Management. New York, Praeger, 1986.

130. Groth CG, Pechet L, Starzl TE: Coagulation during and after orthotopic transplantation of the human liver. Arch Surg 98:31, 1969.

131. Comp PC, Esmon CT: Initiation of clot lysis in plasma by activated protein C. Circulation 58:(Suppl II)210, 1978.

132. Thurer RL, Lytle BW, Cosgrove DM, et al: Autotransfusion following cardiac surgery: A randomized, prospective study. Ann Thorac Surg 27:500, 1979.

133. Kang YG, Navalgund A, Russell M, et al: Antifibrinolytic therapy during liver transplantation (abstract). Anesthesiology 63:A92, 1985.

134. von Kaulla KN, Kaye H, von Kaulla E, et al: Changes in blood coagulation, before and after hepatectomy or transplantation in dogs and man. Arch Surg 92:71, 1966.

135. Carmichael FJ, Lindop MJ, Farman JV: Anesthesia for hepatic transplantation: Cardiovascular and metabolic alterations and their management. Anesth Analg 64:108, 1985.

136. Marquez J: Citrate intoxication during hepatic transplantation. In Winter PM, Kang YG (eds): Hepatic Transplantation: Anesthetic and Perioperative Management. New York, Praeger, 1986.

137. Kahn RC, Jascott D, Carlon GC, et al: Massive blood replacement: Correlation of ionized calcium, citrate, and hydrogen ion concentration. Anesth Analg 58:274, 1979.

138. Howland WS, Bellville JW, Zucker MB, et al: Massive blood replacement: Failure to observe citrate intoxication. Surg Gynecol Obstet 105:529, 1975.

139. Abouna GM, Aldrete JA, Starzl TE: Changes in serum potassium and pH during clinical and experimental liver transplantation. Surgery 69:419, 1971.

140. Tullock WC, Pinsky MR, Shaw BW Jr: Metabolic changes during the anhepatic phase of liver transplantation (abstract). Anesthesiology 61:A271, 1984.

141. Aldrete J, Clapp HW, Starzl TE: Body temperature changes during organ transplantation. Anesth Analg 49:384, 1970.

142. Shapiro MJ, Wood RP, Shaw BW Jr: Postoperative care of liver transplantation patients. In Winter PM, Kang YG (eds): Hepatic Transplantation: Anesthetic and Perioperative Management. New York, Praeger, 1986.

143. Jaffers GJ, Cosimi AB: Kidney Transplantation. New York, Grune & Stratton, 1984, p 281.

144. Wood RP, Shaw BW Jr, Starzl TE: Extrahepatic complications of liver transplantation. Semin Liver Dis 5:377, 1985.

145. Calne RY, Williams R, Lindrop M, et al: Improved survival after orthotopic liver grafting. Br Med J 283:115, 1981.

146. Starzl TE, Iwatsuki S, Shaw BW Jr, et al: Orthotopic liver transplantation in 1984. Transplant Proc 17:250, 1985.

# Appendix A   Protective Measures Against Viral Hepatitis

The following guidelines are suggested for effectively cleaning, sterilizing, and disposing of anesthesia equipment that has come in direct contact with patients with active viral hepatitis. Viral hepatitis is defined as active from the time of diagnosis until the antigens become negative and the antibody becomes positive. Patients with non-A non-B hepatitis are treated the same as patients with hepatitis B.

1. Preparation
   A. All unnecessary equipment is removed from the operating room, and disposable equipment is used whenever possible. If possible, all operating room attire should be disposable.
2. Intraoperative period
   A. Individuals assigned to the room should not leave unless it is absolutely necessary. Before leaving the operating room, disposable cap, face mask, scrub gown, shoe covers, and gloves are disposed of in a double plastic bag marked **Hepatitis Precaution**. Hands are washed immediately with antimicrobial soap.
3. Postoperative period
   A. All disposable items are collected in an impervious plastic bag and marked **Hepatitis Precaution**.

B. The following items are washed in antimicrobial soap and water and sent for ethylene oxide sterilization: metal connecting tubes, face mask, head strap, laryngoscope, McGill forceps, blood pressure cuff, blood pump, temperature probe, precordial and esophageal stethoscopes, and PEEP valve.

C. Parts of the anesthesia gas machine and ventilator that come in direct contact with the patient are sterilized with ethylene oxide. These are the $CO_2$ absorber, directional flow valves, and ventilator bellows and cap.

D. The following equipment is washed with 5 per cent hypochlorite (1:10 dilution of household bleach) for an exposure time of 30 minutes when there are major blood spills and 5 minutes for other surfaces: arm boards, anesthesia cart, intubation cart, anesthesia gas machine, ventilator stand, blood warmer, inspired gas humidifier, and all other major equipment inside the operating room, including vital sign monitor and cables.

# Appendix B   Anesthesia for Liver Transplantation Protocol

1. Preparation
   A. Drugs. Sodium bicarbonate, calcium chloride, Normosol solution, albumin, Solu-Medrol, furosemide, mannitol, insulin, potassium chloride, Neo-Synephrine, epinephrine, dobutamine, Pitressin, nitroglycerin, verapamil, dextrose 5 per cent in water, dextrose 20 per cent, epsilon aminocaproic acid.
   B. Equipment. Humidifier in anesthesia machine with compressed air mixture, PEEP valve, heating mattress, neuromuscular monitor, nasogastric tube, two blood pumps, mass spectrometer, monitor of core temperature, roller rapid infusion pump, arterial line, and Swan-Ganz catheter with permanent mixed venous oxygen saturation monitor, four intravenous infusion sets, two IMED pumps.

C.  Inform the blood bank.
2. Patient is in the operating room
   A.  Standard or rapid-sequence anesthesia induction, muscle relaxation, anesthesia with isoflurane without nitrous oxide, insertion of all necessary lines.
3. Surgery
   A.  Stage 1 (Preanhepatic Phase) main problems
       (1) Clotting abnormalities (treat with fresh frozen plasma, platelets, cryoprecipitate, and calcium, according to laboratory data and thromboelastography).
       (2) Metabolic acidosis (treat with sodium bicarbonate).
       (3) Hyperpotassemia (if calcium is greater than 4 mEq/L, diuresis is necessary; treat with furosemide, calcium chloride, sodium bicarbonate, and, if needed, insulin plus glucose).
       (4) Right lobe exposure (inferior vena cava compression, kinking of pericardium, potassium liberation from anoxic liver, air embolism).
   B.  Stage 2 (Anhepatic Phase) main problems
       (1) Decrease in venous return, filling pressure, and cardiac output (treat with volume, calcium chloride, and sodium bicarbonate).
       (2) Metabolic acidosis (treat with sodium bicarbonate).
       (3) Hypocalcemia (treat with calcium chloride).

   (4) Clotting abnormalities (treat with fresh frozen plasma, platelets, cryoprecipitate, and calcium, according to laboratory data and thromboelastography).
   (5) Pulmonary edema (treat with calcium chloride, PEEP and dopamine; increased filling pressures are sometimes needed to keep aterial pressure adequate).
   C.  Stage 3 (Postanhepatic Phase) main problems
       (1) Hypopotassemia (prevent and treat with calcium chloride, sodium bicarbonate, and, if needed, insulin plus glucose).
       (2) Metabolic acidosis (treat with sodium bicarbonate).
       (3) Increase in pulmonary artery and filling pressures, decrease in arterial pressure and cardiac output (treat with dopamine, calcium chloride, and dobutamine, if needed).
       (4) Clotting abnormalities and bleeding (treat with blood replacement, fresh frozen plasma, platelets, and cryoprecipitate under control of thromboelastography).
       (5) Air embolism (treat with PEEP; try to aspirate air from Swan-Ganz catheter).
       (6) Pulmonary edema (treat with calcium chloride, PEEP, and dopamine; increased filling pressures are sometimes needed to keep arterial pressure adequate).

# 9

# *Replantation of Severed Limbs*

JOHN P. EBERT

*Any fool can cut off a leg—it takes a surgeon to save one.*

GEORGE G. ROSS (1834–1892)

A successful replantation of an amputated upper extremity in 1962[1] was the first obvious example that severed body parts could be viably and functionally reattached. Since that time, the numbers of qualified microvascular surgeons as well as centers with facilities suitable for replantation programs have steadily increased. The capability of anastomosing blood vessels as small as 0.3 mm in diameter has not only initiated a new era in surgical therapy, but has also exposed several social, economic, and psychological issues concerning its use. The techniques that enable the surgeon to reanastomose tiny blood vessels and thereby reperfuse an amputated body part demonstrate technical triumph, but in some ill-chosen circumstances represent an incredible economical cost to society, an unreasonable physiological risk to the patient, and the beginning of a life with a useless, painful, and troublesome extremity. Successful replantation requires a team composed of surgeons, anesthesiologists, psychiatrists, nurses, physiotherapists, and emergency room personnel. This team must be available 24 hours a day, 365 days per year, and must be fully aware that the majority of the work demanded will be tedious, exhausting, of long duration, and will most commonly begin in the late afternoon and span upward of 24 hours. Although the majority of cases offer the prospect for successful reperfusion, less than 50 per cent represent reasonable chances for a complete functional recovery. In determining the success or failure of our efforts, the same objective criteria should be employed for patients undergoing replantation as those applied to patients undergoing other types of organ transplantation, that is, organ function. The question is no longer can it be replanted, but should it be replanted. "A stiff, insensitive finger may be a tribute to technical skills, but it is also a monument to poor judgment."[2] The objectives of this discourse are to put the results of replantation into perspective and to present the available data and controversies that direct our anesthetic conduct.

## PERSPECTIVES ON FUNCTIONAL RECOVERY

Replantation is the surgical restoration of a lost organ or appendage to its original site

187

in the same patient.[3] Revascularization, on the other hand, is the re-establishment of arterial circulation to a part that has been incompletely amputated.[4] This chapter will deal exclusively with the problems associated with replantation. For our purposes, considerations operant in replantation are also applicable in composite grafting, or free vascularized tissue transfer, with the possible exception that there are often additional positioning and technical problems associated with composite grafting. Successful replantation of several organs, including the upper[5] and lower extremities,[6] penis,[7] lip,[8] ear,[9,10] scalp,[11,12] and spleen[13] have been described. Upper extremity replantation is by far the most common autotransplantation procedure, with a worldwide incidence of 1 to 10 replants per 100,000 population, extrapolated from reports of several large series.[14]

The importance of intimal integrity of veins and arteries of sufficient length cannot be overstated, for any significant defect will result in an increased incidence of thrombotic complications. In certain grafts, such as composite grafts of the face (i.e., nose and lip), venous channels are notably small, multiple, and functionally inaccessible for reanastomosis. Even in circumstances in which sufficient venous drainage was absent, unconventional therapy such as the use of leeches has been employed in the early postoperative period, culminating in an ultimately successful outcome.[8] Although the majority of attention has been focused on microvascular techniques enabling reperfusion of amputated parts, results in terms of function are not restricted merely to the presence or absence of circulation. In cases of replantation of thumbs or fingers, intact circulation with absence of sensory function, or nonunion of the fracture site, will render the whole procedure useless. Likewise, replantation of the penis without the return of sensory and sexual functions would be an equally disappointing result. Unlike other forms of organ transplantation that rely primarily on adequate circulation in the absence of rejection for their functional survival, successful replantation of an amputated body part necessitates the recovery of normal function in all of the heterogeneous tissues present in the amputated part, such as bone, muscle and nerve. It is helpful to put the anatomical and physiological consequences of reimplantation into perspective. Factors that favor or discourage

good functional recovery may be found in Tables 9–1 and 9–2. Although children pose more technical difficulties because of their size, the potential for a functional outcome is greatest in them because of their ability to relearn and adapt to their injuries. Therefore, all amputations in children should be considered for replantation. It is generally felt that single-digit replantations, except for the thumb, are not rewarding, and this is particularly true for the index finger because the end product is often a stiff and unusable liability for the entire hand. The exception to this rule may be the amputation of digits distal to the proximal interphalangeal joint where good function and excellent cosmetic restoration can be obtained. Revascularization should be performed in incomplete amputations, if there is a reasonable chance for functional integrity. Amputation sites proximal to the proximal interphalangeal joints,

### TABLE 9–1. Conditions Favoring Extremity Replantation

A. Anatomical
1. Distal to proximal interphalangeal joint
2. Thumb
3. Multiple digits
4. Palm, wrist or distal forearm
5. Incomplete
B. Type
1. Guillotine
C. Associated factors
1. Children
2. Motivation
3. Employed
4. Extenuating circumstances
5. Proper preservation

### TABLE 9–2. Factors Discouraging Extremity Replantation

A. Anatomic
1. Lower extremity
2. Single digits
3. "No man's land"
4. Proximal forearm and arm
B. Type
1. Avulsion
2. Crush
C. Contributing factors
1. Compromising medical illness
2. Lack of motivation, psychosis
3. Advanced age
4. Long ischemia time

but distal to the metacarpophalangeal joints, are referred to as no man's land, so that replantation is recommended at this location only in extreme circumstances. Conversely, amputations through the palm, and at the wrist, including the distal forearm, have a reasonable chance for a good result and therefore may be aggressively pursued. Proximal forearm and arm amputations are associated with adequate perfusion, but dreadful functional outcomes. Reamputation has been the final procedure after an initially successful, arduous vascular repair in some of these cases.[15] Although successful replantations of lower extremities have been reported, an equivalent functional result can be achieved at lower risk with prosthetic devices than with surgery. Replantation of salvage parts leading to a better prosthetic fit have been also described.[16] Nonmicrovascular penile repairs have culminated in limited sexual function and the development of urethral fistulas, and have dictated the recommendation of microsurgical replantation in all feasible circumstances. Even though hair growth may not return to normal in all cases of scalp replantation, this undertaking is associated with a lower incidence of infection and better coverage of the calvarium than conventional techniques. Cosmetic restoration must be considered foremost in replantation of tissues of the head.

Any discussion of anatomy of amputated parts would be incomplete without a discussion of functional results as they relate to the type of amputation. Guillotine amputations are associated with a survival rate of better than 90 per cent, with functional result approaching normality in most distal amputations. Injuries caused by compression have an outcome that is likely compromised. In either local or diffuse crush injuries, the contact surface is much greater than in guillotine amputation, and therefore the bone, skin, nerve, and vascular destruction is so extensive that serious loss of length and technical difficulties compromise the results. Avulsion amputations are the most unfavorable, and their prognosis is at best guarded with respect to both survival and function.

Good functional outcomes rely on good judgment that applies not only to the anatomical lesion itself, but also addresses psychological and motivational aspects of the candidate for replantation. At one extreme there is the victim of self-mutilation who may anatomically present optimal technical conditions, but may exhibit behavior that is so noncompliant that any form of therapy is doomed to failure.[17] These patients are often schizophrenics who, following rapid neuroleptic treatment and unwaveringly firm and aggressive psychiatric intervention, may accept operative treatment and exhibit reasonable functional results. The overall psychological profile of patients requiring replantation reveals characteristics that may come as a surprise to some. Although many amputations occur in job-related situations, one study has documented that psychiatric intervention was warranted in 60 per cent of these patients; 33 per cent showed evidence of preaccident psychopathology; 20 per cent suffered from a substance abuse disorder; and 50 per cent reported a stressful life event within the year antedating the accident.[18] With these facts in mind, it is not unexpected that excellent functional results are seen in less than 40 per cent of these patients[15] even though a solid anatomical repair is obvious and healing is complete in a much higher percentage. For these reasons the inclusion of psychiatric consultants on the replantation team would enhance hopes for functional recovery.

In the final analysis, the decision regarding replantation for all patients must be individualized. The motivation and strong wishes of the patient may override other considerations such as advanced age and medical infirmities. Extenuating circumstances, such as occupational requirements (e.g., the index finger of a physician) or appearance (e.g., the ring finger of an adolescent female) may influence the decision to replant a part. For valid informed consent the patient must understand that surgery is not a miraculous overnight cure, and the period of rehabilitation will be long and will require extensive cooperation. The operative procedure, including anesthetic risks and those associated with blood transfusions, should neither be minimized nor overlooked. The return to work or to gainful employment may be delayed up to six months and regrettably, may never occur for some patients. Patients must be willing to undertake these risks and must be motivated to participate in the treatment plan before the enormous and expensive machinery of a replantation team is started in motion.

A great deal of progress has been made since the first reports of an arm replantation by Malt and McKhann,[1] and the hand replant by Chen.[19] In 1965, Kleinert and Kasden[20] documented the first successful anastomosis of digital vessels in a devascularized thumb, and in 1968, Komatsu and Tamai,[21] from Japan, published the first account of successful replantation of an amputated thumb. In these early days, it appeared that survival of the digit was the most important end point, and little emphasis was placed on other, possibly more important, considerations such as sensibility, cold intolerance, recovery time, eventual function, and, most importantly, time lost from work and the potential for return to work. The disability time averages six months in patients who have successful replantations. It is indefinite when outcome is poor. Functional results have been emphasized to this point because these factual data must be understood by the anesthesiologist before informed cost-benefit decisions can be made. Function and benefits should outweigh the risks and financial costs before a decision is made to undertake replantation.

## ORGAN PRESERVATION

Another notable difference between replantation and other forms of transplantation is that organ harvesting is usually a self-inflicted phenomenon. This procedure is unplanned, often undertaken in unsterile conditions, and preservation procedures are unavailable. How long the amputated part can withstand ischemia depends on multiple factors, including the temperature, muscle mass, and time. With prolonged ischemia, cellular adenosine triphosphate is depleted, resulting in failure of the sodium pump and inability of the cell to regulate its volume. This is undoubtedly responsible for the swelling of epithelial and perivascular cells, resulting in the postischemic vascular obstruction. The major limiting process occurs not in the larger vessels but in the microcirculation and is mainly responsible for the "no-reflow phenomenon" or high vascular resistance after a prolonged period of warm ischemia.[22]

Preservation of the amputated part should be directed toward maintenance of the microvascular competence and cellular integrity during this ischemia. Although several methods of preservation have been tried, cooling, not freezing, has emerged as the most easily achieved and efficacious means of sustaining integrity of the amputated part.[23] This cooling results in a state of metabolic suspension in which cellular activity decreases with decreasing temperature, resulting in generalized depression of metabolism, decreased oxygen utilization, and diminution of production of toxic metabolic by-products. This reduction is intimately associated with the decrement in temperature, such that oxygen consumption is lowered by 84 per cent at 20°C and 96 per cent at 10°C.

Hypothermic preservation of the extremities has not achieved the same success as preservation of red blood cells. This should be attributed to the inability of surface cooling to result in the rapid lowering of the tissue's core temperature. While surface cooling has not exhibited the same success for composite tissues as for red cells, skin, and sperm, it can be credited with reliable preservation of tissues, such as digits, scalp, and ear, for up to 24 hours, and bulkier tissues with larger amounts of muscle mass, such as forearms, for up to 10 hours. It seems that the muscle fibers in the amputated limb are more sensitive to ischemia than any of the other tissues. Disturbances in the microcirculation of the muscle have been confirmed within 30 minutes of removal of the limb. For these reasons the amputated tissue should be gently cleaned and irrigated with saline solution, wrapped in sterile, dry gauze, and placed in a sterile plastic container or plastic bag. The part is then placed in a styrofoam container filled with ice in separate plastic bags. The amputated part should not come in direct contact with the ice, for this may result in tissue freezing, which would compromise revascularization attempts. The cooling of a partially amputated devascularized extremity is equally important.[24] The wound is also flushed with sterile saline, wrapped in dry gauze, and splinted. The appendage is then wrapped with plastic bags containing ice, which should be secured in place until the part is examined by the replantation team. The concept of controlled digital hyperthermia using coils and a roller pump for external cooling has been described[25] and is intriguing, but its efficacy and facility have not been documented.

## REPLANTATION AND ASSOCIATED COMPROMISE

Amputation of even one digit is thought of by most patients as a life-threatening incident. While no amputation should be considered a trivial event, many are associated with

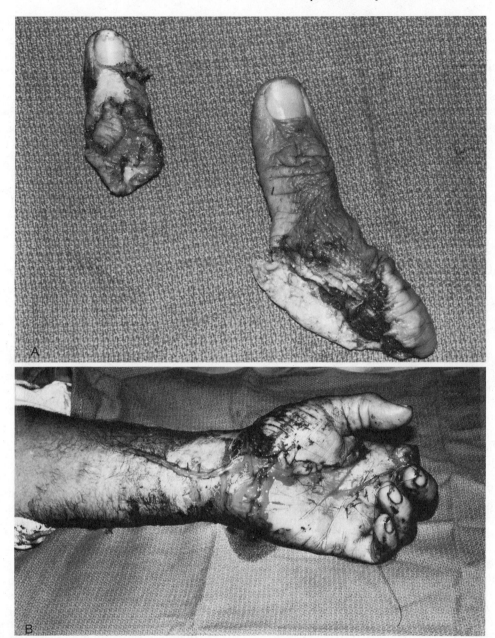

**Figure 9–1.** *A*, Amputated left thumb and index finger. *B*, Replanted thumb. Replantation of the index finger was not undertaken.

other trauma that is truly life threatening. Scalp and ear avulsions may coexist with closed head injuries, while patients with hand and forearm amputations incurred in motor vehicle accidents may have concomitant blunt chest and abdominal trauma. One case report described an intraoperative death due to catastrophic intra-abdominal hemorrhage occurring during the operative replantation procedure.

A thorough, thoughtful, and comprehensive assessment of the patient is necessary before any replantation procedures are entertained. A carefully obtained history, a complete physical examination, and evaluation of important data, including the appropriate roentgenograms, ECG, and laboratory data, such as hemoglobin concentration, hematocrit value, coagulation profile, and blood chemistry, are imperative. Blood should be typed and crossmatched, and the blood bank should be alerted to the possibility that blood loss may exceed 10 units. Because substance abuse has been documented in 20 per cent of these patients,[18] a drug screening at the time of admission is appropriate. These recommendations are made neither for the sake of completeness nor as lip service to some standard of care in anesthesiology. They are made because the anesthesiologist, who is to initiate emergency anesthesia that may last 24 hours, must be data rich and informed. The blood loss at the scene of the injury is often quite significant, regardless of the pulse rate and arterial blood pressure at the time of admission to the hospital. Underestimation could be an important mistake.

## PREANESTHETIC THOUGHTS

Unless the amputation was self-inflicted, these patients usually find themselves unexpectedly in a large medical facility needing major medical care. They customarily experience pain and are quite scared. Their last meal was more often than not in temporal proximity to their injury. The risk of an acid aspiration containing food particles is not insignificant. If administered intravenously 90 minutes before the induction of anesthesia, a single dose of cimetidine has an excellent (i.e., 90 per cent) chance of raising the gastric pH above the critical level of 2.5.[26,27] Oral doses have less chance of being effective.[28] The same dose should be repeated at least every six hours to reduce the risk of acid aspiration at the time of extubation and postoperatively. Metoclopramide may facilitate gastric emptying and, it is hoped, reduce gastric volume;[29] however, the efficacy of this drug in this circumstance has not been fully documented.[30]

Psychotic patients who have self-inflicted injuries must be immediately assessed by a psychiatrist experienced in these matters. Failure to perform surgery can be interpreted either as denying a mentally incompetent patient medical treatment or as violating an individual's right to refuse treatment. The psychiatrist's contribution to this circumstance is invaluable.[17] The anesthesiologist should be aware of the psychotropic drugs administered and suggested for continued therapy through the procedure.

For nonpsychotic patients the preoperative visit can contribute significantly to reducing their anxiety. Pain usually may be relieved with small doses of narcotics and additional anxiety managed with judicious doses of a drug like diazepam. The need for fluid resuscitation and antibiotics dictates the establishment of intravenous access, and this should be used as the route for premedication, especially cimetidine, in deference to others. Unless for some reason the ischemic time has been dangerously long, there is little need to rush to the operating room; therefore, preparations may be made in an orderly fashion and management protocols carefully formulated.

## THE ANESTHETIC

Although the part or parts to be reattached may be small, the anesthetic is not. Because there are few descriptions in the literature depicting the anesthetic management of these patients, much of the following will be taken from personal experience and application of existing data. These are long procedures, and most of the considerations described herein have much to do with any anesthetic for a long operation. Over protracted periods, major changes can occur insidiously, unobserved by all but the most vigilant of anesthesiologists. The replantation anesthetic protocol near the end of this chapter summarizes the following considerations.

Even though blood loss can be significant, exceeding 7500 ml in some circumstances, this loss may occur so insidiously that it goes unnoticed for some time, unless it is anticipated and monitored appropriately. These patients may thoughtlessly be given large volumes of crystalloid solutions, culminating in increased intravascular volume, considerable fluid translocation, and, regrettably, the development of edema that may compromise the perfusion of the replanted part. For these reasons, crystalloid infusions should be carefully titrated to objective signs of effective intravascular volume, such as urine output and/or the cardiac index–pulmonary artery occluded pressure relationship. In the abient sence of pulmonary artery catheterization, a urine output of $0.5 \text{ ml·kg}^{-1}\text{·hr}^{-1}$ is sufficient. Excesses have been reported[31] and may result in the detrimental features already mentioned. In the absence of hypoglycemia, glucose infusions are avoided, because of injury-induced gluconeogenesis and glycogenolysis.[32] Glucose administration may result in osmotic diuresis and negatively influence the accuracy of the urine output as a monitor of intravascular volume. All infusions should be warmed; however, if benign hyperthermia develops, continued warming would obviously be inappropriate. In the presence of slow and insidious loss of blood, serial hematocrit monitoring is invaluable. In a healthy, normothermic, and nonalkalemic patient with adequate cardiac output, hematocrits ranging from 25 to 30 per cent in the face of normal intravascular volume should result in adequate oxygen delivery and improved rheological properties. Some coexisting factors may dictate the maintenance of higher hematocrit values. These hematocrit determinations can be made as frequently as every half-hour; however, the interval should not exceed two hours. Commonly, these hematocrits are measured on the same sample used for the determination of arterial blood gases. Likewise, the acid-base status and gas exchange are assessed by serial analysis of arterial blood samples. The negative effect of acidosis on reperfusion[33] and the well-known influence of alkalemia on blood flow recommend the maintenance of physiological levels of $pH_a$ and $Pa_{CO_2}$. Ventilation in the supine position, especially with an oxygen-enriched mixture of anesthetic gases, results in progressive decrease in the functional residual capacity.[34] This phenomenon is reflected in steady decreases in $Pa_{O_2}$, and can be avoided through the use of low-dose positive end-expiratory pressure.[35] Maintenance of airway humidification is an important physiological adjunct.[36] Serum concentrations of sodium and potassium can drastically change during long procedures; therefore, serial determinations of these (usually every two hours) as well as blood glucose concentrations are well advised. Hyponatremia is linked to gastric decompression and hypotonic fluid administration, while hypokalemia may result from homologous blood transfusion. Supplementation may be easily effected through the infusion of normal saline with potassium chloride, if needed. If intravenous regular insulin therapy is required for the treatment of hyperglycemia, more frequent determinations of glucose and electrolyte concentrations are indicated.[37] Those patients who have elevated serum ethanol concentrations at the time of injury often manifest hyperglycemic, osmotic, and hormonally induced diuresis. In these circumstances, serial measurements of urine as well as serum osmolality should be

made. We have measured serum colloid-osmotic pressures in the past and have witnessed their decline during these procedures, but have been unable to pinpoint any physiological abnormality directly emanating from this low value. This experience has been supported by others, and we have discontinued the regular use of this measurement in this group of patients.

As far as cardiovascular monitoring is concerned, arterial and central venous cannulation with continuous pressure transduction are employed in all patients. In young and healthy patients, with excellent right ventricular function and compliant pulmonary circulation, the central venous pressure may be low in the absence of decreased intravascular volume. Therapy should not be based on this low value. If any question arises throughout the procedure concerning cardiac performance, the state of the circulation, or the effective intravascular volume, pulmonary arterial cannulation is recommended.[38] Because coronary artery disease is not restricted to male patients over the age of 40 years, both lead II and lead $V_5$ are continuously monitored for arrhythmic and ischemic changes respectively.

The best anesthetic management of these patients is debatable. Support for both regional and general forms of anesthesia exist, and just as the decision to replant is individualized, so should the anesthetic management. Practically, regional anesthesia may be appropriate only for procedures confined to the extremities. If there is a serious question whether the replantation of a thumb or hand will be possible, the procedure may be initiated using a brachial plexus block, especially in a patient with a full stomach. A continuous brachial plexus block using the axillary route has been advocated most often; however, it requires the elicitation of a paresthesia for successful completion.[39] A supraclavicular approach not relying on a paresthesia has likewise been described.[40] Either block is initiated before the beginning of the procedure, and the catheter is secured in place with both suture and betadine dressing. It is our habit to attach a Cobe connector with a three-way stopcock to this catheter, maintaining a sealed system between injections. Intravenous general anesthesia without endotracheal intubation as supplementation of a block is an ill-advised alternative. Heavy sedation in the presence of a full stomach also may precipitate aspiration. In these situations, as well as in very long procedures or in those in which vein harvesting from another location is necessary, a thoughtfully planned general anesthetic is an appropriate complement to the regional technique. The beneficial effects of the sympathetic block are appreciated by some surgeons, and in these cases, the blocks should be continued and more local anesthetic administered at regular intervals. The draping and tourniquet make the axilla somewhat inaccessible intraoperatively; therefore, a supraclavicular block using the first rib as a landmark may be a reasonable and effective alternative for continuation throughout the operation.

The general anesthesia, which may last for a day or more, is a commitment of considerable proportions. In the presence of a full stomach, a rapid induction intubation sequence is followed. Nitrous oxide is avoided because of its vasoconstrictive effects, its influence on postoperative nausea and vomiting, its bone marrow depression and resulting leukopenia, and its toxic effects on the methionine-synthetase enzyme system. Air is used instead, and the $F_{I_{O_2}}$ adjusted to the target $Pa_{O_2}$. Five cm $H_2O$ of positive end-expiratory pressure is employed to maintain the physiological functional residual capacity unless there is a coexisting head injury or other contraindication. To predictably provide anesthesia in the absence of nitrous oxide, a volatile anesthetic must be employed. Narcotics may be used for supplementation. Clear appreciation of the uptake and distribution of volatile inhalational anesthetics is essential for the safe conduct of anesthesia for a long procedure. The uptake of these drugs decreases over time in the vessel-rich groups as well as in the muscle groups. To prevent ever increasing end-tidal concentrations of the volatile agent and excessive organ-based accumulations, the inhaled concentration must be synchronously reduced. If not, prolonged emergence may be the consequence.[31] A mass spectrometer, or some other form of gas analyzer that continuously measures the end-tidal concentration of anesthetic agents, is an invaluable adjunct in these protracted operations. It is our practice to use a closed-system anesthetic technique so that trends in oxygen consumption may be appreciated, the anesthetic agents will not be needlessly wasted, and airway dehydration and heat loss will be prevented.[41]

Every volatile anesthetic available in the United States today undergoes biotransformation to xenobiotics. Metabolism is greatest for halothane (approximately 20 per cent) and least for isoflurane (0.5 per cent). Less biotransformation has its benefits, since the xenobiotics associated with halothane and enflurane may have toxic manifestations if the concentrations are high enough. Aside from the hepatic toxicity that may stem from the reductive metabolism of halothane, breakdown of this compound may give rise to psychoactive levels of bromine.[42] Likewise, enflurane biotransformation can result in inorganic fluoride levels of 50 $\mu M \cdot L^{-1}$ following as little as 4.0 MAC-hours of administration.[43] However, the renal concentrating defect accompanying prolonged enflurane anesthesia is probably not of major importance, while prolongation of awakening has been reported with this anesthetic when it was employed for replantation.[31] It should be pointed out that end-tidal anesthetic concentration was not measured, and objective evidence of anesthetic depth was not described in this report.

Isoflurane may represent a superior alternative, and anecdotal support exists for it.[44] In most circumstances, isoflurane can be considered the anesthetic of choice; however, some reservations concerning myocardial perfusion in patients with coronary artery disease have stimulated caution and employment of alternative anesthetics in these situations.[45,46]

Hypothermia and its attendant vasoconstriction make it an unwanted visitor during these procedures, but hyperthermia is a more often encountered, and an equally disconcerting alternative. Both benign[47] and malignant hyperthermia[48] have been described during replantation. Malignant hyperthermia has a well-defined cause, and the diagnosis and treatment are discussed in detail elsewhere.[48] The causes for benign hyperthermia may vary from inadequate convective heat loss caused by the occlusive drapings to infection emanating from the site of the injury. Whatever the cause, malignant forms must be ruled out and the appropriate therapy to maintain normothermia initiated. Measurement of core temperature using an esophageal thermistor probe is the monitoring method of choice. A location of the tip in the caudad one third of the esophagus is thought to be optimal.[49] It is likely that ambient temperature is the single most important influence on the body temperature of uncovered patients;[50] however, other factors, such as a warming-cooling mattress, circuit humidifiers, and fluid warmers, may also have a telling effect[51] and should enable the anesthesiologist to achieve normothermia in the replant patient during operation.

Positioning of a patient on an operating table for a 24-hour procedure so that position-related injury is avoided is no easy task. In procedures not involving the head, a foam rubber headrest is used to prevent pressure-induced alopecia. A foam rubber mattress, in conjunction with the water mattress for heating and cooling, has been effective in preventing pressure-induced lesions of the torso. The extremities not prepared in the surgical field are maintained in a physiological position and are well padded. For scalp, ear, and lip replantation, the head is often supported on a neurosurgical headrest and the operating table reversed so that the surgeons may sit comfortably with their legs under the table during these long operations.

When the conditions that appropriately trigger transfusion have been met, provided normovolemia has been maintained, red blood cells reconstituted with normal saline or Normosol-R should be appropriately infused. Although disseminated intravascular coagulation has been described in association with extremity replantation,[52] clotting abnormalities usually should not result either from the procedure itself or from dilution, if the transfused volume is less than 15 units. For a more in-depth discussion of blood transfusion and its ramifications, the reader is referred to Chapter 11.

Occasionally adjuvant drugs are required or requested intraoperatively. If it is expected that a higher mean arterial pressure would enhance perfusion, a drug such as dopamine in a dose of less than 10 $\mu g \cdot kg^{-1} \cdot min^{-1}$ is advised, while the use of vasoconstrictors like phenylephrine and norepinephrine is discouraged. Rheomacrodex, low molecular weight dextran, has received considerable support for its enhancement of flow characteristics in replant recipients. In many centers, infusion of this solution in a dose of 0.5 ml·kg$^{-1}$·hr$^{-1}$ is part of the intraoperative and postoperative protocol.[53] There is some experimental evidence of improved postanastomosis perfusion in heparinized animals,[54] but conclusive data are absent in humans. If heparinization is employed, the effects of heparin should be monitored by means of the activated coagulation time, partial thromboplastin time, or

heparin activity. Because of the open vascular planes of the penis, heparinization in penile replantation is to be avoided.

## POSTOPERATIVE CARE

Postoperatively, vigilant monitoring and supportive care must be continued until the patient is completely awake. Careful weaning from supportive ventilation is advisable, especially if neuromuscular blocking drugs have been employed, if the patient has pre-existing pulmonary compromise, or if narcotic analgesics supplemented the anesthetic. Extubation can be optimally effected when normothermia has been achieved and the potential for shivering minimized. Supplemental oxygen to maintain the desired level of $Pa_{O_2}$ should be administered. Analgesics should be given generously, but judiciously, to minimize the vasoconstrictive pain response, although an effective regional block may obviate this. Rheomacrodex in association with low-dose aspirin for antithromboxane effects are used as adjunctive antithrombotic therapy. Heparin is employed only if additional exploration for thrombosis is necessary. The measurement of postoperative skin temperatures of the replanted organ[55] remains the mainstay of monitoring postoperative replant viability. Newer measurements of transcutaneous $P_{O_2}$[56] and hydrogen washout[57,58] have also been employed. The transcutaneous $P_{O_2}$ monitoring has been associated with skin burns, especially in the poorly perfused replant; however, the hydrogen washout method is repeatable, reliable, accurate, and quantitative, but has the drawback that it is an invasive method requiring implantation of a platinum electrode at the surgery site. There is some evidence suggesting that the earlier the diagnosis of postreplant thrombosis, the better the chances for salvage. These methods may be well worth the risk.

## SUMMARY AND CONCLUSIONS

Replantation of the entire scalp is an essential procedure with both a cosmetic and physical outcome worthy of the arduous endeavor. The small venous channels of the ear make this replantation difficult, albeit medical and cosmetic indications encourage attempts whenever possible. Replantation of the amputated penis deserves considerable latitude as far as indications are concerned,

## Replantation Anesthetic Protocol

1. **Monitors—noninvasive**
   a. ECG ($V_5$, II)
   b. Usual (BP cuff, PCS)
   c. Esophageal thermistor probe
   d. Mass spectrometer
2. **Monitors—invasive**
   a. Systemic arterial cannula ⎫
   b. Central venous cannula ⎬ transduced
   c. Pulmonary arterial catheter (as needed)
   d. Urinary catheter
   e. Nasogastric catheter
3. **Laboratory determinations**
   a. ABG ⎫
   b. $N^+$, $K^+$ ⎪
   c. Glucose ⎬ At least q 2 hours
   d. Osmolality ⎪ More often, if conditions
   e. Hematocrit ⎭ dictate
   f. Coagulation profile-q 12 hours
4. **Thermal devices**
   a. Blood and fluid warmers
   b. Mattress
   c. Circuit humidifiers
5. **Fluids**
   a. Non-glucose-containing crystalloids
   b. Blood and components
   c. Rheomacrodex
6. **Positive end-expiratory pressure**
7. **Physiological position**
   a. Foam rubber headrest
   b. Soft mattress
   c. Plenty of padding
8. **Drugs**
   a. Anesthetic (local and general)
   b. Heparin
   c. Insulin
   d. Potassium chloride
   e. Dopamine (infusion, pump)
   f. Vasodilators (nitroglycerin, sodium nitroprusside)
9. **Avoid**
   a. $N_2O$
   b. Extensively biotransformed anesthetics
   c. Acidemia
   d. Alkalemia
   e. Hypocapnia
   f. Oral airway
   g. Excessive cuff pressure

and free tissue transfers are appropriate for repair of defects whenever medical and surgical indications for this therapy coexist. Steadily improving functional results are being demonstrated by some centers for extremity replantation through improved patient selection. In the absence of clear-cut criteria, it is essential that the financial burden, as well as the practical expectations of functional return, be understood. Whether to replant an amputated part in a patient who, because of advanced age or physical infirmity, has little chance of ever returning to the work place is an emerging concern worthy of our attention.

Considerable emphasis in this chapter has been given to the prognosis for return of function following replantation, the psychological aspects associated with and responsible for it, and the impact of this surgery on society in terms of both temporal and financial expenditures. The reason for stressing these issues in an anesthesia-related text is so that the anesthesiologist can, as an integral and necessary part of this team, make judicious and data-based contributions that culminate in a successful replant endeavor.

## REFERENCES

1. Malt RA, McKhann CF: Replantation of severed arms. JAMA 189:716, 1964.

2. Nahai F, Jurkiewicz MJ: Microsurgery: Replantation and free flaps. Adv Surg 17:73, 1984.

3. Gallico GG, Stirrat CR: Extremity replantation. Surg Annu 15:229, 1983.

4. Hamilton RB, O'Brien BM, Morrison WA, MacLeod AM: Replantation and revascularization of digits. Surg Gynecol Obstet 151:508, 1980.

5. Kutz JE, Hanel D, Scheker L, Lopez G: Upper extremity replantation. Orthop Clin N Am 14: 873, 1983.

6. Kusunoki M, Toyoshima Y, Okajima M: Successful replantation of a leg—A 7 year follow-up. Injury 16:118, 1984.

7. Strauch B, Sharzer LA, Petro J, Greenstein B: Replantation of amputated parts of the penis, nose, ear and scalp. Clin Plast Surg 10:115, 1983.

8. Holtje WJ: Successful replantation of an amputated upper lip. Plast Reconstr Surg 73:664, 1984.

9. Pennington DG, Lai MF, Pelly AD: Successful replantation of a completely avulsed ear by microvascular anastomosis. Plast Reconstr Surg 65: 820, 1980.

10. Salyapongse A, Maun LP, Suthunyarat P: Successful replantation of a totally severed ear. Plast Reconstr Surg 64:706, 1979.

11. Odland M, Van Beek A, Hubble B: Management of scalping injuries. Minn Med 65:671, 1982.

12. Tantri DP, Cervino AL, Tabbal N: Replantation of the totally avulsed scalp. J Trauma 20:350, 1980.

13. Velcek FT, Jongco B, Shaftan GW, et al: Post-traumatic splenic replantation in children. J Pediatr Surg 17:879, 1982.

14. Cunningham BL, Shons AR: Upper extremity—Replantation surgery. Minn Med 65:463, 1982.

15. Stromberg BV: Microsurgery and replantation in the upper extremity. J S C Med Assoc 80:63, 1984.

16. Colen SR, Romita MC, Godfrey NV, Shaw WW:

Salvage replantation. Clin Plast Surg 10:125, 1983.

17. Strain JJ, DeMuth GW: Care of the psychotic self-amputee undergoing replantation. Ann Surg 197:210, 1983.

18. Schweitzer I, Rosenbaum MB: Psychiatric aspects of replantation surgery. Gen Hosp Psychiatry 4:271, 1982.

19. Gonzalez ER: China; rest of technical world share replantation data. JAMA 242:1593, 1979.

20. Kleinert HE, Kasdan ML: Anastomosis of digital vessels. J Ky Med Assoc 63:106, 1965.

21. Komatsu S, Tamai S: Successful replantation of a completely cut off thumb. Plast Reconstr Surg 42:347, 1968.

22. Strock PE, Majno G: Vascular responses to experimental tourniquet ischemia. Surg Gynecol Obstet 129:309, 1969.

23. Razaboni R, Shaw WW: Preservation of tissue for transplantation and replantation. Clin Plast Surg 10:211, 1983.

24. Morgan RF, Reisman NR, Curtis RM: Preservation of upper extremity devascularizations and amputations for replantation. Am Surg 48:481, 1982.

25. Caffee HH, Hankins T: Controlled digital hypothermia. Plast Reconstr Surg 69:1013, 1982.

26. Maliniak K, Vakil AH: Pre-anesthetic cimetidine and gastric pH. Anesth Analg 58:309, 1979.

27. Coombs DW, Hooper D, Colton T: Pre-anesthetic cimetidine alteration of gastric fluid volume and pH. Anesth Analg 58:183, 1979.

28. Coombs DW, Hooper D, Colton T: Acid-aspiration prophylaxis by use of preoperative oral administration of cimetidine. Anesthesiology 51:352, 1979.

29. Manchikanti L, Marrero TC, Roush JR: Preanesthetic cimetidine and metoclopramide for acid aspiration prophylaxis in elective surgery. Anesthesiology 61:48, 1984.

30. Schmidt JF, Jorgensen BC: The effect of metoclopramide on gastric contents after preoperative ingestion of sodium citrate. Anesth Analg 63:841, 1984.

31. Caplan RA, Long MC: Prolonged anesthesia—Management and sequelae of a two-day general anesthetic. Anesth Analg 63:353, 1984.

32. Madsen SN, Engquist A, Badawi I, Kehlet H: Cyclic AMP, glucose and cortisol in plasma during surgery. Horm Metab Res 8:483, 1976.

33. Dell PC, Seaber AV, Urbaniak JR: The effect of systemic acidosis on perfusion of replanted extremities. J Hand Surg 5:433, 1980.

34. Rehder K, Sessler AD, Marsh HM: General anesthesia and the lung. Am Rev Resp Dis 112:541, 1975.

35. Bindsleu L, Hedenstierna G, Santesson J, Norlander O, Gram I: Airway closure during anaesthesia and its prevention by positive end expiratory pressure. Acta Anaesthiol Scand 24:199, 1980.

36. Chalon J, Patel C, Ali M, et al: Humidity and the anesthetized patient. Anesthesiology 50:195, 1979.

37. Walts LF, Miller J, Davidson MB, Brown J: Perioperative management of diabetes mellitus. Anesthesiology 55:104, 1981.

38. Shanahan PT: Replantation anesthesia. Anesth Analg 63:785, 1984.

39. Matsuda M, Kato N, Hosoi M: Continuous brachial plexus block for replantation in the upper extremity. Hand 14:129, 1982.

40. Hempel V, van Finck M, Baumgartner E: A longitudinal supraclavicular approach to the brachial plexus for insertion of plastic cannulas. Anesth Analg 60:352, 1981.

41. Lowe JH, Ernst EA: The quantitative practice of anesthesia. Baltimore, Williams and Wilkins, 1981.

42. Mazze RI, Calverley RK, Smith NT: Inorganic fluoride nephrotoxicity: Prolonged enflurane and halothane anesthesia in volunteers. Anesthesiology 46:265, 1977.

43. Cousins MJ, Greenstein LR, Hitt BA, Mazze RI: Metabolism and renal effects of enflurane in man. Anesthesiology 44:44, 1976.

44. Pearson J: Prolonged anesthesia with isoflurane. Anesth Analg 64:92, 1985.

45. Reiz S, Balfors E, Sorensen MB, et al: Isoflurane—A powerful coronary vasodilator in patients with coronary artery disease. Anesthesiology 59:91, 1983.

46. Merin RG, Lowenstein E, Gelman S: Is anesthesia beneficial for the ischemic heart? III. Anesthesiology 64:137–140, 1986.

47. Fraser JG: Iatrogenic benign hyperthermia in children. Anesthesiology 48:375, 1978.

48. Murphy AL, Conlay L, Ryan JF, Roberts JT: Malignant hyperthermia during a prolonged anesthetic for reattachment of a limb. Anesthesiology 60:149, 1984.

49. Whitby JD, Dunkin LJ: Temperature differences in the oesophagus. Br J Anaesth 40:991, 1968.

50. Morris RH, Kumar A: The effect of warming blankets on maintainence of body temperature of the anesthetized, paralyzed adult patient. Anesthesiology 36:408, 1972.

51. Roizen MF, Sohn YJ, L'Hommedieu CS, et al: Operating room temperature prior to surgical draping: Effect on patient temperature in recovery room. Anesth Analg 59:852, 1980.

52. Hales P, Pullen D: Hypotension and bleeding diathesis following attempted arm replantation. Anaesth Intensive Care 10:359, 1982.

53. Weiland AJ, Villarreal-Rios A, Kleinert HE, et al: Replantation of digits and hands: Analysis of surgical techniques and functional results in 71 patients with 86 replantations. J Hand Surg 2:1, 1977.

54. Vlastou C, Earle AS: Intraoperative heparin in replantation surgery—An experimental study. Ann Plast Surg 10:112, 1983.

55. Vilkki SK: Postoperative skin temperature dynamics and the nature of vascular complications after replantation. Scand J Plast Reconstr Surg 16:151, 1982.

56. Keller HP, Lanz U: Objective control of replanted fingers by transcutaneous partial $O_2$ ($PO_2$) measurement. Microsurgery 5:85, 1984.

57. Smith AR, Sonneveld GJ, Kort WJ, van der Meulen J: Clinical application of transcutaneous oxygen measurements in replantation surgery and free tissue transfer. J Hand Surg 8:139, 1983.

58. Glogovac SV, Bitz DM, Whiteside LA: Hydrogen washout technique in monitoring vascular status after replantation surgery. J Hand Surg 7:601, 1982.

# 10

# *Skin Transplantation*

JAMES D. PEARSON
NEELAKANTAN SUNDER
J. A. JEEVENDRA MARTYN

## ANATOMY AND PHYSIOLOGY OF THE SKIN

Skin covers the surface of the body and forms an extensive physical barrier protecting the body from the environment. The three major layers are the epidermis, the dermis, and the subcutaneous tissue. The epidermis forms the outer covering. Deep to the epidermis, the dermis, made of dense fibroelastic connective tissue, forms the principal layer of the skin. Beneath the dermis is the subcutaneous tissue composed of areolar and adipose tissue.

### Epidermis

The epidermis is stratified squamous epithelium consisting of a horny zone that is constantly shed from the body and a germinative zone that is responsible for the production of new cells. The relative thickness of the zones may vary in different parts of the body.

The germinative zone consists of a basal layer (stratum basale) and a prickly layer (stratum spinosum). The cells of stratum basale undergo continual mitosis, supplying new cells to replace the surface layers, and hence it is also known as stratum germinativum. The horny zone has a granular layer (stratum granulosum), a clear layer (stratum lucidum), and a horny layer (stratum corneum) (Fig. 10–1).[1–3]

**Stratum Basale.** The deepest layer is composed of columnar or cylindrical cells that show many mitotic figures as they divide to form new cells. The ends of these cells that are in contact with the basement membrane have toothlike projections that anchor it to the underlying dermis. These newly formed cells are pushed toward the surface and form the next layer.

**Stratum Spinosum.** This layer consists of polygonal cells that adhere to each other at points called desmosomes. The cytoplasm of these cells contains minute fibrils, some of which are oriented toward the desmosomes; called tonofibrils, they appear to be running between the cells.

**Stratum Granulosum.** This layer consists of flat cells that contain numerous large granules composed of keratohyalin, a substance that is transformed into keratin in more superficial layers.

**Stratum Lucidum.** The granules from the previous layer have been converted into an achromatic substance, eleidin. The nuclei and the cell boundaries have disappeared.

**Stratum Corneum.** The outermost layer consists of several layers of cells that have

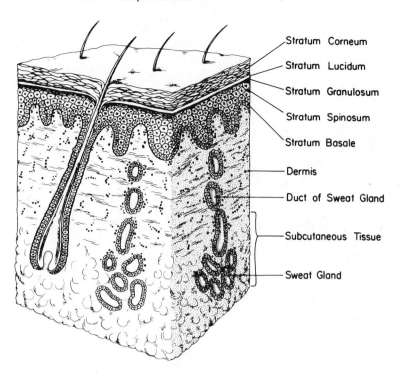

Stratum Corneum

Stratum Lucidum

Stratum Granulosum

Stratum Spinosum

Stratum Basale

Dermis

Duct of Sweat Gland

Subcutaneous Tissue

Sweat Gland

**Figure 10–1.** Anatomy of the skin. See text for details.

undergone cornification. In the most superficial part of this layer the cells have been converted to squamous plates of scales fused together as a result of the transformation of the eleidin of the clear layer into keratin. The most superficial cells slough off or desquamate and are replaced by new ones. The thickness of this layer depends on the trauma an area is subjected to. Melanin, the pigment in the epidermis of the skin, is found primarily in stratum basale.

## Dermis

The dermis is a tough elastic layer composed of collagen and elastic fibers and a gel of mucopolysaccharide called the ground substance. The dermis varies greatly in thickness. At its outermost surface it establishes the topography of the basal surface of the epidermis. This portion constitutes the papillary part of the dermis (stratum papillare), which makes close contact with the functioning surface epithelium and encloses superficial elements of the microcirculation of the skin. It consists of relatively cellular, loose connective tissue with collagen and elastic fibers that are smaller and fewer than found in the remaining deeper reticular dermis (stratum reticulare). In the reticular portion of the dermis, the collagen and elastic fibers are more dense, the fibers are thicker,

and there are relatively fewer cells and less ground substance. The collagen fibers provide high resistance to breakage under mechanical stress, and the elastic fibers restore the resting condition when deforming loads are removed. The mucopolysaccharides, by virtue of their viscous properties, contribute resistance to compression of the skin and, by virtue of their elastic properties, contribute to the restoration of the sets of fibers after deformation.

The dermis also encloses a cellular system of nerves, vessels, glands, and appendages. The cell population includes fibroblasts, tissue and perivascular macrophages, and the mononuclear element of the reticuloendothelial system.

## Blood Supply and Lymphatic Drainage of the Skin

The epidermis is avascular, but the dermis has a rich blood supply. Arteries from the superficial fascia enter the lower dermis and by repeated subdivisions form arterioles and capillaries that are arranged in superficial and deep plexuses parallel to the skin surface. Vertical and oblique communicating vessels link the two plexuses. From these arise the microcirculatory units that attend to the metabolic demands of the dermis, glands, and appendages. In addition to this, there are numerous arteriovenous anastomoses that can regulate the blood flow into the skin. The blood is drained through small venules into the veins in the superficial fascia. A well-developed system of lymphatics arises from the papillary dermis and drains into subcutaneous lymphatic trunks.

### Innervation of the Skin

Skin contains an extensive network of neural receptors and free nerve endings that transmit information from the environment to the central nervous system. It is still not clear if specific nerve endings produce specific sensations. In addition, there are adrenergic nerves to the erector pili muscles, adrenergic and possibly cholinergic fibers to smooth muscles of the small blood vessels, and cholinergic fibers to sweat glands.

### Sweat Glands and Sebaceous Glands

Sweat glands are found in the skin of all parts of the body except the red surface of the lips. The secretory portion of the gland is located deep in the dermis and the ducts pursue a spiral course through the dermis and epidermis to open on the surface of the papillary ridges. Their primary role is thermal regulation. Sebaceous glands are lipid-producing branched acinar glands found in association with hair follicles. The secretory product, sebum, consists of lipid droplets that contain free fatty acids, wax, and sterol esters. The function of the sebum in humans is not clearly defined.

### Subcutaneous Tissue

Beneath the dermis is a highly variable adipose tissue layer, the subcutaneous tissue. The dermis and subcutaneous tissue have an intricate pattern of vasculature, lymphatic drainage, and neuroreceptor mechanisms.

### Skin and Thermal Regulation

The human body is able to maintain normothermia over a wide range of temperature conditions. Body heat production is fairly constant. Heat dissipation and conservation are controlled by altering skin blood flow, which influences heat loss by convection, radiation, and evaporation. Heat loss by radiation depends on the blood flow to the skin. Vasoconstriction of arterioles and capillaries limits blood flow and conserves heat. Heat loss by evaporation, exclusive of sweating, is minimized by the limited permeability of the epidermis. Sweating is a powerful mechanism for heat loss. High ambient temperatures in association with sweating can lead to significant hypovolemia.

### Functions of the Skin

The physical and chemical properties of the skin protect the body from (1) loss of water, electrolytes, and proteins, (2) invasion by microorganisms, (3) toxic and foreign substances, (4) injury, (5) ultraviolet radiation, and (6) electrical injury. In addition, the skin participates in the production of vitamin D and maintenance of normothermia.

**Protection from Loss of Water.** The stratum corneum acts as a barrier to the loss of plasma and its constituents. Water moves from the hydrated stratum corneum to the epidermis by passive diffusion without active transport of electrolytes. The water loss through normal adult skin is about 500 ml/24 hr.[4] Skin loss of 50 per cent in an adult can increase this loss of water to more than 2 L per day. In addition to water, electrolytes and plasma proteins are lost. Not only are body components lost through the open skin wound, but substances, e.g., topical antibiotics, can be absorbed through the skin, resulting in toxic levels or reaction.[5]

**Protection from Invasion by Microorganisms.** The stratum corneum is a good barrier against invasion by microorganisms. The destruction of skin and the resultant exudate that occurs as a result of passive diffusion and the inflammatory process form a medium for the growth and multiplication of microorganisms. The release of vasoactive substances causes thrombosis and ischemia of the zone immediately beyond the burn. This can result in further necrosis of tissue with a potential for growth of anaerobic organisms.

**Protection from Foreign and Toxic Substances.** Permeability of skin to drugs and toxic substances is dependent on the hydration and thickness of the skin. The capacity of the skin to absorb various substances is now used for drugs such as nitroglycerin. When the skin is partially damaged this capacity may be increased. However, when there is severe damage to the skin, absorption is variable, depending on whether thrombosis or hyperemia of the blood vessels is present.

**Protection of Deeper Tissues from Injury.** The elastic nature of the skin allows considerable stretch during blunt trauma. Similarly, the presence of subcutaneous tissue and fat protects the deeper tissues from mechanical trauma. A complex network of nerve endings provides the necessary sensation for voluntary and involuntary responses to noxious stimuli.

**Protection from Ultraviolet Radiation.** Melanin in the epidermis and stratum corneum absorbs harmful ultraviolet radiation.

**Protection from Electrical Injury.** The skin offers high resistance to the flow of electrical current. Normal skin has a resistance of 1.9 megaohms to 1.0 volt direct current.[6] When the skin is moist, this resistance is decreased to 0.7 megaohms. When the stratum corneum is damaged, it is decreased further to 0.005 megaohms. Potential problems related to this might include the placement of electrocardiographic and diathermy ground pads over burned areas.

**Production of Vitamin D.** The skin can synthesize vitamin D.[7] This source probably plays an important role only in patients who do not have adequate dietary intake of vitamin D. There is now some evidence that the skin may be involved in other physiological roles, including the immune response.

**Maintenance of Normothermia.** Skin can gain or lose heat by convection, radiation, or conduction, depending on the blood flow. A denervation-like phenomenon after a burn causes profound vasodilatation and increased blood flow to the injured area. Normal vasoconstriction to cold does not occur.[8] Thus, patients with skin loss are quite prone to hypothermia. This is compounded further by evaporative water loss, which causes further cooling, reinforcing the importance of maintaining a warm and humid environment for these patients.

## PATHOPHYSIOLOGY OF THE BURNED SKIN

Injury to the skin destroys cells and disrupts surface continuity. As the normal wound healing process begins, the body attempts to heal the wound by intricate mechanisms occurring in definite phases. Complete wound healing occurs by either primary or secondary intention. However, wound skin loss leads to healing by unstable epithelialization, resulting in severe contractures. In these instances, skin grafting is required for reasonable physiological and anatomical healing. Extensive skin loss occurs most commonly with thermal injuries.

Burn injuries are classified as either partial thickness or full thickness, according to the depth of cell destruction. The superficial, partial-thickness wound usually involves the epidermis and parts of the dermis. The deep, partial-thickness wound usually involves the entire epidermis and dermis, leaving the subcutaneous tissues and the appendages unharmed. Full-thickness burns, by definition, involve all skin layers, thereby precluding spontaneous restoration of the skin.

Immediately after burning occurs, local thrombosis leads to cessation of arterial and venous blood flow. This is followed by neovascularization and formation of granulation tissue. Drying and infection stop circulation, which may cause further damage.

Burning causes immediate loss of capillary integrity, leading to an increase in permeability that results in continuous loss of fluid from the wound surface during the resuscitation phase. This leads to large volume losses from the extravascular and intravascular spaces. Leakage of plasma proteins also occurs in the area of the burn. Thus, massive edema formation occurs within the burned tissue, particularly in the subcutaneous tissue deep to the surface burn. In patients with larger burns (more than 30 per cent of the body surface area [BSA]) the hypoproteinemia occurring during the resuscitation phase results in edema at sites distant from the burn.[9,10] This massive fluid leakage leads to large fluid deficits, requiring aggressive fluid resuscitation.[11]

The burn wound characteristically has (1) a zone of coagulation, the site of irreversible cell destruction; (2) zone of stasis, which if allowed to become dry and infected will cause further damage; and (3) zone of hyperemia, which is the site of minimal involvement and early spontaneous recovery.

Striking changes occur in the blood and plasma. Immediate destruction of red cells is dependent on the severity and extent of the burn. In addition, the red cells in a burned patient also have a reduced life span.[12] The cellular transmembrane potentials also change after thermal injury. The potentials decrease from $-90$ mV to $-60$ mV in cells in the postburn period as a result of marked increases in intracellular sodium. The increase in cellular osmolarity leads to an increase in intracellular water.[11]

The hypermetabolic phase begins about 48 hours after a burn. As the cardiac output increases, there is a selective increase in blood flow to the altered microvasculature. This extraordinarily selective flow and serum leakage through the thermally injured vasculature results in great wound losses and marked disturbances of body fluids, electrolytes, serum proteins, and metabolic substrates. Depression of the immune system may occur because of loss of immune factors through the damaged membranes. Factors released from the burned tissue may also depress the immune system.[13] The hypermetabolic state is accompanied by increased levels of circulating catecholamines, loss of nutrients through the wound, and decreased food intake. A negative nitrogen balance leads to muscle protein breakdown, weakness, and weight loss in the patient in the postburn period. The necrotic tissue is bathed with nutrients and is an excellent culture medium for harmful bacteria. Wound infection is common.

## PATHOPHYSIOLOGY OF THE BURNED PATIENT

Not only does a surface burn destroy skin, but the postburn state alters metabolic, respiratory, cardiovascular, renal, gastrointestinal, hepatic, and immune system function. If a system is not involved in the primary disease process, then it may be involved in the body's response to the injury.

### Metabolic Changes

The hallmark of the postburn state is increased metabolism. Catecholamines and cortisol levels are elevated sharply. Plasma ACTH is also increased in the postburn state.[14] Hyperglycemia results from impaired glucose uptake by the tissues, despite increased insulin levels.[15] Protein catabolism, lipolysis, and gluconeogenesis increase, and skeletal muscle protein undergoes proteolysis, providing amino acids for hepatic gluconeogenesis and protein synthesis.[16] Quantitatively the increase in metabolic rate is greater after severe burn injury than after any other insult. All metabolic fuel pathways are utilized. Calorie requirement is partially met by oxidation of fat, representing about 24 per cent of the total body weight and providing a high energy source. However, "fat can be burned only in the fire of carbohydrate." Total carbohydrate stores are small, providing less than 1500 total calories. Protein, about 16 per cent of the body weight, is catabolized to supply fuel and carbohydrate intermediates.[17] Albumin concentration uniformly decreases, as in all acute disease processes, but especially in the postburn state as albumin leaks out of the injured vasculature. Plasma protein binding of certain drugs diminishes, increasing the free fraction of albumin-bound drugs such as warfarin, dilantin, sulfonylurea, and diazepam. On the other hand, alpha-acid glycoprotein concentrations are increased in the postburn state, and therefore the free fraction of drugs such as lidocaine, propranolol, and the tricyclic antidepressants, which bind predominantly to the alpha-acid glycoprotein in human plasma, may decrease[18] (Fig. 10–2). As in other critical illnesses,[19] total and ionized calcium concentrations decrease as the size

**Figure 10–2.** Free fraction of imipramine from burn patients (*left*) is lower than in healthy controls. The percentage of unbound diazepam in all samples from burn patients is higher than in those from healthy controls. (From Martyn JAJ, Abernathy DR, Greenblatt DJ: Plasma protein binding of drugs after severe burn injury. Clin Pharmacol Ther 35:535, 1984, with permission of the authors and publisher.)

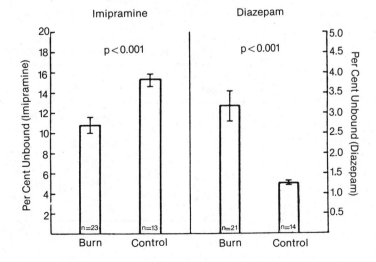

of the burn increases. This uniform decrease in serum calcium concentration is independent of protein concentration.[20]

Thus it is easy to understand how severe thermal injury with fright and pain, circulatory and pulmonary complications sometimes leading to shock and hypoxia, long-term tremendous loss of water and heat, and wound infection and sepsis activates the hormones of stress (catecholamines), the storage hormone (insulin), and the permissive hormones (glucagon, growth hormone, and glucocorticoids).[16,17]

### Respiratory Function

In recent years, improved and aggressive fluid replacement has decreased the immediate mortality from shock, but pulmonary complications can become the major cause of immediate morbidity and mortality if such patients are not managed aggressively. Despite the availability of antibiotics and pulmonary therapy, pulmonary complications continue to be a leading cause of death in burned patients.

The initial lung and airway injuries depend on the type of fire and the duration of exposure to the thermal environment. Lung injury due to inhalation of smoke is characterized by several stages during the first 24 hours. In stage 1, smoke inhalation causes profound hypoxemia associated with acidosis. These changes are secondary to the presence of noxious gases and carbon monoxide and to a decrease in oxygen in the ambient air. In stage 2, immediately following the inhalational injury, hypoxic hypoxemia continues. In addition, cardiac output may be severely depressed, possibly reflecting an increase in pulmonary vascular resistance caused by cerebral hypoxia or hypoxic pulmonary vasoconstriction. Physiological dead space increases, and pulmonary compliance decreases. Stage 3 of the injury, which involves the next 2 to 24 hours, is associated with clearance of the carbon monoxide. Hypoxemia may worsen because of atelectasis of injured alveoli and because of interstitial edema. This is reflected by a decrease in compliance and altered ventilation-perfusion ratios. Most patients who survive this stage do well if they have no other injuries. During stage 4 the patient may develop bacterial pneumonia, adult respiratory distress syndrome, or pulmonary edema.[21]

Efficient cooling of hot gases by the upper air passages makes thermal injury below the vocal cords uncommon. However, steam and noxious fumes can damage airways distally. Stridor, hoarseness, and difficulty with phonation demand prompt and aggressive action, because thermal injury to the hypopharynx or glottis may be followed in several hours by airway obstruction and rapid asphyxiation.[22] When the injury is severe, sloughing of the tracheal mucosa occurs, and the dislodged mucosa may cause segmental or lobar atelectasis.[23]

Carbon monoxide poisoning is a major cause of early mortality following exposure to fire. This odorless, nonirritating gas results from incomplete combustion of carbon-containing materials. In comparison to oxygen, carbon monoxide has 200 times greater affinity for hemoglobin, making small concentrations of carbon monoxide lethal.[22,24] Because of this marked affinity for hemoglobin, a carbon monoxide concentration of 0.1 per cent in room air produces equal blood concentrations of oxyhemoglobin and carboxyhemoglobin, resulting in 50 per cent reduction in oxygen-carrying capacity[22] (Table 10–

**TABLE 10–1.  Carbon Monoxide Poisoning**

| Carboxyhemoglobin Level (%) | Severity | Symptoms |
| --- | --- | --- |
| 20 | Mild | Headache, mild dyspnea, visual changes, confusion |
| 20–40 | Moderate | Irritability, diminished judgment, dimness of vision, nausea, easy fatigability |
| 40–60 | Severe | Hallucinations, confusion, ataxia, collapse, coma |
| 60 | Fatal | |

From Trunkey DD: Inhalational injury. Surg Clin North Am 58:1133, 1978, with permission of the author and publisher.

1). Because the carotid bodies respond to changes in the partial pressure of oxygen, not oxygen content, a carbon monoxide–intoxicated person may have profound reduction in tissue oxygen delivery and yet have no increase in minute ventilation until lactic acidosis develops. Carbon monoxide also shifts the oxygen-hemoglobin dissociation curve to the left, and the lowered $P_{50}$ of carboxyhemoglobin decreases tissue oxygen availability (Fig. 10–3). Carbon monoxide intoxication is treated with increased inspired concentrations of oxygen, decreasing the half-life of carbon monoxide from four hours to one hour. One hundred per cent oxygen may be required to maintain reasonable oxygen delivery.

Combustion of structural materials and home furnishings produces complex organic acids, aldehydes, and noxious gases. These substances reduce bacterial clearance and mucociliary transport and cause peribronchial edema of the mucosal tissue.[22] One of these chemicals, acrolein, in a concentration of 5.5 ppm, produces severe irritation of the upper respiratory tract. Pulmonary edema occurs at 10 ppm. Noxious gases from the pyrolysis of man-made polymers include hydrogen cyanide, hydrochloric acid, and sulfuric acid. Combustion of some plastics also produces benzene. Since benzene is an anesthetic, this may allow the corrosive acids and aldehydes to pass down the respiratory tract into the alveoli for absorption. Phosphorus-fire retardants in plastics may produce even more toxic gases, including phosgene and related substances.[21]

Of all hospitalized burned patients, 15 to 25 per cent develop some pulmonary complications in which mortality is 50 to 90 per cent.[23] Pneumonia is the primary cause of death in 4.8 per cent of all burned patients. The ratio of airborne to hematogenous pneumonia is about 2 to 1. The burn wound, infected veins, peritonitis secondary to intestinal perforation, and peripheral burn abscesses are the primary sources of bacteria causing hematogenous pneumonias.[25]

Pulmonary function tests in burned patients without inhalation injury reveal an increased respiratory rate. Minute ventilation increases by the third postburn day, rising to a maximum in approximately five days, and then gradually decreases. These changes are associated with appreciable changes in static compliance, forced vital capacity, and lung clearance index. FVC, $FEV_I$, and $FEV_{III}$ vary significantly, indicating that there are substantial respiratory abnormalities associated with a large burn, even in the absence of inhalation injury.[26]

The reported incidence of pulmonary embolism in burned patients varies widely and may reach 30 per cent, reflecting the extent the diagnosis is sought. Minidose heparin therapy is probably justified, since burned patients are often confined to bed for prolonged periods. However, gastrointestinal bleeding and coagulopathies, which are common in burned patients, may contraindicate this therapy.[22]

In conclusion, carbon monoxide poisoning, tracheobronchitis, and chemically induced pulmonary edema may result from direct burn injury. Pneumonia, adult respiratory distress syndrome, pulmonary congestion, and pulmonary emboli complicate the burned patient's recovery. Pulmonary complications develop in about 30 per cent of burned patients and must be treated aggressively. Patients who are involved in a closed-space fire and those who have a burn involving 50 per cent or more of their surface area, seem to be at greatest risk of developing pulmonary complications.

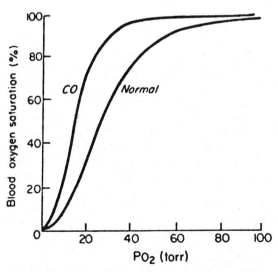

**Figure 10–3.** Oxygen-hemoglobin dissociation curve. Note the "shift to the left," i.e., the lowered $P_{50}$ for COHb, which results in decreased tissue oxygen availability. (From Fein A, Leff A, Hopewell PC: Pathophysiology and management of the complications resulting from fire and the inhaled products of combustion. Crit Care Med 8:94, 1980, with permission from the authors and publisher.)

## Cardiovascular Function

As the pulmonary system, the cardiovascular system undergoes immediate and delayed changes in response to a burn. The immediate changes occur in cardiac output, volumes of vascular compartments, and vascular permeability. Animal studies demonstrate a marked immediate increase in vascular permeability in the area of the burn. The destruction of the semipermeable qualities of the vascular tree leads to tremendous transvascular loss of fluid, electrolytes, and proteins. Though most prominent in the area of the burn, this increase in vascular permeability becomes generalized in patients with burns greater than 30 per cent BSA. Except for this early transient change in permeability, which is probably caused by histamine and other vasoactive substances, the edema developing in nonburned soft tissues does not appear to be due to altered membrane permeability, but rather to the severe hypoproteinemia.[9,10] This redistribution of body fluids, the visual manifestation of which is tissue swelling, is essentially complete within 24 hours, the greater proportion having occurred in the first 12 hours.[24]

Cross-perfusion techniques between burned and normal animals demonstrate the presence of a substance that depresses myocardial contractility. Exposure of isolated papillary muscle to plasma from burned animals results in immediate cessation of myocardial contraction. This substance is readily dialyzable and has a molecular weight less than 1000.[27] In burned patients, despite normal filling pressures, left ventricular stroke work index may be markedly decreased. On the second day, however, it returns to normal values without an increase in pulmonary capillary wedge pressure[28] (Fig. 10-4). In a most recent study, thermal trauma to the anesthetized dog resulted in an immediate decrease in cardiac output and an increase in peripheral vascular resistance with no changes in mean arterial blood pressure. Intravenous administration of verapamil, 1 mg·kg$^{-1}$ resulted in a decrease in peripheral resistance and a rapid increase in cardiac output. Mean arterial pressure fell, but returned to the pre-verapamil values within 30 minutes[29] (Fig. 10-5). Thus, in the first 24 hours, cardiac output is depressed by reasons other than changes in blood volume.[30] Other factors that decrease cardiac output include increased viscosity, hormonal effects, and vasoconstriction.[31]

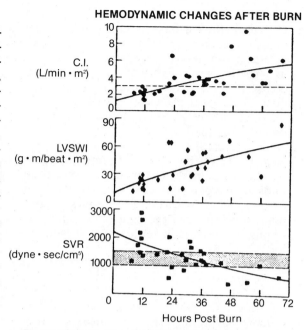

**HEMODYNAMIC CHANGES AFTER BURN**

**Figure 10–4.** Cardiac index (CI), left ventricular stroke work index (LVSWI), and systemic vascular resistance (SVR) as a function of time after thermal injury. Solid lines = quadratic regression curves, fitted to the data by least square routine; dashed line, top panel = normal value of CI; shaded area, bottom panel = normal range of SVR. (From Aikawa N, Martyn JAJ, Burke JF: Pulmonary artery catheterization and thermodilution cardiac output determination in the management of critically burned patients. Am J Surg 135:811, 1978, with permission of the authors and publisher.)

Once resuscitation is complete, cardiac output usually returns to normal values within 36 hours if circulating volume has been adequately restored. In the early resuscitation phase, crystalloid administration may approach or exceed 4 ml·kg$^{-1}$% BSA$^{-1}$ burn. In elderly patients or patients with previous myocardial dysfunction, cardiac function may deteriorate despite proper resuscitation. Hypertonic saline and colloids may be useful in the resuscitation phase to limit the infusion volumes.[10]

After the immediate phase of resuscitation, cardiac output increases to meet the patient's increased oxygen consumption caused by the increased metabolic rate. Increased metabolic rate and utilization of calories continue despite placing the burned patient in a thermally neutral environment.[32] Thus, heat loss through the burn wound, whether or not calorie production follows, is not the sole cause of hypermetabolism. A cold environment

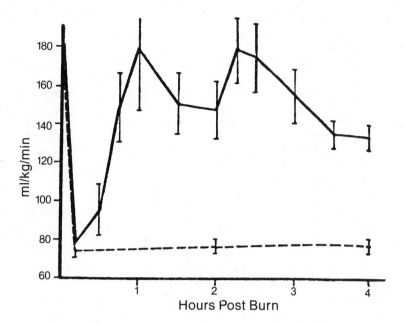

**Figure 10–5.** Effects of verapamil on cardiac output after thermal trauma. Ordinate: cardiac output in $ml \cdot kg^{-1} \cdot min^{-1}$. Abscissa: post-burn time in hours. Solid line represents animals receiving verapamil, 1.0 $mg \cdot kg^{-1}$ at 0.5 hour and 0.5 $mg \cdot kg^{-1}$ at 2.0 hours after burn. Dashed line represents untreated animals. Each point represents the mean of 6 treated and 14 untreated animals. Bars represent standard error of the mean. (From Hilton JG: Effects of verapamil on thermal trauma depressed cardiac output in the anaesthetized dog. Burns 10:313, 1984, with permission of the author and publisher.)

only adds further stress to the already hypermetabolic burned patient. Burned patients have tremendously increased cardiac output and oxygen consumption with decreased systemic and pulmonary vascular resistances. The arteriovenous oxygen content difference can be low, normal, or high.[33] The systemic vascular resistance often drops to 350 $dynes \cdot sec \cdot cm^{-5}$, and cardiac output may exceed 18 $L \cdot min^{-1}$ (Gregoretti S, Gelman S, Dimick AR, unpublished data). This hyperdynamic state is also characteristic for septic shock. In fact, the resting body temperature of most burned patients is approximately 38°C. In this situation the combination of hyperthermia and hyperdynamic circulation may mask developing sepsis.

Blood viscosity increases acutely, remaining high for four to five days after the initial injury, in spite of a usual decrease in hematocrit value. The platelet count decreases in the first week and then slowly increases and remains elevated for three weeks; platelet adhesiveness is almost doubled. Factors V and VIII are also increased four to eight times; regression does not take place until the third postburn month. However, the only findings peculiar to the burned patient are an increase in fibrin split products lasting for three to five days and a consistent increase in blood viscosity.[31]

The tremendous total body oxygen requirements place significant demands on the myocardium. If the myocardium is unable to respond to these demands, the patient may lapse into a low cardiac output state and eventually die.

## Renal Function

The failure of kidney function, which can be detrimental in patients with severe burns, is secondary to circulatory changes. In Great Britain, renal failure was at one time more common and is documented to occur in a widely ranging frequency of 1.3 per cent of total admissions to 15.3 per cent of burns over 15 per cent BSA.[31] The American experience is different, and the reasons for this discrepancy are relatively simple: The British resuscitate their burned patients with less fluid and at a much slower rate than Americans. Depressed renal clearances in all patients with burns of over 40 per cent BSA have been documented in both countries and are directly correlated with low cardiac output and increased peripheral vascular resistance secondary to hypovolemia. Renal function usually improves with volume resuscitation and improvement in cardiac output.

Generalized dysfunction of the proximal renal tubule appears to be characteristic of severe burn injury. The increased excretion of uric acid, phosphate, and several low molecular weight proteins has been demonstrated in most burned patients. The observations are not related to increased serum levels of the compounds, but rather to increased membrane permeability. Increased urinary glucose excretion occurs despite serum glucose concentrations of less than 200 mg per dl and suggest a lowered renal threshold for glucose filtration. Patients who die usually exhibit the most marked abnormalities of proximal tubular function, although the normal fractional clearances of specific substances are occasionally encountered.[34] On the other hand, glomerular function can be increased in the hypermetabolic phase of burn injury, resulting in enhanced elimination of drugs by this route (antibiotics, cimetidine).[35,36]

A special caveat with respect to fluid resuscitation following electrical injury must be made. Cutaneous burns following electrical injury are obvious at the entry and exit points, but the severe damage to deep muscle groups between these points may not be apparent. Intravascular myoglobin precipitates in the renal tubules. Forced diuresis with mannitol and alkalinization of the urine with intravenous sodium bicarbonate prevents precipitation of these hemochromogens in the renal tubules.[37]

In summary, renal function usually responds to adequate volume resuscitation; however, if hypoperfusion persists (e.g., myocardial necrosis or sepsis), then renal function may deteriorate.

## Gastrointestinal Function

The gastrointestinal tract is often involved in the secondary stress response. Diffuse erosive gastritis develops as early as five hours after injury and may be found in 83 per cent of burned patients. Acute ulcers are identified in 26 per cent of these patients.[38] Histological examinations of these lesions suggest primary ischemia either by opening of submucosal shunts or local vasoconstriction. Treatment includes oral antacids, histamine$_2$ receptor antagonists, and early enteral feedings, whenever possible. Adynamic ileus, secondary to decreased perfusion, intestinal edema, and hypokalemia, may accompany the phase of burn resuscitation. Adynamic ileus usually responds to fluid resuscitation, potassium replacement, and nasogastric suctioning.

## Hepatic Function

Hepatic metabolism changes dramatically after thermal injury. Twenty-five per cent BSA third-degree burns to rats have shown hepatic histological abnormalities and alter-

ations in protein, carbohydrate, and lipid content in the liver lasting 45 days after the burn.[17] Thermal injury produces a dose-related and time-dependent depression of the *in vivo* and *in vitro* hepatic microsomal drug metabolism in the Sprague-Dawley rat. Decreased concentrations of total hepatic protein and increased weight of the liver and spleen have been documented along with a slower weight gain in the burned animals. These effects reach peak between five and ten days after the injury. Also, the livers of some human burned victims have been shown to be swollen, congested, and infiltrated by fat.[39] A direct correlation has been found between impairment of liver function tests, such as prothrombin time or Bromsulphalein clearance, and the extent of thermal injury.[40] Studies have also shown impaired metabolism of drugs inactivated by the liver, implying that the usual therapeutic doses may result in drug toxicity when administered to severely burned patients. Therefore it is not surprising that smaller amounts of barbiturate anesthetics and oral anticoagulants are required in these patients.[41]

The immediate effect of hypovolemic shock on hepatic function has been elucidated. In one study, six adult female baboons were subjected to 50 per cent BSA third-degree burns. The animals were resuscitated, using the Parkland formula, only after the muscle transmembrane potential difference (TPD) had fallen to $-70$ mV (normal, $-90$ mV). Liver TPD decreased from $-46.2$ mV to $-22$ mV during burn shock. Volume resuscitation returned the liver TPD to normal values. Hepatic adenosine triphosphate and glucose 6-phosphatase content did not change. Serum lactate rose threefold. Marked hepatocyte depolarization indicated severe cellular derangement. Maintenance of normal intracellular adenosine triphosphate excludes energy depletion as the mechanism of this cell dysfunction. The findings are consistent with failure of active ion transport or changes in cell membrane permeability. In burn shock, hepatocyte dysfunction, as assessed by TPD, improves but is not normalized by volume resuscitation of 18 hours' duration. This early primary membrane derangement may be responsible for late changes in hepatocyte function.[42]

## Immune System

Infection is the most frequent cause of morbidity and mortality in the extensively burned patient. The susceptibility to infection increases in a sigmoid dose-response fashion as the burn size increases. This burn-related impairment of host resistance is multifactorial. The denatured protein of the burn eschar provides a rich diet for microorganisms. Also, the relatively avascular burned tissue places the microorganism beyond the reach of host defense mechanisms and systemic antibiotics.[25] Offending organisms may be gram positive, gram negative, or fungal. The elimination of prophylactic systemic antibiotics in burned patients has decreased the incidence of fungal infections. Systemic antibiotics are now used only to treat documented bacterial infections. Impaired phagocyte function appears to correlate most closely with the onset of sepsis.[43] Therapy usually consists of topical and/or systemic antibiotics and early wound debridement. Early burn excision with wound closure has been reported to reverse many of the developing immunological defects.[44] The anesthesiologist should always remember the immunocompromised state of the patient. Thus the administration of drugs, anesthetics, and fluids, as well as the insertion of intravascular catheters, should be performed as aseptically as possible.

## HISTORY OF SKIN TRANSPLANTATION

It is said that the tilemaker caste in India recorded the earliest reports of skin grafting. They utilized free grafts of skin, including the subcutaneous fat, taken from the gluteal region after it had been beaten with wooden slippers until a considerable amount of swelling had taken place.

The father of plastic surgery, Gaspare Taglicozzi (1546–1599) is said to have performed some interesting grafts of noses. Hoaffacker, the surgeon of the duelist students in Heidelberg in the eighteenth century, put 16 noses back in place with varying degrees of success. G. Baronio published the first treatise on experimental plastic surgery in 1804. He demonstrated a possibility of successful free full-thickness autografting in sheep. Bunger, in 1823, moved grafts from the thigh to the nose, and Mason of Boston repeated the same procedure in 1843. The first grafting of epidermis was performed by the Swiss surgeon Reverdin in 1869. He reported transferring two small pieces of skin in a patient who had lost the skin of his thumb. Each of these was a thin bit of skin about 2 sq mm placed upon the granulated surface of the injured part. At the time of his fundamental discovery, Reverdin was a house physician on Guyon's service at the Hospital Necker in Paris. In 1872 Ollier reported success with larger and thicker pieces of skin. Thiersch, in 1874, described the use of thicker pieces of skin. He deliberately transferred some dermis along with the epidermis.

In Glasgow, Scotland, in 1875, Wolfe reported the plastic repair of a defect of the lower eyelid with a free full-thickness graft from the arm. This is probably the first report of a full-thickness graft. In 1914 John Staige Davis of Baltimore described what he called the small, deep graft. This work was based upon Reverdin's idea, but instead of the thinnest bit of superficial skin, he included the full thickness of skin. The graft proved to be of great practical value and became known as the pinch graft. Prior to 1930 the pinch graft was the prime method of skin coverage for full-thickness burns. After the area was allowed to granulate, pinch grafts were placed over the surface. These grafts could be obtained under local anesthesia from almost any area of the body; however, the success rate was poor, usually because of infection or because the grafts were placed too far apart.

Sheet grafts were taken by a variety of plastic surgeons who learned to use the long, thin knife. The Ferris Smith knife was popular in the United States. A similar knife with a roller in front became known in England as the Humby knife. Blair and Brown of St. Louis became very adept at cutting grafts with the free-hand technique they taught to a large number of plastic surgeons in their training program. Later a suction retractor was placed in front of the knife to make it easier to cut the skin. In 1939 the currently popular drum type of dermatome was developed by Padgett and Hood at the University of Kansas. The electric dermatome conceived by a young surgeon, Harry M. Brown of Indianapolis, while he was a Japanese prisoner in World War II, was one of the great advances in the treatment of burns. With this instrument sheets of skin 3 inches wide could be cut with great ease. Many physicians who previously had been unable to obtain skin for coverage with other dermatomes, or by the free-hand method, utilized this new instrument. The Brown dermatome was modified in 1965 by Hargest, who replaced the electric motor and cable with an air-driven motor that increased the speed of the blade and made a smoother cut.[45]

In the 1960's skin from dogs and pigs came into use as biological dressings for burns. Porcine heterografts are now popular as temporary coverage for granulating wounds because the optical properties allow visualization of the healing, grafted skin. Human allograft along with immunosuppressive therapy has also been used successfully while waiting for donor sites to become reusable.[46]

In 1981 a bilayer artificial skin was developed and successfully used in patients.[47] This concentrated on dermal reconstruction with a copolymer fiber of collagen and glycosaminoglycan covered by a Silastic sheet to provide an outer barrier. This promoted formation of neodermis without inflammation, and the Silastic sheet provided a good physical barrier. Later the Silastic sheet is removed and epidermal graft is placed for epithelialization.[48] One limitation of this technique is that ultimately the Silastic layer has to be removed and epidermal graft placed on it. Another is that it is still not commercially available. Although this form of coverage shows great promise, the test of time will verify its usefulness.

Sheets of epithelial cells can be cultured from human epidermal cells taken from a small skin biopsy sample.[49] Generation of permanent epidermis has been shown in small wounds in both children and adults. Recently Gallico et al. reported successful use of autologous cultured human epithelium in two children with more than 90 per cent skin loss due to burns.[50] This technique is not presently available on a wide scale.

## SURGICAL PROCEDURE

Early debridement of burns with split-thickness skin grafting has emerged as the standard of care to prevent excessive scar formation that occurs when grafting is postponed. Also, debridement of the dead tissue and replacement with healthy skin leaves fewer areas for infection and may remove tissue responsible for impairment of the immune system. With this approach the burned patient is often brought to the operating room within three to four days after the initial injury and may be in the acute resuscitation phase.

The surgical procedure consists of excision and then grafting. First, the injured tissue must be excised. This can be tangential excision with an air-driven dematome, or a Goulian or Watson knife. This technique shaves very thin layers of burn eschar down to viable tissue and therefore is useful with relatively shallow and moderately deep burns in which deep excision is not needed. Deep, fascial excision is necessary for patients with deep burns. An electrocautery knife ("hot knife") with coagulation and cutting controls helps decrease bleeding. A tourniquet may be applied to an extremity during excision to reduce blood loss. Close communication between the anesthesiologist and the surgeon as to the extent of the debridement is a must.

Donor skin to be applied to the burn area is usually obtained with the air-driven dermatome. A true split-thickness graft is obtained by cutting through half of the dermis. The ideal areas for donor skin are the thighs, abdomen, buttocks, chest, and back. Other sites might include the head, arms, and posterior area of the thighs. Sites may be reused, if necessary, once healing has taken place. Once the donor skin has been removed, brisk bleeding may occur, and epinephrine in a 1:10,000 solution may be applied to the dermis to control the hemorrhage. Interestingly enough, serum epinephrine levels may increase tenfold and may persist for several hours after application of the sponges.[51]

The donor skin is then passed through a Tanner mesher to allow expansion of the sheet skin to cover a larger area. The mesher ratio is variable; a higher mesh ratio is used as less skin is available. Sheet skin is preferred for the face, neck, and hands. The skin graft is secured with staples or sutures.

Of note: The donor site is usually prepared by injecting saline (0.9 per cent) into the subcutaneous tissues to provide a firmer base for the dermatome. The patient may receive 2000 ml of crystalloid in this manner, and this may affect intraoperative volume status.

## PREOPERATIVE EVALUATION OF THE BURNED PATIENT

### Laboratory Studies

A complete preoperative evaluation of the burned patient includes all laboratory studies. Hematocrit should be 30 per cent in the young burned patient and possibly 35 per cent in the older burned patient to ensure adequate oxygen-carrying capacity in light of the marked increase in minute oxygen consumption. Liver function should be studied carefully, as alkaline phosphatase and glutamic-oxaloacetic transaminase (GOT) may be increased during total parenteral nutrition. Burn patients may have hepatic dysfunction secondary to chronic ethanol consumption. The prothrombin time and partial thromboplastin time should be determined, and if these values are abnormal, a search should be made for the cause. It is important to realize that hepatic function must be decreased approximately 90 per cent before any change in the prothrombin time occurs. Platelet count is decreased in the early phase, but later rises to values above normal.[13] White blood cell count can also decrease and later is often elevated to 12,000 to 15,000 per ml. If the white cell count approaches 20,000 to 25,000 per ml, a search must be made for a site of infection. However, the presence of infection does not preclude surgery, since surgical cleansing of the infected burn wound will improve the situation. Total parenteral nutrition and resistance to insulin often result in hyperglycemia, and additional insulin may be required. Renal function is evaluated by means of the blood urea nitrogen and creatinine concentrations. Although renal dysfunction is rare in patients who survive the initial shock from the burn, elevation of BUN and creatinine levels can occur with sepsis.

### Chest Roentgenogram

A chest roentgenogram should be obtained and examined closely for cardiomegaly, redistribution of pulmonary blood flow, pneumonia, and pneumothorax. Correctable conditions should be treated preoperatively.

### Electrocardiogram

A preoperative ECG usually reveals sinus tachycardia. Myocardial ischemia, left ventricular hypertrophy, bundle-branch block, sinus arrhythmia, or premature ventricular contractions should be sought, and further investigation of an abnormal ECG should be completed before surgery.

### Physical Examination

Examination of the burned patient before the operative procedure should be directed to several specific systems. Attention should be paid to the airway; if the endotracheal tube is in place, correct position of the tube and competence of the cuff should be confirmed. The tube must be secured, because loss of the airway may lead to rapid deterioration

and quick reintubation may be impossible. Mouth scarring or neck contractures may necessitate fiberoptic intubation. Otherwise, examination of the patient should consist of assessing the chest wall burn and decrease in chest wall compliance. Comparison of body weight to baseline values may help determine the fluid status. Auscultation of the lungs may reveal pneumonia or pulmonary edema. The respiratory rate and heart rate may help judge the hyperdynamic state. Plans must be made ahead of time for placement of the blood pressure cuff, ECG electrodes, and intravascular catheters.

### Drugs

The medication record should be examined closely to determine the requirements for narcotics and sedatives. Unusually large doses of narcotics may suggest a certain resistance during surgery. Antihypertensive medications should be continued through the day of surgery. Other cardiac medications such as beta blockers, calcium channel blockers, or digoxin should be continued through the day of surgery. Cimetidine therapy should not be interrupted.

### ANESTHETIC CONSIDERATIONS

1. Premedication of the burned patient should help allay the anxiety associated with the planned procedures and help prevent discomfort during transport to the operating room. Oral or intravenous administration of diazepam ($0.1$ mg·kg$^{-1}$), triazolam ($0.004$ mg·kg$^{-1}$), or lorazepam ($0.02$ mg·kg$^{-1}$) are all good choices to calm the anxious patient. Triazolam has potent amnestic effects and should be useful if fiberoptic intubation is planned. Intramuscular or intravenous morphine sulfate ($0.1$ mg·kg$^{-1}$) might be given, as the transfer to the operating room may be painful. Oral cimetidine ($4$ to $10$ mg·kg$^{-1}$) and metoclopramide ($10$ mg) are useful to promote gastric emptying.

2. The area and the approximate percentage of BSA burn that will be grafted must be known to the anesthesiologist to plan intraoperative fluid and blood administration.

3. The intraoperative position of the patient must also be known preoperatively. If the prone position is necessary, appropriate rolls and padding devices should be available. As always, the eyes, ears, and nose must be protected from excessive pressure. There is the possibility of airway edema re-

sulting from the prone position as well as from the large volume of administered crystalloids. Simple laryngoscopy during extubation should be considered. If there is edema of the face or glottis, extubation should be postponed.

4. Intravenous access is certainly a problem in these patients, since the arms are often damaged, scarred, or will undergo grafting. One or two large-bore intravenous lines are needed to meet requirements for blood and fluid replacement. Central venous cannulation may be necessary and can be accomplished through the external jugular, internal jugular, or subclavian vein. The femoral vein has also been used quite successfully in these patients.

5. An appropriate-sized blood pressure cuff should be placed on the arm or leg. All devices should be sterile to prevent cross-contamination of the immunosuppressed burned patient. An arterial cannula often must be placed because a blood pressure cuff cannot be used. Arterial or central venous catheterization may be performed through burned or freshly grafted tissue. Arterial line monitoring is also useful for serial hematocrit, pH, and arterial blood gas determinations.

6. The esophageal stethoscope is a very useful monitor of cardiac and respiratory sounds. An ECG may be obtained in several ways: Needle electrodes may be used if the areas where ECG pads are normally placed are involved in the burn. The needle electrodes for ECG monitoring must be used with caution if burn excision requires the use of electrocautery. Adequate patient electrical grounding should prevent all problems, and the modern operating room (which is electrically isolated by a transformer) adds further safety. Kates et al. described ECG electrodes secured to an esophageal stethoscope.[52] If standard electrical safety guidelines are followed, the use of esophageal leads should pose no additional risk to the noncardiac patient.[52] Alternatively, the ECG pads can be stitched to the patient after induction of anesthesia.

7. A Foley catheter should be placed in a patient who is to undergo burn grafting greater than 20 per cent of BSA. Inadequate monitoring of fluid load and urine output may lead to perioperative renal dysfunction, which can be detrimental in the burned patient.

8. End-tidal $CO_2$ monitoring is extremely useful, since altered chest mechanics and increased metabolic rate may require greater minute ventilation to ensure adequate $CO_2$ elimination. The end-tidal $CO_2$ varies as the dead space changes and usually serves as a reference to the arterial $CO_2$ tension. Controlled ventilation is probably the best method to ensure adequate ventilation of these patients, since narcotics, inhalational anesthetics, and nitrous oxide depress ventilation. Oxygenation may be impaired by pneumonia or pulmonary edema. The pulmonary edema may be secondary to increased vascular permeability during resuscitation or due to increased hydrostatic pressures during mobilization of edema fluid. Any of these conditions may necessitate high inspired oxygen concentration and positive end-expiratory pressure.

9. Intraoperative hypothermia occurs in most patients and contributes to a decrease in oxygen consumption.[53] In this regard the burned patient represents a unique subgroup for several reasons.[54] The wound deprives the patient of the usual skin lipids that prevent evaporative heat and water loss. In addition, the vessels in the area of the burn are unable to constrict appropriately in response to cold. The patient must generate 0.58 calories of energy per gram of water that evaporates; a 50 per cent BSA burn is associated with a loss of 88 gm of water per hour. This equals approximately 2300 calories per day for evaporative heat loss. The increased heat production is associated with an endogenous reset in metabolic activity and is further influenced by environmental conditions. Extensively burned patients cannot overcome the cold stress by increasing functional heat insulation; the decrease in body temperature is usually compensated for by the costly metabolic activity of shivering. In addition, the tremendous postoperative shivering may dislodge the fresh graft. This is, of course, not to mention the harmful effects of dry anesthetic gases on the ciliated epithelium of the tracheobronchial tree.[55] Therefore, anesthesia circuit humidifiers that can actively heat the airway, warmed intravenous fluids, and warm operating rooms are no longer a luxury but a necessity in the care of burned patients to prevent intraoperative hypothermia. The use of closed-circuit anesthesia, which preserves heat and humidity, might be an alternative.

10. Intraoperative blood loss may be brisk and is difficult to estimate. Losses may

approach one to two blood volumes as the deep burn tissue is excised. It is virtually impossible to estimate blood loss by weighing the sponges; therefore, serial hematocrit determinations along with measurement of urine output and/or central venous pressure monitoring may be necessary. In patients older than 50 to 55 years of age with more than 30 to 40 per cent BSA burn, monitoring, using a pulmonary artery catheter, might be required. Packed red blood cells diluted with normal saline are the choice for blood replacement. Platelet counts should be determined and the condition treated appropriately if thrombocytopenia is confirmed. During plasma and colloid infusions, the already low calcium levels can decrease, further resulting in hypocalcemic cardiac disorders. Determinations of ionized calcium concentrations as well as observation of the QT intervals are helpful in guiding calcium replacement therapy.

11. The "nothing-by-mouth time" should be kept to a minimum (approximately four to six hours) because of the hypermetabolic state and the tremendous need for energy. If the operation is to be in the afternoon, then a high-calorie, liquid breakfast for the patient is reasonable.

12. If the patient is not to be awake for intubation or fiberoptic intubation is not planned, fentanyl, diazepam, and thiopental are all useful drugs for induction of anesthesia in the burned patient. If hypovolemia is suspected, then ketamine or etomidate may be substituted for thiopental. Adequate preoxygenation in the burned patient is always encouraged.

13. Muscle relaxants are often used in these patients to facilitate endotracheal intubation. Succinylcholine may lead to severe hyperkalemia in burned patients, and therefore the drug is contraindicated at all times, except possibly on the first postburn day.[56] The development of hyperkalemia in burned patients may be due to muscle membrane damage or increased sensitivity to succinylcholine related to disuse atrophy. Burned patients move little because of severe pain and maintain poor muscle tone. The effect of this relative disuse of nerves and muscles is aggravated by inanition. Atrophy and increased sensitivity may develop, resulting in increased potassium release following the administration of succinylcholine. Muscle potassium efflux, resulting in a decrease in muscle potassium content of about 1 per

cent, is sufficient to increase serum potassium to 10 $mEq \cdot L^{-1}$. This value is generally associated with cardiac depression severe enough to produce circulatory arrest.[57] Indirect evidence suggests that this sensitivity to succinylcholine may persist for a period beyond complete healing of the burn.[58]

Nondepolarizing muscle relaxants are the relaxants of choice. Burned patients demonstrate hyposensitivity to all of the nondepolarizing muscle relaxants and require much larger doses of the drug than nonburned patients. $ED_{95}$ for twitch depression for pancuronium is two and one-half times greater in burned children than in non-burned children (0.13 $mg \cdot kg^{-1}$ vs 0.05 $mg \cdot kg^{-1}$).[59] Comparable results have been observed with dimethyltubocurarine ($ED_{95}$ is 0.81 $mg \cdot kg^{-1}$ in burned children compared with 0.32 $mg \cdot kg^{-1}$ in non-burned children). Similar observations hold true for d-tubocurarine, which shows a rightward shift by a factor of 3 in the dose-response curve for burned patients (Fig. 10–6). Burned patients ($>$ 33 per cent BSA) show decreased sensitivity to atracurium and prolonged time for maximal twitch depression development.[60] However, regardless of the larger dose requirements, the speed of recovery from neuromuscular blockade in burned patients is comparable to that in non-burned patients.[59] Also, neuromuscular blockade is easily antagonized by usual doses of cholinesterase inhibitors.

An alternative to a single muscle relaxant is the combination technique that decreases the total dose of each drug. Only 0.04 $mg \cdot kg^{-1}$ of pancuronium with 0.16 $mg \cdot kg^{-1}$ of dimethyltubocurarine is required to obtain 95 per cent twitch depression in burned patients with greater than 70 per cent BSA burn. The total dose in "relaxant units" is cut in half with this technique (Fig. 10–7). This method may limit side effects of muscle relaxants and potential overdose. The mechanism for the potentiation is unclear, but is probably related to the combined postjunctional effect of pancuronium and the prejunctional effect of dimethyltubocurarine.[61] The resistance to nondepolarizing muscle relaxants may persist for months after the burn has healed.[58]

Complete recovery from neuromuscular blockade is seen in burned patients at serum concentrations of muscle relaxants that cause 100 per cent twitch depression in normal patients. This indicates that neither increased excretion nor metabolism is respon-

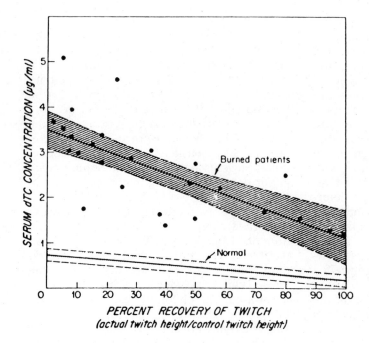

**Figure 10–6.** Relationship between (y) serum *d*-tubocurarine (dTC) concentration and (x) percent recovery of the twitch response ($r = 0.72$, $p < 0.001$). The equation for the regression line is: $y = 3.44 - 0.022x$. The regression for normal patients is at the bottom of the graph. The 95 per cent confidence bands for the mean serum concentrations for normal subjects and burned patients are shown by the shaded areas. There is no overlap of the bands. (From Martyn JAJ, Szyfelbein SK, Ali HH, Maheo RS, Savarese JJ: Increased *d*-tubocurarine requirement following major thermal injury. Anesthesiology 52:352, 1980, with permission of the authors and publisher.)

sible for these effects.[62] Loss of muscle relaxant through the burned tissue and increased volume of distribution are not apparent, so the evidence points to abnormal pharmacodynamics at the neuromuscular junction. Further information is necessary.

14. Anesthesia can be maintained by one of several techniques relying on an inhalational anesthetic such as isoflurane, enflurane, or halothane. A narcotic-nitrous oxide technique is also useful. Burned patients receive multiple anesthetics: Note that re-

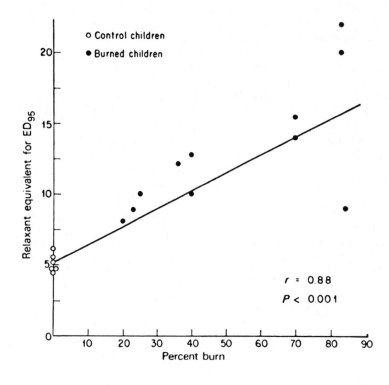

**Figure 10–7.** Relationship between the muscle relaxant dose requirement and the magnitude of burn. A dose of pancuronium 0.005 mg·kg$^{-1}$ was considered to be equipotent to dimethyltubocurarine 0.02 mg·kg$^{-1}$, and each dose was defined as being equal to one relaxant equivalent. (From Satwicz PR, Martyn JAJ, Szyfelbein SK, Firestone S: Potentiation of neuromuscular blockade using a combination of pancuronium and dimethyltubocurarine. Br J Anesth 56:479, 1984, with permission of the authors and publisher.)

peated halothane anesthesia has not been accompanied by apparent complications in burned patients.[63] The use of nitrous oxide is not contraindicated as long as adequate oxygenation is maintained. There is, however, some concern over possible pollution of the operating room because the nitrous oxide will leave the blood stream and diffuse into the operating room from the freshly debrided tissue.[64] The metabolism of enflurane with the release of inorganic fluoride ions into the blood stream is also a concern. Inhalational anesthetics, particularly isoflurane, cause systemic vasodilation and could possibly lead to increased blood loss with skin debridement. So far, however, this has not been documented. It is important to remember that surgeons may use epinephrine-soaked sponges to control bleeding, and patients may develop a tenfold increase in epinephrine concentration following application of these sponges.[51] This hypercatecholaminemia persists for at least an hour after the sponges are removed. The use of halothane may be relatively contraindicated when these sponges are to be used. The patient's pathophysiology will usually dictate the type of anesthetic, but the narcotic-nitrous oxide technique is probably the most common.

Fentanyl or sufentanil as a bolus or infusion provides stable hemodynamics and profound analgesia that lasts into the early recovery period.[65] Although fentanyl in a total dose of 10 to 20 $\mu g \cdot kg^{-1}$ or sufentanil in a total dose of 2 to 3 $\mu g \cdot kg^{-1}$ is useful for these operations, narcotic administration should be individualized according to clinical needs.

15.  In the recovery room, the goals are timely extubation, fine tuning of the volume status, adequate pain relief, and restoration of normothermia. If arterial blood gases and ventilatory parameters are acceptable, early extubation can be accomplished. Crystalloids and packed red blood cell transfusions may be necessary. Narcotics such as morphine and meperidine are useful for pain relief. Active patient warming with infrared lamps, blankets, or a warmed water mattress decrease shivering. Hemodynamically stable and comfortable, the patient is transferred to the floor or to the intensive care unit.

Metabolic, cardiovascular, respiratory, renal, gastrointestinal, and immune system derangements occur as a result of thermal injury. The preoperative evaluation should assess the status of each organ system in preparation for anesthesia. The anesthetic plan should be tailored to the individual needs of the patient as well as the general considerations particular to the burned patient.

## REFERENCES

1.  Scothorne RJ: Peripheral nervous system. In Hamilton WJ (ed): Textbook of Human Anatomy. St. Louis, CV Mosby Company, 1976, p 706.
2.  Clementine CD (ed): The integument. In Anatomy of the Human Body. Philadelphia, Lea & Febiger, 1985, p 1345.
3.  Odland GF, Short JM: Structure and development of the skin. In Fitzpatrick TB (ed): Dermatology in General Medicine. New York, McGraw-Hill Book Company, 1971, p 39.
4.  Scheuplein RJ, Blank IH: Permeability of skin. Physiol Rev 51:702, 1971.
5.  Martyn JA: Drug therapy in burned patients. Anesthesiology. In press.
6.  Blank IH: What are the functions of skin lost in burn injury that affect short- and long-term recovery. J Trauma 24:S10, 1984.
7.  Holick MF, MacLaughlin JA, Clark MB, et al: Photosynthesis of previtamin $D_3$ in human skin and the physiologic consequences. Science 210:203, 1980.
8.  Aulick LH, Wilmore DW, Mason AD Jr, Pruitt BA Jr: Depressed reflex vasomotor control of burn wound. Cardiovasc Res 16:113, 1982.
9.  Demling RH, Kramer G, Harms B: Role of thermal injury-induced hypoproteinemia on fluid flux and protein permeability in burned and non-burned tissue. Surgery 95:136, 1984.
10.  Demling RH: Burns. N Engl J Med 313:1389, 1985.
11.  Baxter C: Fluid volume and electrolyte changes of the early postburn period. Clin Past Surg 1:693, 1974.
12.  Loebl EC, Baxter CR, Curreri PW: The mechanism of erythrocyte destruction in the early post-burn period. Ann Surg 178:681, 1973.
13.  Heideman M: The effect of thermal injury on hemodynamic respiratory variables in relation to complement activation. J Trauma 19:239, 1979.
14.  Brizio-Molteni L, et al: Prolactin, corticotropin, and gonadatropin concentrations following thermal injury in adults. J Trauma 24:1, 1984.
15.  Thomas R, Aikawa N, Burke JF: Insulin resistance in peripheral tissues after a burn injury. Surgery 86:742, 1979.
16.  Wilmore DW, Aulick LH, Becker RA: Hormones and the control of metabolism. In Fischer JE (ed): Surgical Nutrition. Boston, Little, Brown and Company, 1983, p 65.
17.  Arturson MGS: Metabolic changes following thermal injury. World J Surg 2:203, 1978.
18.  Martyn JAJ, Abernathy DR, Greenblatt DJ: Plasma protein binding of drugs after severe burn injury. Clin Pharmacol Ther 35:535, 1984.
19.  Drop LJ, Laver MB: Low plasma ionized calcium and response to calcium therapy in critically ill man. Anesthesiology 43:300, 1975.
20.  Szyfelbein SK, Drop LJ, Martyn JAJ: Persistent ionized hypocalcemia. Crit Care Med 9:454, 1981.
21.  Trunkey DD: Inhalational injury. Surg Clin North Am 58:1133, 1978.

22. Fein A, Leff A, Hopewell PC: Pathophysiology and management of the complications resulting from fire and the inhaled products of combustion. Crit Care Med 8:94, 1980.

23. Teixidor HS, Novick G, Rubin E: Pulmonary complications in burn patients. J Can Assoc Radiol 34:264, 1983.

24. Lamb JD: Anaesthetic considerations for major thermal injury. Can Anaesth Soc J 32:84, 1985.

25. Pruitt BA, McManus AT: Opportunistic infections in severely burned patients. Am J Med 76:146, 1984.

26. Whitener DR, Whitener LM, Robertson KJ, Baxter CR, Pierce AK: Pulmonary function measurements in patients with thermal injury and smoke inhalation. Am Rev Respir Dis 122:731, 1980.

27. Moati F, Sepulchre C, Miskulin M, et al: Biochemical and pharmacological properties of a cardiotoxic factor isolated from the serum of burned patients. J Pathol 127:147, 1978.

28. Aikawa N, Martyn JAJ, Burke JF: Pulmonary artery catheterization and thermodilution cardiac output determination in the management of critically burned patients. Am J Surg 135:811, 1978.

29. Hilton JG: Effects of verapamil on thermal trauma depressed cardiac output in the anaesthetized dog. Burns 10:313, 1984.

30. Porter JM, Shakespeare PG: Cardiac output after burn injury. Ann R Coll Surg Engl 66:33, 1984.

31. Moncrief JA: Burns. N Engl J Med 288:444, 1973.

32. Caldwell FT, Bowser BH, Crabtree JH: The effect of occlusive dressings on the energy metabolism of severely burned children. Ann Surg 193:579, 1981.

33. Martyn JAJ, Aikawa N, Wilson RS, Szyfelbein SK, Burke JF: Extrapulmonary factors influencing arterial oxygen tension to inspired oxygen concentration in burn patients. Crit Care Med 7:492, 1979.

34. Lindquist J, Drueck C, Simon NM, Elson B, Hurwich D, Roxe D: Proximal renal tubular dysfunction in severe burns. Am J Kidney Dis 4:44, 1984.

35. Martyn JAJ, Abernathy DR, Greenblatt DJ: Increased cimetidine clearance in burned patients. JAMA 253:876, 1985.

36. Sawchuk RJ, Rector TS: Drug kinetics in burn patients. Clin Pharmacokinet 5:548, 1980.

37. Reaves LE, Antonacci AC, Shiver GT: Fluid and electrolyte resuscitation of the thermally injured patient. World J Surg 7:566, 1983.

38. Czaja AJ, McAlhany JC, Andes WA, Pruitt BA: Acute gastric disease after cutaneous thermal injury. Arch Surg 110:600, 1975.

39. Czaja AJ, Rizzo TA, Smith WR, Pruitt BA: Acute liver disease after cutaneous thermal injury. J Trauma 15:887, 1975.

40. James GW: The anemia of thermal injury: Studies of liver function. J Clin Invest 30:191, 1951.

41. Fruncillo RJ, DiGregorio GJ: The effect of thermal injury on drug metabolism in the rat. J Trauma 23:523, 1983.

42. Shires GT, Albert SA, Illner H, Shires GT: Hepatocyte dysfunction in thermal injury. J Trauma 23:899, 1983.

43. Alexander JW, Ogle CK, Stinnett JD, MacMillan BG: A sequential, prospective analysis of immunologic abnormalities and infections following severe thermal injury. Ann Surg 188:809, 1978.

44. Echinard CE, Sajdel-Sulkowska E, Burke PA, Burke JF: The beneficial effects of early excision on clinical response and thymic activity after burn injury. J Trauma 22:560, 1982.

45. Artz C, Moncrief J, Pruitt B: Burns: A Team Approach. Philadelphia, WB Saunders Company, 1979.

46. Burke JF, Quinby WC, Bondoc CE, et al: Immunosuppression and temporary skin transplantation in the treatment of massive third degree burns. Ann Surg 182:183, 1975.

47. Burke JF, Yannas IV, Quinby WC Jr, et al: Successful use of physiologically acceptable artificial skin in the treatment of extensive burn injury. Ann Surg 194:413, 1981.

48. Burke JF, Yannas IV: Artificial skin—A bioabsorbable skin replacement. In Pruitt B, Andrew F (eds): Proceedings of the International Burn Research Conference, San Antonio, Texas, April 1984. Fort Sam Houston, United States Army Institute of Surgical Research, 1983, p 174.

49. O'Connor NE: Grafting of burns with cultured epithelium prepared from autologous epidermal cells: II. Intermediate term results on three pediatric patients. In Hunt TK, Heppenstall KB, Pines E, Rovee D (eds): Soft and Hard Tissue Repair: Biological and Clinical Aspects. New York, Praeger Scientific, Vol 2, p 283.

50. Gallico GG III, O'Connor NE, Compton CC, Kehinde O, Green H: Permanent coverage of large burn wounds with autologous cultured human epithelium. N Engl J Med 311:448, 1984.

51. Timonen RM, Pavlin EG, Haschke RH, Heimbach DM: Epinephrine levels pre and post application of topical epinephrine during burn surgery. Anesthesiology 57:A138, 1982.

52. Kates RA, Zaidan JR, Kaplan JA: Esophageal lead for intraoperative electrocardiographic monitoring. Anesth Analg 61:781, 1982.

53. Pavlin EG, Yazakis S, Heimbach D: The effects of ketamine and neuroleptanesthesia on oxygen consumption and cardiac output in the hypermetabolic burned patient. Anesthesiology 55:A190, 1981.

54. Wilmore DW, Mason AD, Johnson DW, Pruitt BA: Effect of ambient temperature on heat production and heat loss in burn patients. J Appl Physiol 38:593, 1975.

55. Chalon J, Loew DA, Malebranche J: Effects of dry anesthetic cases on tracheabronchial ciliated epithelium. Anesthiology 37:338, 1972.

56. Tolmie JD, Joyce TH, Mitchell GD: Succinylcholine danger in the burned patient. Anesthesiology 28:467, 1967.

57. Gronert GA, Theye RA: Pathophysiology of hyperkalemia induced by succinylcholine. Anesthesiology 43:89, 1975.

58. Martyn JAJ, Matteo RS, Szyfelbein SK, Kaplan RF: Unprecedented resistance of neuromuscular blocking effects of metocurine with persistence after complete recovery in a burned patient. Anesth Analg 61:614, 1982.

59. Martyn JAJ, Goudsouzain NG, Matteo RS, Lin LMP, Szyfelbein SK, Kaplan RF: Metocurine requirements and plasma concentrations in burned pediatric patients. Br J Anaesth 55:263, 1983.

60. Dwersteg JF, Pavlin EG, Heimbach D: Burn patients are resistant to atracurium. Anesthesiology 63:A338, 1985.

61. Satwicz PR, Martyn JAJ, Szyfelbein SK, Firestone

S: Potentiation of neuromuscular blockade using a combination of pancuronium and dimethyltubocurarine. Br J Anaesth 56:479, 1984.

62. Martyn JAJ, Szyfelbein SK, Ali HH, Maheo RS, Savarese JJ: Increased d-tubocurarine requirement following major thermal injury. Anesthesiology 52:352, 1980.

63. Gronert GA, Schaner PJ, Gunther RO: Multiple halothane anesthesia in burn patients. JAMA 205:878, 1968.

64. Rose DJA: Percutaneous nitrous oxide loss during surgery for major burns. Anaesthesia 39:604, 1984.

65. Gregoretti S, Vinik HR: Sufentanil pharmacokinetics in burn patients undergoing skin-grafting. Anesth Analg 65:S64, 1986.

# 11

# *Blood Transplantation— Blood Transfusion*

JOHN P. EBERT

*Blood transfusion is neither a panacea nor a last rite.*

ANONYMOUS, LANCET 1:288, 1951

The fact that blood is necessary for the healthful continuation of life in the human organism is well known; however, the indications for and the sequelae associated with this homologous organ transplantation are less clearly defined. The scientific basis and clinical practice of blood transfusion are exhaustively reviewed elsewhere,[1,2] and a discussion of all aspects of transfusion therapy is beyond the scope of this chapter. It will be my goal to concisely present the indications, benefits, risks, alternatives, and imponderables associated with this form of therapy as it relates to the specialty of anesthesiology.

## "TRANSFUSION TRIGGER"

Although the delivery of oxygen to tissues is a multifactorial issue, it is distressing to realize that the most common single factor, or "transfusion trigger," that precipitates initiation of a blood transfusion for a patient by an informed health care professional is still the absolute level of the preconceived "safe" hematocrit at the time that the decision is made. The physiological basis for oxygen delivery, the ability for an individual patient to compensate for anemia, and the metabolic burden and benefits associated with transfusion should provide a basis for the proper initiation of therapy.

The concept that oxygen delivery is dependent on the oxygen content of arterial blood and the cardiac output is well known. Physiologically, in a patient with a hemoglobin concentration of 15 gm·dl$^{-1}$ and a cardiac output of 5 L·min$^{-1}$, the oxygen availability exceeds physiological oxygen consumption by a factor of four. Under most circumstances, oxygen is loosely and reversibly bound to the hemoglobin molecule, indicated by a low $P_{50}$ (the partial pressure of oxygen at which hemoglobin is 50 per cent saturated) on the sigmoid oxygen-hemoglobin dissociation curve. Factors such as hyperthermia, acidemia, and increased levels of 2,3-diphosphoglycerate (2,3-DPG) facilitate the unloading of oxygen to the tissues. The importance of the $P_{50}$ may be further underscored by the increased mortality and lower cardiac output seen in an animal with low $P_{50}$ exposed to experimentally induced hypovolemic shock.[3] The presence of anemia *per se*

219

is not life threatening because of important compensatory responses, which include lowered viscosity and improved flow characteristics of blood that serve to maintain oxygen delivery.[4] This principle is the foundation for perioperative hemodilution techniques favored by some. Tissue blood flow and oxygen transport are also preserved in normovolemic anemia by increased myocardial contractility and cardiac output, decreased systemic vascular resistance, and increased oxygen extraction, frequently culminating in lowered mixed venous oxygen tensions.[5] The differential diagnosis of a decreased mixed venous oxygen tension includes arterial desaturation, impairment of cardiac output, decreased $P_{50}$ (leftward shift of the $O_2$-Hb dissociation curve), decreased red blood cell mass, and increased global oxygen consumption. The overall stability of the patient and the ability for compensation by other systems, evaluated in part by the level of the mixed-venous oxygen tension, should collectively serve as the appropriate transfusion trigger rather than a preconceived notion of adequate hematocrit or hemoglobin concentration.[6] A mixed-venous oxygen tension of 25 mmHg is thought to represent a "critical" value designating maximal compensation, requiring immediate attention and therapy.

The response of the coronary circulation and the myocardium to a stressful situation such as hemorrhagic shock, anemia, globally increased oxygen demand, and altered oxygen-hemoglobin affinity, deserves special mention. The human heart functions physiologically near the lower limit of coronary sinus oxygen tensions, so it relies heavily on factors that increase myocardial oxygen supply (e.g., coronary vasodilatation) during times of stress.[7] Compensatory extraction mechanisms are, obviously, nonexistent. In circumstances such as severe coronary artery disease, in which the coronary vasculature is unable to dilate and increase myocardial blood flow in response to increased needs, other factors such as increased hemoglobin concentration and decreased hemoglobin-oxygen affinity must be provided to prevent a myocardial oxygen supply–demand imbalance.

Thus, the appropriate key triggering transfusion necessitates the understanding of oxygen transport (i.e., oxygen loading, blood flow, hemoglobin mass, hemoglobin-oxygen affinity, and tissue demands). The adequacy of oxygen transport, as indicated by the mixed-venous oxygen tension and the patient's compensatory reserves, should also be evaluated. It may be easily seen that the most commonly employed transfusion trigger, namely, the hemoglobin concentration, is only one of many factors that should be included in the algorithm leading to blood transfusion. Because of the risks and hazards associated with blood transfusion, it is not inconceivable that the physician may one day be ultimately held responsible for pulling the wrong trigger.[8]

## OXYGEN DELIVERY, THE TRIGGER, AND BLOOD STORAGE AND PRESERVATION

From the moment that donated blood is transferred into the polyvinylchloride bags intended for its storage, structural and metabolic changes develop. These changes have been termed the storage lesions of stored blood.

The solutions added to donated blood have properties that both maintain the blood in an anticoagulated state and preserve the integrity of the blood cells. Whole blood may be stored at 4°C in either acid citrate dextrose (ACD) or citrate phosphate dextrose (CPD) for 21 days or in a CPD anticoagulant supplemented with adenine and additional glucose (CPDA-1) for 35 days. The citrate of these preparations chelates the calcium present in blood, disrupting the clotting mechanism and increasing the red blood cell pH, thereby stimulating red cell glycolysis to maintain the level of adenosine triphosphate (ATP) and 2,3-DPG necessary for red cell viability and function. The glucose in this preservative is utilized by the anaerobic metabolism of the red cell resulting in the production of lactate, while the phosphate contributes to the maintenance of the pH of the blood as well as the red cell ATP and 2,3-DPG levels. CPD has largely replaced ACD as the anticoagulant of choice because of the improved levels of 2,3-DPG associated with this method of preservation. These anticoagulants preserve the viability of the red blood cells; however, they do not maintain red cell function, platelet viability or function, granulocyte viability or function, or physiological plasma levels of labile clotting proteins. These added substances seem to preserve the oncotic and immunological proteins and perhaps plasma fibronectin, an important opsonic protein. To prolong the shelf life, ad-

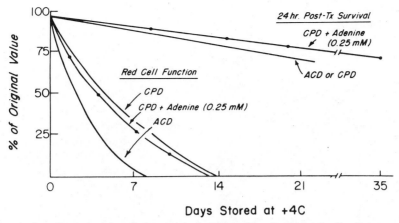

**Figure 11–1.** Twenty-four–hour post-transfusion survival and function of red blood cells after storage in acid-citrate-dextrose (ACD) or citrate-phosphate-dextrose (CPD) anticoagulant for as long as 21 days and in CPD plus 0.25 mM adenine for as long as 35 days. The units were stored at 4°C as whole blood or as a red blood cell concentrate with a hematocrit value of 70 V per cent. (From Valeri CR, Valeri DA, Dennis RC, Vecchione JJ, Emerson CP: Biochemical modification and freeze preservation of red blood cells. Crit Care Med 7:440, 1979, with permission.)

ditional glucose and adenine are added to the CPD anticoagulant, enabling blood to be stored at 4°C for 35 days. Although there is controversy concerning the methods for determining the post-transfusion survival of stored red blood cells,[9,10] it was hoped that the addition of adenine and glucose to the CPD anticoagulants would maintain red cell ATP levels for longer periods, permitting longer survival of the transfused red blood cells (Fig. 11–1). There is some evidence, however, that 24-hour post-transfusion survival of cells stored as red cell concentrates in CPDA-1 for 35 days is unacceptably low (approximately 60 per cent). This method of preservation is also associated with more rapid deterioration of 2,3-DPG levels than CPD anticoagulant blood. New anticoagulants, namely, CPDA-2 and CPDA-3, contain even more adenine and glucose. This results in maintenance of red cell APT levels for longer periods, but is also associated with the scourge of more rapid deterioration of red blood cell 2,3-DPG (Fig. 11–2). Levels of 2,3-DPG increase slightly during the first two days of storage at 4°C in CPD anticoagulant and then decrease linearly thereafter, culminating in levels of approximately 10 per cent of normal at three weeks.[11] In solutions containing adenine, the 2,3-DPG levels do not measurably increase, and the deterioration is even more rapid, with only negligible levels existent at 28 days. Storage of blood with higher hematocrit values (i.e., 80 per cent)

results in the maintenance of higher levels of 2,3-DPG[11] (Fig. 11–3) at the expense of poorer post-transfusion red blood cell survival.

Transfusion of blood depleted of 2,3-DPG will understandably result in a lowering of the $P_{50}$ of the recipient's blood. This change occurs in proportion to the extent and rate of blood replacement as well as to the duration of the storage. The storage lesion of depleted 2,3-DPG content is reversible upon reinfusion, and varies with several factors in the recipient, including the arterial pH, inorganic phosphate level, and the adequacy of systemic oxygenation. At best, regeneration of levels of 2,3-DPG in cells requires several hours for even half completion, and at least 24 hours for full completion. This period may be considerably extended when the homologous transfusion volume is large and rapidly administered. This means that in surgical patients requiring massive transfusions, enhanced hemoglobin-oxygen affinity may have a potential for serious compromise.

In spite of the obvious theoretical importance of transfusion of blood with impaired oxygen transport capabilities, it has been surprisingly difficult to document detrimental effects directly attributable to this defect.[12,13] The responses compensating for anemia include increased cardiac output and enhanced hemoglobin desaturation, and these are undoubtedly essential in the face of low levels of 2,3-DPG in patients receiving massive

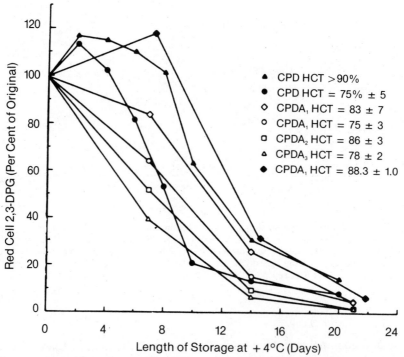

**Figure 11–2.** The 2,3-DPG levels of red cell concentrates stored at 4°C in CPD, CPDA-1, CPDA-2, or CPDA-3. (From Valeri CR: Use of rejuvenation solutions in blood preservation. Crit Rev Clin Lab Sci 17:304, 1982, with permission.)

transfusion. When incredible transfusion volumes are required, as in hepatic transplantation, compensation may be overwhelmed, even in the presence of a healthy circulatory system. Furthermore, it is intuitively sound to expect even more significant compromise in patients in whom compensation is limited. In an elderly patient with decreased myocardial contractility, fixed cardiac output, and coronary or cerebral vascular disease of

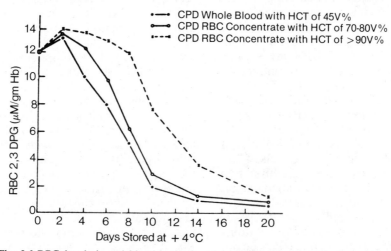

**Figure 11–3.** The 2,3-DPG levels in red blood cells stored in citrate-phosphate-dextrose as whole blood with a hematocrit value of 45 V per cent or as a red blood cell concentrate with a hematocrit value of 70 to 80 V per cent, or of greater than 90 V per cent. Neither the whole blood nor the red blood cell concentrate was mixed during liquid storage at 4°C. (From Valeri CR: Use of rejuvenation solutions in blood preservation. Crit Rev Clin Lab Sci 17:306, 1982, with permission.)

variable severity, a large volume transfusion over a short interval may not culminate in encouraging results. Presently, therapeutic goals in these patients should include maintenance of normothermia, warming of transfused blood, avoidance of alkalemia, and use of recently donated or rejuvenated blood, if available.[14]

Rejuvenation solutions for either outdated or currently preserved whole blood have been developed, tested, and are presently available.[11] Red blood cells stored with a hematocrit value of 80 per cent in CPDA-1 at 4°C for 35 days, biochemically treated with PIPA (a solution containing pyruvate, inosine, disodium phosphate, and adenine), then frozen, washed, and stored at 4°C for 24 hours have a 24-hour post-transfusion survival of 80 per cent and an index of therapeutic effectiveness of about 72%. More important benefits of rejuvenation may include improvement in levels of 2,3-DPG to as high as 300 per cent of normal, resulting in enhanced oxygen transport, as well as restoration of the ATP level with satisfactory post-transfusion survival. The importance of rejuvenation may also be found in its potential for the resuscitation of outdated blood, thereby preserving and enhancing the therapeutic efficacy of this resource, especially in times of blood shortage. Rejuvenation of old blood has the added benefits of reducing red blood cell sodium toward normal and returning the red blood cell morphology to that of the biconcave disc, but it has little influence on the restoration of red blood cell potassium concentrations. Deficits of this process include increased handling of the blood with added risks of contamination and the increased expense of added solutions, freezing, and time. A carefully controlled prospective investigation comparing conventional transfusion therapy to the use of rejuvenated blood may further elucidate the impact of this storage lesion on the recipient's physiology.

## CONSEQUENCES OF PRESERVED BLOOD INFUSION

Although not having as great an impact on the recipient's homeostasis as the oxygen transport lesion of storage, several other changes associated with storage deserve mention. In each unit of blood, there is an intentional excess of citrate that avidly binds calcium both *in vivo* and *in vitro*. Upon infusion of this citrated blood, the response in the recipient is mobilization of ionized calcium and metabolic conversion of citrate. The metabolism of citrate is affected by tissue perfusion, acid-base status, and the rate limitations of aconitase, an enzyme responsible for metabolism of citrate to cisaconitic acid and isocitric acid. During a rapid transfusion, citrate administered in the homologous blood may outstrip the recipient's metabolic capabilities, resulting in transitory depression of the levels of ionized calcium in the serum due to chelation of calcium by citrate. Mobilization of calcium is dependent on endogenous parathormone secretion, which profoundly influences the release of calcium from bone. Mobilization, however, may play only a minor role in the restitution of the ionized calcium levels, for the blood flow to bone is dramatically reduced during hemorrhagic hypotension, requiring massive transfusion. Ionized calcium concentrations were transiently decreased during the peak blood replacement rate of 33 $ml \cdot kg^{-1} \cdot hr^{-1}$ in patients receiving massive transfusions.[15] Soon after the transfusion was discontinued the level of ionized calcium increased almost to its baseline level and was accompanied by a lower hydrogen ion concentration. Hemodynamic stability was maintained throughout despite significant prolongation of the corrected QT intervals ($Q_o$-$T_c$) both during and after transfusion. These data suggest that as long as the intravascular volume is maintained, calcium therapy is unnecessary during massive blood replacement unless extenuating circumstances coexist, such as the anhepatic state during hepatic transplantation or a profound hypoperfusion state. The dangers of administration of exogenous calcium salt, even in the presence of low levels of ionized calcium, should neither be overlooked nor underestimated.[16]

Despite a pH of 6.7 of three-week old citrated blood, metabolic acidemia, as a direct result of the infusion of this acid load is seldom manifest. Seriously injured, metabolically acidemic patients studied during the Vietnam conflict responded to the infusion of this acid load in the transfused blood by resolving the pre-existing metabolic acidemia.[17] This metabolic correction even occurred in some patients whose systemic arterial hypotension was not completely corrected by the transfusion therapy. Only those patients in whom hemorrhage could not be controlled during the course of transfusion exhibited worsening of the acid-base condition, which was undoubtedly associated with the hypoperfusion state rather than as the result of the transfusion. Furthermore, alkalizing therapy in this group of patients was also futile. Even more noteworthy, in elective surgery massive transfusion in a patient with stable circulation is associated with a tendency toward metabolic alkalemia, not acidemia. With this in mind, it is justifiable to recommend bicarbonate therapy only if arterial blood sampling indicates the development of metabolic acidemia.

During storage, potassium progressively leaks from red blood cells because of impairment of the intracellular sodium-potassium pump linked to depletion of ATP during cold temperature storage. This may lead to an excess concentration of potassium in the plasma of about 25 mEq per liter. Intuitively one would estimate that infusion of 10 units of blood in an average-sized adult would result in the administration of roughly 75 mEq of potassium. These calculations have led some to speculate that hyperkalemia may be a serious consequence in the massively transfused patient; however, in reality, just the converse is true. Following transfusion, these viable red cells act as sponges for potassium, simultaneously extruding sodium and reversing the lesion that took place with storage.[18] The alkalemia that commonly accompanies massive transfusion acts to further lower the serum potassium concentration. Logic and data indicate that hypokalemia rather than hyperkalemia should be anticipated.[19] When the transfusion recipient may already be hyperkalemic or there may be inability to excrete potassium, the risk of hyperkalemia may be eliminated by infusion of red cell concentrates rather than whole blood, since the excess potassium is limited to the plasma.

The transfusion of cold blood, which is stored at 4°C, often results in the development of hypothermia in the recipient.[20] This hypothermia may be exaggerated by cold ambient temperatures and viscera exposed at operation. Problems associated with hypothermia include the leftward shift of the oxygen-hemoglobin dissociation curve, further release of potassium from intracellular compartments, impairment of the metabolism of citrate and lactate resulting in metabolic acidemia, a detrimental effect on the clotting system, and the danger of ventricular arrhythmias at core temperatures less than 30°C: Although concrete proof underscoring

the need for warming of blood is lacking, the theoretical potential for harm is so apparent that every effort should be made to warm blood prior to infusion, especially in the patient requiring massive blood replacement.

Despite considerable increases in both phosphate and ammonia during storage, infusion of blood containing these substances represents little risk to the average patient, with the possible exception of patients with defects in phosphate metabolism. Although the ammonia present in stored blood may reach a concentration as high as $1 \ mg \cdot dl^{-1}$, this may be easily handled by patients with adequate hepatic function. On the other hand, patients undergoing hepatic transplantation may represent a group at greatest risk. Their preoperative ammonia levels may be elevated already, homologous blood transfusion may be massive, and hepatic function may be absent or impaired during operation.

Particulate matter, consisting of conglomerates of platelets, leukocytes, and fibrin particles ranging in size from 2 to 200 $\mu$ may be found in a unit of blood in amounts approaching a net weight of 10 gm. Evidence clearly supports the need for a standard 170 $\mu$ transfusion filter to remove large clots, but data upholding the need for the filtration of these microaggregates is still controversial. A multimillion dollar industry has been developed to cure a disease whose existence is circumstantial and whose cause is undocumented. The target of the controversy lies in the respiratory failure or adult respiratory distress syndrome (ARDS) that occurs in some traumatized patients following massive transfusion. Although considerable debris exists in most units of blood stored for longer than 48 hours, some patients who have received massive transfusions without microfiltration have exhibited very little change in arterial oxygenation postoperatively.[21] The matter is further complicated by the fact that shock, tissue trauma, and sepsis may generate an appreciable amount of microaggregate debris that obviously cannot be filtered.[22] Accurately differentiating the effects of the primary disease from exogenously administered microaggregates is currently impossible. Moreover, microfiltration may additionally represent an adverse effect in the massively traumatized patient if it delays the resuscitative effort, resulting in a longer period of hypoperfusion.[23] Furthermore, in patients receiving less than massive transfusions, the use of microaggregate blood filters does not seem to provide any significant, conclusively proven, clinical benefit.[24] The added expense of these devices in these days of cost containment, coupled with technical disadvantages, represent additional negative features. Based on the data available, routine and unrestricted use of microaggregate blood filters cannot be recommended, even for massive blood transfusion. The evidence supporting the use of these devices in patients with pre-existing pulmonary disease is likewise insufficient.[25]

Blood stored in polyvinylchloride bags accumulates approximately 0.25 mg of the plasticizer di-2-ethyl-hexo phthalate (DEHP) per 100 ml of blood per day of storage. As a result of the pervasive presence of plastics in our society, levels of this plasticizer have been documented in patients who have not received transfusion. Much higher levels of the plasticizer are found in platelet concentrates maintained at 22°C for three days. Evidence to date indicates that these plasticizers are well tolerated in large amounts when infused into adults; however, the safety of these substances in the pediatric population has yet to be proven.

One of the most distressing and frustrating problems facing the clinician is the development of diffuse bleeding during or after the infusion of massive quantities of homologous blood. At times it appears that a vicious cycle has developed in which more bleeding causes more transfusions, resulting in even more bleeding. In the absence of an immediate hemolytic transfusion reaction, the coagulopathy in this circumstance can be ascribed to either dilution or the injury itself, or to both.

Studies in battle casualties suggest that in the most severely wounded patients, trauma and shock produce an initial phase of hypercoaguability followed by a phase of hypocoaguability. This hypocoaguable phase probably indicates disseminated intravascular coagulation (DIC). A scientific discussion of the ramifications of DIC is beyond the scope of this chapter, however; in short, it is a clinicopathological syndrome of variable expression resulting from uncontrolled, simultaneous activation of the coagulation and fibrinolytic systems.[26] It is a disorder secondary to some underlying pathological process that is usually confined to trauma, shock, and sepsis and leads to the main clinical feature of this process: bleeding. No single laboratory test is pathognomonic for the disorder; however, a low fibrinogen concentration, usually in combination with thrombocytopenia, is thought to provide the best evidence for the syndrome. Thromboelastography can be very helpful in diagnosis and treatment of DIC. This topic is described in more detail in Chapter 8 on liver transplantation. Resolution of the underlying pathological process is the primary treatment of the disorder. DIC may be corrected through synchronous control of the hemorrhage and transfusion of large quantities of blood. This therapy was effective in combat casualties even though the transfused blood was deficient in factors and platelets. Heparinization in this environment, especially in the hands of the uninitiated, represents a dangerous intervention with the potential for great confusion. It is not recommended.

It is obvious that DIC must be separated from dilutional causes in patients requiring a blood transfusion. Small-volume blood transfusion should not pose concern regarding coagulation; however, patients receiving massive transfusion deserve more attention. In a group of combat casualties from Vietnam, significant microvascular bleeding tendencies occurred after the administration of roughly 20 units of blood.[27] The platelet count decreased but was uniformly higher than that predicted strictly from a washout equation. Platelet mobilization from the spleen and possibly premature release of marrow platelets may have prevented the platelet counts from falling to anticipated levels. Bleeding in most of these patients responded to infusion of fresh blood. In others, fresh frozen plasma (FFP) therapy normalized the coexisting abnormal prothrombin and partial thromboplastin times, but did not affect the microvascular bleeding.

This study suggests that thrombocytopenia, rather than the dilution of clotting factors, should be the first consideration in these patients.[27] *In vitro* quantitation of labile clotting factor activity revealed expected rapid decreases over time; however, *in vivo* factor levels were well maintained in spite of the transfusion of an average of 33 units of blood per patient.[28] Those individuals with low clotting factor levels usually displayed coexistent decreased fibrinogen and platelet concentrations, indicative of DIC. Although the quantitative platelet counts in patients who developed abnormal bleeding did not directly correlate with the bleeding tendency, this bleeding was responsive to the infusion of platelet concentrates in six of eight patients. In most, the thrombocytopenia was combined with a prolonged bleeding time, representing the additional factor of platelet dysfunction. This abnormal platelet activity may culminate in defective hemostasis even when counts exceed $100,000 \cdot mm^{-3}$. Not unlike the previously described study, the prothrombin and partial thromboplastin times were predictive of bleeding only when they exceeded the control by 150 per cent.

Other investigations have corroborated thrombocytopenia as the most likely cause of microvascular bleeding associated with massive transfusion,[29] even in patients with severe liver injuries.[30] Although dilutional thrombocytopenia seems to be the predominant cause of microvascular bleeding in patients receiving large volume transfusion, diagnosis and treatment of any coagulation abnormality must be based on quantifiable laboratory data. Hysterical shotgun therapy is not likely to be effective, so guidelines have been formulated from existing data. A prolonged bleeding time in a patient with a platelet count in excess of $100,000 \cdot mm^{-3}$ following massive transfusion indicates an adequate concentration of dysfunctional platelets and should dictate the infusion of platelet concentrates. A platelet count of less than $100,000 \cdot mm^{-3}$ is an obvious indication for platelet therapy. Prolongation of the prothrombin or partial thromboplastin time is not, *per se*, an indication for infusion of FFP. The indiscriminate use of this substance carries with it considerable risk and little chance of solving the hemostatic defect.

A recent consensus development statement from the NIH,[31] precipitated by the accelerated and often indiscriminate use of FFP over the last 10 years, clearly defines the indications and risks for this form of therapy. The panel's current recommendations and indications for FFP include: (1) replacement of isolated factor deficiencies when specific component therapy is neither available nor appropriate, (2) reversal of warfarin effect, (3) treatment of hemostatic abnormalities associated with massive transfusion that are caused principally or solely by factor deficiencies, (4) source of antithrombin III, (5) treatment of immunodeficiencies in infants, and (6) treatment of thrombotic thrombocytopenic purpura. It can be seen that the empirical administration of FFP with blood transfusions is neither supportable nor acceptable. Aggressive treatment of the underlying cause should be the primary goal; however, if necessary, and with vigilant observation, FFP and platelet concentrates may be carefully infused. If any deterioration in coagulation intervenes, this therapy should be discontinued.

## BLOOD FRACTIONATION

There is little question that the age of component therapy is here. Because of recently developed fractionation procedures, countless patients with leukemia, overwhelming infection, and acute and chronic coagulopathies have been positively influenced and many ultimately saved. Critics claim that the component philosophy leads to a shortage of whole blood, resulting in the need for more plasma to reconstitute red blood cell concentrates, which leads to a further shortage of whole blood, and the creation of a vicious cycle.[32] The expense of fractionation should likewise not be forgotten. On the other hand, it is unreasonable and philosophically unsound to recommend the use of whole blood for every patient requiring transfusion simply because whole blood was the substance originally lost. This type of replacement philosophy would be very ineffective in the treatment of diarrhea and is equally unsound in many circumstances in which transfusion is required. Few would argue against the use of whole blood for the resuscitation of the exsanguinating patient.[33] The viscous nature of red blood cell concentrates and the time needed for reconstitution of these products may represent a real threat for patients with severe hemorrhagic shock.

A reasonable stance recommends the availability of whole blood for patients who may experience massive, especially rapid, blood loss. Conversely, the transfusion of packed red blood cells is unquestionably superior to the administration of whole blood in patients who are normovolemic with a contracted red blood cell mass, in those experiencing moderate blood loss, in individuals with decreased cardiac compliance who may poorly tolerate an increase in blood volume, and in patients in whom the intake of citrate should be restricted. The viscous nature and the poor flow characteristics of this preparation highly recommend its reconstitution with crystalloids. Calcium-containing solutions such as Ringer's lactate have the potential for antagonizing the *in vitro* citrate anticoagulation resulting in clot formation. Aqueous dextrose-containing solutions cause hemolysis because of their hypo-osmolar nature.[34] Saline solutions, either with or without dextrose, as well as Normosol-R pH 7.4 may be safely employed as diluents for packed erythrocyte reconstitution.[35] The administration of FFP for either reconstitution or hypocoagulation prophylaxis is discouraged. Use of plasma for these purposes represents the added danger of disease transmission and unnecessary treatment of a condition that is not even present.

## SAFETY AND HAZARDS OF HOMOLOGOUS BLOOD

With all of its limitations and sequelae, homologous blood transfusion is a safe, essential lifesaving therapy with an extremely high therapeutic index. The review of the Bureau of Biologics has documented an incidence of transfusion-associated fatalities of less than 1 per 400,000 units of blood transfused. Despite this low incidence of mortality associated with blood transfusion, adverse effects should be addressed. They may be broadly categorized under the headings of disease transmission and transfusion reactions.

With the exception of gross bacterial contamination of blood for transfusion, the pathophysiological changes of transmitted disease secondary to blood transfusion are variably delayed. Transmission of cytomegalovirus (CMV) infection, malaria, and the acquired immune deficiency syndrome (AIDS) has been linked to transfusion, but post-transfusion viral hepatitis still remains the most common, fatal, infectious complication of blood transfusion. **Post-transfusion hepatitis** (PTH) develops in approximately 7 per cent of all transfusion recipients. Non-A, non-B (NANB) hepatitis accounts for approximately 90 per cent of these cases, while type B hepatitis is responsible for the remainder. Exclusion of commercial donor blood and that positive for the hepatitis B surface antigen (HB$_s$Ag) has resulted in a marked decrease in the occurrence of type B hepatitis among transfusion recipients. While screening for the HB$_s$Ag has decreased the incidence of hepatitis B in the patients receiving transfusions, it does not appear to have markedly decreased the total overall incidence of post-transfusion hepatitis. Even the ultrasensitive methods of testing HB$_s$Ag, such as radioimmunassay, are not sensitive enough to determine and eliminate all car-

riers of type B hepatitis from the blood donor population. Some blood donors capable of transmitting hepatitis B may have anti-HB$_c$ as the only serological marker of this disease.[36] Less than 0.1 per cent of volunteer donor blood has detectable levels of anti-HB$_c$, in the absence of anti-HB$_s$. To eliminate all donor blood that is potentially infectious would require performance of three separate serological tests, the expense of which seems prohibitive when one realizes that this still only accounts for less than 10 per cent of PTH.

Non-A, non-B post-transfusion hepatitis accounts for the lion's share of the problems. The difficulty with NANB hepatitis lies in the fact that there is no presently available serological marker for the disease,[37] that the disease may be caused by more than one agent, and that 80 per cent of the patients who contract the disease are anicteric.[38] The importance of this disease should not be underestimated. Testing donor blood for serum alanine aminotransferase (ALT) has been advocated. However, studies have demonstrated that 70 per cent of post-transfusion hepatitis would not be prevented by this ALT testing and, on the other hand, that transfusion of 70 per cent of donor blood with an elevated ALT level did not result in post-transfusion hepatitis.[39] For this reason, routine testing for ALT has not been advocated as the means for reducing the incidence of NANB hepatitis. The risk of developing NANB hepatitis increases in direct proportion to the number of units of blood and blood products transfused. Some evidence suggests that transfusion of blood with detectable levels of anti-HB$_s$ is associated with a greater risk of development of NANB hepatitis, and the possibility that anti-HB$_s$ may represent a marker in donor populations, indicating blood that carries an increased risk of NANB hepatitis.[40] Presently, the data are not convincing enough to routinely screen donors and delete those with positive anti-HB$_s$. Even though the course of NANB hepatitis may be affected by prior treatment with either normal gamma globulin or hepatitis B immunoglobulin, transfusion recipients should not routinely receive an immune serum globulin preparation prior to transfusion. These risks may be reduced to some extent by removal of viruses in the washing and freezing process of some blood preparations, but the extent of this reduction is not known. At the present time, deferral of donors is probably the best means of reducing the incidence of this disease. Efforts are currently being directed at the deferral of paid donors and any donor who has ever been implicated in the development of post-transfusion hepatitis in the past. The development of a serological test to detect past or present infection is a high priority, and the production of a vaccine that would prevent the disease would be an outstanding accomplishment indeed. The absence of these underscores the need to vigorously pursue other means to prevent the disease, and the anesthesiologist may be influential in this regard by using homologous blood transfusions only when the improvement in oxygen transport is outweighed by these risks.

The recognition of **AIDS** seems to have created more hysteria than understanding in both the medical community and the general population. It is now clearly established that this syndrome is caused by a human T-cell lymphocyte-tropic retrovirus. This agent has been termed human T-cell lymphotropic virus (HTLV-3) to distinguish it from the HTLV-1, which is the etiologic agent for adult T-cell lymphoma, and from the HTLV-2, which has been linked to a T-cell variant of hairy-cell leukemia. An essentially identical retrovirus was isolated and was named the lymphadenopathy-associated virus (LAV). The virus associated with this syndrome is referred to as HTLV-3/LAV.[41] Mathematical modeling has suggested that the most likely mean incubation period for adults is five years. Once this disease is clinically manifest, the immune systems of patients afflicted with it are characterized by functional deficits in virtually all limbs. The first case of AIDS associated with blood transfusion was diagnosed in 1982. Subsequent cases and the donors have demonstrated that the syndrome is transmissible via blood and blood products. It is imperative to recognize that asymptomatic persons can be long-term carriers of the virus and can transmit the HTLV-3/LAV. It should be emphasized, however, that transfusion-associated AIDS is an extremely rare phenomena: Only 194 cases have been identified to date, while more than 3,000,000 people receive blood per year, and greater than 10 million units of blood are transfused yearly. Additionally, of these 194 documented cases, 46 per cent of the patients received blood products for "unknown reasons." This sobering fact underscores the need for solid and thoughtful clinical judgment in choosing the transfusion trigger. Inappropriate judgment may result not only in serious patient morbidity but in the added potential for legal liability. It would be especially disheartening to know that you were responsible for a patient contracting a life-threatening disease secondary to a transfusion that was of more benefit to the transfusionist than to the patient.

Complications of more immediate concern to the anesthesiologist are the immunologically mediated transfusion reactions. Immediate hemolytic transfusion reactions (IHTR's) comprise the majority of fatalities reported following transfusion-related complications.[42] Most of these reactions resulted from the infusion of ABO incompatible blood administered as a result of clerical errors– half from the misidentification of blood samples and half from the failure to identify the proper recipient at the time of transfusion. The importance of following the accepted procedures of fastidiously identifying the recipient, assuring that the donor blood was intended for and matched to the recipient, and certifying that the blood type and Rh are identical and that the antibody screened negative prior to transfusion cannot be underestimated. If symptoms such as fever, chills, chest pain, arterial hypotension, flushing, or hemoglobinuria develop, an IHTR should be suspected. In the anesthetized patient, DIC and hemoglobinuria may be the only signs. A positive direct Coombs test, indicating that the transfused cells are coated with a recipient's alloantibody, and the presence of hemoglobin in the patient's serum or urine are diagnostic of an IHTR. Support of the circulation, identification and treatment of the coagulation abnormalities, and maintenance of urine flow are the essential therapeutic goals. In some cases, hemodilution and exchange transfusion have been lifesaving after other conservative, supportive treatments had failed.[43] The efficacy and contribution of drug-induced diuresis in this circumstance has been questioned.

A delayed hemolytic transfusion reaction (DHTR) may occur from 3 to 21 days following a crossmatch-compatible transfusion as a secondary immune response.[44] A DHTR is not the result of a clerical error and may not, in fact, be preventable, because antibodies either may not be present or they are below detectable levels at the time of the initial crossmatch. Initially donor cells survive well, but after a variable delay they undergo hemolysis. This phenomenon usually occurs as an unexplained post-transfusion decrease in the hematocrit value with alloantibodies sometimes undetectable for as long as 72 hours after the reaction. Both immediate and delayed hemolytic transfusion reactions may occur less frequently after transfusion of red blood cells than whole blood.[45]

Pulmonary edema associated with blood transfusion in the absence of hypervolemia was first described in 1951. Since then, several reports of leukoagglutinin-induced noncardiogenic pulmonary edema have appeared.[46,47] While leukoagglutinins in the recipient's plasma directed against donor granulocytes can result in a reaction, it is commonly only febrile and minor in nature. The pulmonary compromise in patients exhibiting a severe insult is caused by passive transfer from the donor to the recipient of an agglutinating antibody directed against human leukocyte antigens (HLA), granulocyte-specific antigens, or both. This transfer usually leads to prompt neutropenia, typical signs of a transfusion reaction (fever, chills, pain), and, finally, overt pulmonary dysfunction and pulmonary edema. The postulated pathophysiology of this pulmonary dysfunction is a complement C5a-mediated pulmonary leukocyte aggregation and leukostasis.[48] While leukostasis by itself is not a trivial event, the pulmonary endothelial damage and subsequent alveolar flooding result from the increased adhesiveness of these complement-activated granulocytes and their production of oxygen radicals that increase endothelial and epithelial permeability. The treatment of this type of pulmonary edema should include supportive measures specifically intended for increased-permeability types of pulmonary edema, as well as inhibition of the ongoing pathological process. Treatment should consist of steps that improve gas exchange and ventilation-perfusion relationships (i.e., increased $F_{IO_2}$ and PEEP) and of interventions that concurrently reduce pulmonary hydrostatic pressure, thereby decreasing the gradient influencing the movement of fluid into the alveoli. Large doses of corticosteroids may be administered in the hopes of interrupting this pathophysiological process, as recent evidence indicates that pharmacological doses of these drugs can prevent aggregation of granulocytes exposed to C5a *in vitro* and can inhibit granulocyte production of superoxide.[49]

Human post-transfusion graft-versus-host disease (GVHD) has emerged as an entity worthy of great concern. Human GVHD is the clinical manifestation of the graft-versus-host reaction in man. It occurs following the infusion of immunocompetent cells into a recipient who is incapable of rejecting these cells. This entity is probably not an uncommon cause of mortality in patients with cell-mediated immunological deficiencies who have received transfusion of a blood product.[50] The acute form of the disease is seen in at least 70 per cent of recipients of allogenic bone marrow transplants, and it causes death in individuals with primary immunodeficiencies who receive viable allogenic lymphocytes. It is clinically manifested by high fever, diarrhea, anorexia, nausea, vomiting, erythematous maculopapular skin rash, hepatomegaly, increased liver enzymes, and pancytopenia. Reaction usually occurs within a week after the introduction of immunologically competent lymphocytes into the immune-deficient host. Death is usually the result of overwhelming infection and sepsis. Mortality in this circumstance is between 90 and 100 per cent. A chronic form of the disease has also been identified. The safest blood products that can be administered to immunocompromised patients are packed red blood cells, whole blood, platelet concentrates, and granulocyte concentrates that have been irradiated with an optimal dose of 3500 to 5000 rads. Those patients who are at greatest risk of GVHD should receive irradiated blood products.

## METHODS OF REDUCING THE USE OF HOMOLOGOUS BLOOD TRANSFUSION

Much has already been said concerning the necessity of fastidious attention to detail in the transfusion of homologous blood to reduce the potential risks and complications. Implementation of a developed guideline[51,52] for transfusion therapy lowers excessive crossmatching, decreases the outdating of blood, decreases patient charges and laboratory costs, and allows for appropriate and efficient allocation of technician time. An added benefit may be the lessened chance for clerical and technical errors. This guideline recommends a **typing and screening procedure** consisting of ABO-Rh typing and screening for unexpected antibodies within 48 hours of anticipated surgical procedures for which the expected blood usage is less than one unit. This typing and screening procedure has been shown to be 99.99 per cent effective in preventing the transfusion of incompatible blood.[53] If, by chance, blood for transfusion would be needed urgently, the initial portion of the major crossmatch verifying ABO compatibility and detecting any high-titer antibodies against low-incidence antigens could be performed within one minute and the blood released as "emergency blood." The full crossmatch would be completed in the meantime. Experience has reinforced the safety and efficiency of this procedure; however, this is only a suggested guideline influenced by a multitude of factors and should not be considered a hard and fast rule.

The limited shelf life of liquid preserved blood, the finite number of donors, periodic and unpredictable shortages of whole blood, and the possibility of disease transmission from blood products are drawbacks deserving consideration. The search for **blood substitutes** has been encouraged by these disadvantages. When it was learned that red cell membrane contaminants, and not the hemoglobin molecule itself, possessed renal and coagulation system toxicity, interest developed in stroma-free hemoglobin as a resuscitation fluid. High oxygen affinity and rapid plasma disappearance of the infused hemoglobin (i.e., two to four hours) represented major limitations for the usefulness of this substance as a resuscitation fluid. With use of both intermolecular and intramolecular cross-linking, and compounds analogous to 2,3-DPG, a **modified hemoglobin** has been developed with both lower oxygen affinity and longer vascular retention time than native hemoglobin.[54] Unmodified hemoglobin solution at a concentration of 7 $gm \cdot dl^{-1}$ has the same oncotic pressure as human plasma (i.e., 25 mm Hg). Increases in the plasma concentration of this substance could result in intracellular and interstitial dehydration. Further work has led to development of the pyr-poly-hemoglobin that does not present the oncotic pressure restriction of the unmodified hemoglobin solutions. A concentration of this substance of 13 to 14 $gm \cdot dl^{-1}$ results in oncotic pressure of 25 mm Hg and possesses a plasma half-disappearance time of 25 hours. These results seem promising and demonstrate our proximity to fulfilling the objectives of developing a blood substitute that could be used as blood replacement therapy.[55] Research and development of synthetic erythrocytes is intriguing, but yet unproven.

The **fluorocarbons** constitute a completely different class of erythrocyte substitute. These substances are inert, and their high solubility for oxygen enables them to transport oxygen in solution. One preparation, Fluosol-DA, is a combination of two fluorocarbon species. This, like other fluorocarbons, is neither soluble in nor miscible with water; therefore, the micelles must be stabilized in a glycerol-containing combination of pluronic-F-68 and egg yolk phospholipid emulsifier. The second drawback of this compound is a basic and important one. The amount of oxygen dissolved in the perfluorochemical micelle is directly proportional to the partial pressure of oxygen and requires an arteriovenous difference of greater than 500 mm Hg to provide 5 ml of oxygen per 100 ml of Fluosol-DA 20 per cent. A smaller arteriovenous difference is required for Fluosol-DA 35 per cent. For adequate tissue oxygen delivery then, the $F_{IO_2}$ must be maintained at 0.75 or greater. This means that at the usual $P_{O_2}$ of ambient air, there is almost no advantage attributable to the fluorocarbons. A third encumbrance is intimately associated with the elimination and deposition of the drug within the body. Although no structural change in the compound occurs *in vivo*, most elimination occurs either through the respiratory tract or by excretion in the sweat. The low vapor pressure accounts for the retention of these chemicals in the reticuloendothelial system, principally within the histiocytes and macrophages of the liver, spleen, and lung.[56] Alternate-pathway activation of complement has been precipitated in some patients by this drug, so test doses must be a part of the protocol for their use. Although these deficits seem considerable, the fluorocarbons may prove a feasible alternative as a resuscitation fluid when blood either is not available or is refused on religious grounds. In addition, the improvement of collateral blood flow and oxygen supply to ischemic areas of the myocardium, resulting from the reduced viscosity and small size of the emulsified fluorocarbon particles in the blood has been demonstrated.[57] These substances, as well as stroma-free hemoglobin,[58] may have important benefits in acute ischemic heart disease as well as in some cases of cerebral ischemia. Within a few years, resolution of many of the previously mentioned deficits of these blood substitutes is anticipated, making available to us at that time safe and effective oxygen-transporting plasma expanders.

Another method obviating the use of homologous blood transfusion is **intraoperative autotransfusion**.[59,60] Advantages claimed for this method include immediate blood availability, blood compatibility, normothermia, fresh red blood cells, lack of disease transmission, and cost-effectiveness. Cited objections to the use of intraoperative autotransfusion are administrative bother and cost; embolization of debris, air, bacteria, or malignant cells; and damage to red blood cells resulting in hemolysis, hemoglobinuria, renal failure and/or a coagulopathy, and increased blood loss in the anticoagulated patient. There is no question that autotransfusion is a cumbersome, inefficient, and potentially dangerous system, and for these reasons it is not intended for use in procedures in which blood loss will be less than 2000 ml. These devices are optimally employed in circumstances in which there is major blood loss, as from liver injury or a ruptured aortic aneurysm, and when the need for blood in large amounts is immediate and lifesaving.

Several autotransfusion systems are presently available, such as the roller pump reservoir system originally sold by Bentley, which allows blood retrieved to be immediately reinfused into the patient following filtration. Discussion of other systems that rely on the collection of whole blood or debris-free, resuspended red blood cells for reinfusion can be found elsewhere. The roller-pump system is somewhat complex, necessitating the full-time presence of a vigilant technician during the autotransfusion process to prevent embolization of air.

The primary effect of autotransfusion on the blood is hemolysis, which results in a reduced hematocrit value, increased levels of urine and plasma hemoglobin, and accumulation of debris in the blood. Most hemolysis takes place prior to reinfusion at the air-blood, blood-tissue, or blood-plastic interfaces, rather than as a direct result of the pumping process itself. Autotransfused blood aspirated from serosal cavities is deficient in fibrinogen, has prolonged prothrombin and partial thromboplastin times, and contains increased levels of fibrin degradation products. Coagulation parameters in autotransfused patients are usually prolonged, although normalization in the early postoperative period is the rule rather than the exception.

A frequent objection to autotransfusion is the need for anticoagulation and the problems that accompany it. Blood obtained from serosal cavities is hypocoaguable, hence the controversy concerning the need for anticoagulation. Critics have legitimate concerns about systemic anticoagulation in bleeding patients, especially those suffering multisystem trauma who may have coexisting closed head injuries and closed fractures. Systemic anticoagulation with heparin in these instances would be disastrous, so other methods have been advocated. The disadvantage of the addition of the anticoagulant CPD to the reservoir is the inability to maintain a steady ratio of CPD to blood aspirated into the reservoir. Variable levels of anticoagulation due to regional heparinization of the reservoir prime and small increments of heparin have received claims of efficacy; however, irrefutable proof is still lacking. Embolization of debris and contamination have surfaced as concerns, but results have been encouraging for the most part. Intraoperative deaths attributable to air embolization have been reported, and the need for an alert technician at all times during operation of the pump cannot be overemphasized.

Without a well-organized transfusion program, potential benefits of this device may be readily transformed into morbidity and mortality. Essential to the success of this program are the full support and cooperation of anesthesiologists, surgeons, hospital administration, and all of the ancillary operating room personnel whose activites may potentially have impact on the use of this device and the patient it serves.

## TRANSFUSION AND TRANSPLANTATION

The last issue in this chapter deals with homologous blood transfusion in patients undergoing organ transplantation. This issue is also discussed in Chapter 1. Prior to 1973 transfusions were avoided in patients anticipating renal grafts because of the fear of immunization of the recipients against antigens present on the donor organ, which was thought to lead to hyperacute graft rejection if the crossmatch between the recipient serum and donor lymphocytes was positive. It was at this time that data surfaced indicating a beneficial effect of prior blood transfusion on graft survival. However, the number of transfusions, the type of transfusions, and the timing and the mechanism of this effect were not completely understood. Patients receiving 20 units of blood before transplantation had graft survival rates that were better than patients receiving fewer transfusions. On the other hand, it was simultaneously demonstrated that upward of 50 per cent of this benefit could be achieved by transfusion of a single unit of blood. Furthermore, the use of leukocyte-free blood resulted in graft survival comparable to that in patients who had not received transfusions. Transfusion of blood matched for HLA-A and HLA-B antigens produced poorer graft survival than transfusion from random, third-party donors. Although the ideal blood preparation has not been fully established, provision of the buffy component of the blood seems to be critical in improving graft survival.[61] Frozen or washed red blood cells do not appear to be effective, while there is recent evidence indicating that platelet transfusions may be as capable as third-party whole blood transfusions. The use of pretransplantation transfusion therapy must be balanced against the risks associated with this therapy.[62] The transmission of hepatitis in transfused blood is dose related; therefore, moderation and good judgment have dictated the practice of using three to five transfusions prior to grafting, thereby achieving most of the beneficial effects and, at the same time, lessening the risk of transmissible disease. Pretransplantation hemotherapy with third-party donor blood has been advocated for anticipated cadaveric transplants, while donor-specific blood transfusions have been associated with improved graft survival in patients receiving living-related donor renal transplants. There seems to be little or no added benefit of transfusions at the time of operation, but they are apparently effective when given at least a few weeks, but not longer than one year, prior to transplantation. The mechanism of this transfusion effect is postulated rather than proven. This transfusion effect can be obtained only in combination with immunosuppression. If immunosuppression is omitted, blood transfusions may result in accelerated rejection. This suggests that transfusions elicit a lymphoblastic response and that the immunosuppression given before transplantation kills the reactive cells (i.e., clonal deletion),

paving the way for the subsequent graft.[63] According to this hypothesis, the transfusions immunize, the graft restimulates the recipient, and the immunosuppressants kill or inactivate the responding clones. An alternative explanation is that transfusion therapy differentiates between high responders who would have a high rate of rejection after subsequent organ transplantation and low responders. It is likely that this selection theory plays only a minor role in the blood transfusion effect.

Although this phenomenon is well documented with regard to renal transplantation, the effect of transfusion therapy on patients subsequently undergoing cardiac transplantation is less solid. Lack of a clearly documented beneficial effect on graft survival, combined with the possibility of post-transfusion sensitization of the recipient and the limited number of organ donors, has precipitated recommendation of avoidance of elective transfusion in patients awaiting cardiac transplantation.[64]

Transfusion of blood in patients awaiting bone marrow transplantation presents a very different situation.[65] Candidates for bone marrow transplantation fall into two distinct categories: those with aplastic anemia and those with malignant hematological diseases. There are some obvious and important differences between these two groups. Patients with iatrogenic bone marrow failure, such as leukemia, are usually immunosuppressed during the periods of chemotherapy and blood transfusion and are therefore less likely to be sensitized to histocompatibility antigens. Patients with aplastic anemia, on the other hand, usually have protracted pancytopenia, may not be immunosuppressed, and therefore have considerable potential for sensitization by blood transfusions. If an HLA-identical family member is available and marrow transplantation is anticipated, blood products should not be transfused unless indicated by urgent medical necessity. Early transplantation should be the goal in these situations, but if transfusions prove necessary, transfusions from close relatives should be avoided because of the possible sensitization of the patient for unknown minor transplantation antigens present in the family. Blood cells from third-party donors should be prepared by machine washing, using large volumes of saline or, if possible, passing through nylon fiber columns or tightly packed cotton fiber filters. When necessary, platelets should also be prepared as leukocyte-poor. In the leukemic patients, on the other hand, the rate of graft rejection has been low following pretransplant blood transfusions, undoubtedly related to the powerful chemotherapy and immunosuppressive regimens usually administered concomitantly with the transfusion therapy. There is no indication for avoidance of transfusion therapy in leukemic patients, but transfusions from family members should be avoided.

## SUMMARY AND CONCLUSIONS

It may seem to the reader that only limitations, risks, and complications of blood transfusion therapy have been mentioned in this discussion. Autologous blood *in vivo* seems to be a perfect physiological substance; however, preparation and transfusion of homologous blood demonstrates our imperfection. Fatalities from hemolytic reactions have decreased, but the pattern of ABO predominance due to clerical error still remains unchanged. Complications from non-red blood cell antibodies are increasingly recognized, and the possibility of the graft-versus-host reaction is an emerging concern. Life-threatening bacterial contamination of blood, although rare, is still encountered, and transmission of hepatitis and transmission of AIDS remain prominent complications. Even with all these risks and deficits, homologous blood for transfusion still represents a lifesaving therapy without rival in medicine. It has been the intention of this discussion to present the facts and controversies related to blood transplantation so that they can be considered in decisions that may enhance the potential for survival and improve the quality of life for patients. This will only be possible if the transfusionist fully understands the substance that he or she intends to give, prospectively takes into account the factors associated with this therapy, and uses this information in a thoughtful manner for the patient's maximal benefit. This is the essence of hemotherapy.

*The trouble is not in science but in the uses men make of it. Doctor and layman alike must learn wisdom in their employment of science, whether this applies to atom bombs or blood transfusion.*

WILDER PENFIELD

## REFERENCES

1. Petz LD, Swisher SN: Clinical Practice of Blood Transfusion. New York, Churchill Livingstone, 1981.
2. Mollison PL: Blood Transfusion in Clinical Medicine, 7th ed. Oxford, Blackwell Scientific Publications, 1983.
3. Malmberg PO, Hlastala MP, Woodson RD: Effect of increased blood-oxygen affinity on oxygen transport in hemorrhagic shock. J Appl Physiol 47:889, 1979.
4. Laks H, Pilon RN, Klovekorn WP, Anderson W, MacCallum JR, O'Connor NE: Acute hemodilution: Its effect on hemodynamics and oxygen transport in anesthetized man. Ann Surg 180:103, 1974.
5. Messmer K. Sunder-Plassmann L, Jesch F, Gornandt L, Sinagowitz E, Kessler M: Oxygen supply to the tissues during limited normovolemic hemodilution. Res Exp Med 159:152, 1973.
6. Gould SA, Rice CL, Moss GS: The physiologic base of the use of blood and blood products. Surg Annu 16:13, 1984.
7. Haddy FJ: Physiology and pharmacology of the coronary circulation and myocardium, particularly in relation to coronary artery disease. Am J Med 47:274, 1969.
8. Miller PJ, O'Connell J, Leipold A, Wenzel RP: Potential liability for transfusion-associated AIDS. JAMA 253:3419, 1985.
9. Mollison PL: Methods of determining the post-transfusion survival of stored red cells. Transfusion 24:93, 1984.
10. Peck CC: Evaluating the survival of stored red cells. Transfusion 24:97, 1984.
11. Valeri CR: Use of rejuvenation solutions in blood preservation. CRC Crit Rev Clin Lab Sci 17:299, 1982.
12. Rice CL, Herman CM, Kiesow LA, Homer LD, John DA, Valeri R: Benefits from improved oxygen delivery of blood in shock therapy. J Surg Res 19:193, 1975.
13. Weisel RD, Dennis RC, Manny J, Mannick JA, Valeri CR, Hechtman HB: Adverse effects of transfusion therapy during abdominal aortic aneurysmectomy. Surgery 83:682, 1978.
14. Valtis DJ, Kennedy AC: Defective gas-transport function of stored red blood-cells. Lancet 1:119, 1954.
15. Kahn RC, Jascott D, Carlon GC, Schweizer O, Howland WS, Goldiner PL: Massive blood replacement: Correlation of ionized calcium, citrate and hydrogen ion concentration. Anesth Analg 58:274, 1979.
16. Carlon GC, Howland WS, Goldiner PL, Kahn RC, Bertoni G, Turnbull AD: Adverse effect of calcium administration. Arch Surg 113:882, 1978.
17. Collins JA, Simmons RL, James PM, Bredenberg CE, Anderson RW, Heisterkamp CA: Acid-base status of seriously wounded combat casualties: II. Resuscitation with stored blood. Ann Surg 173:6, 1971.
18. Valeri CR: Viability and function of preserved red cells. N Engl J Med 284:81, 1971.
19. Wilson R, Mammen E, Walt AJ: Eight years' experience with massive blood transfusions. J Trauma 11:275, 1971.

20. Collins JA: Massive blood transfusion. Clin Haematol 5:201, 1976.

21. Collins JA, James PM, Bredenberg CE, Anderson RW, Heisterkamp CA, Simmons RL: The relationship between transfusion and hypoxemia in combat casualties. Ann Surg 188:513, 1978.

22. Carrico CJ: Pulmonary response to injury. Bull NY Acad Med 55:174, 1979.

23. Collins JA: Does a relationship exist between massive blood transfusions and adult respiratory distress syndrome? If so, what are the best preventive measures? Vox Sang 32:313, 1977.

24. Snyder EL, Hezzey A, Barash PG, Palermo G: Microaggregate blood filtration in patients with compromised pulmonary function. Transfusion 22:21, 1982.

25. Snyder EL, Bookbinder M: Role of microaggregate blood filtration in clinical medicine. Transfusion 23:460, 1983.

26. Bell WR: Disseminated intravascular coagulation. Johns Hopkins Med J 146:289, 1980.

27. Miller RD, Robbins TO, Tong MJ, Barton SL: Coagulation defects associated with massive blood transfusions. Ann Surg 174:794, 1971.

28. Counts RB, Haisch C, Simon TL, Maxwell NG, Heimbach DM, Carrico CJ: Hemostasis in massively transfused trauma patients. Ann Surg 190:91, 1979.

29. Mannucci PM, Federici AB, Sirchia G: Hemostasis testing during massive blood replacement. A study of 172 cases. Vox Sang 42:113, 1982.

30. Clagett GP, Olsen WR: Non-mechanical hemorrhage in severe liver injury. Ann Surg 187:369, 1978.

31. NIH Consensus Development Conference Statement. Fresh frozen plasma: Indications and risks. JAMA 253:551, 1985.

32. Schmidt PJ: Red cells for transfusion. N Engl J Med 299:1411, 1978.

33. Wallas CH: Selected topics in blood component therapy. Prog Clin Pathol 9:47, 1984.

34. Ryden SE, Oberman HA: Compatibility of common intravenous solutions with CPD blood. Transfusion 15:250, 1975.

35. Brown WJ, Kim BS, Weeks DB, Packin CE: Physiologic saline solution, Normosol-R pH 7.4, and Plasmanate as reconstituents of packed human erythrocytes. Anesthesiology 49:99, 1978.

36. Mintz PD: Strategies for the prevention of posttransfusion hepatitis. Ann Clin Lab Sci 14:198, 1984.

37. Bayer WL, Tegtmeier GE, Barbara JAJ: The significance of non-A, non-B hepatitis, cytomegalovirus and the acquired immune deficiency syndrome in transfusion practice. Clin Haematol 13:254, 1984.

38. Shimizu YK, Feinstone SM, Purcell RH, Alter HJ, London WT: Non-A, non-B hepatitis: Ultrastructural evidence for two agents in experimentally infected chimpanzees. Science 205:197, 1979.

39. Aach RD, Szmuness W, Mosley JW, Hollinger FB, Kahn RA, Stevens CE, Edwards BM, Werch J: Serum alanine aminotransferase of donors in relation to the risk of non A, non B hepatitis in recipients. The transfusion-transmitted virus study. N Engl J Med 304:989, 1981.

40. Conrad ME, Knodell RG, Bradley EL, Flannery EP, Ginsberg AL: Risk factors in transmission of non A, non B posttransfusion hepatitis. The role of hepatitis B antibody in donor blood. Transfusion 17:579, 1977.

41. Fauci AS, Masur H, Gelmann EP, Markham PD, Hahn BH, Lane HC: The acquired immunodeficiency syndrome: An update. Ann Intern Med 102:800, 1985.

42. Goldfinger D: Acute hemolytic transfusion reactions—A fresh look at pathogenesis and considerations regarding therapy. Transfusion 17:85, 1977.

43. Seager OA, Nesmith MA, Begelman KA, Cullen P, Noyes W, Modell JH, Moulder PV: Massive acute hemodilution for incompatible blood reaction. JAMA 229:790, 1974.

44. Solanki D, McCurdy PR: Delayed hemolytic transfusion reactions. An often missed entity. JAMA 239:729, 1978.

45. Milner LV, Butcher K: Transfusion reactions reported after transfusions of red blood cells and of whole blood. Transfusion 18:493, 1978.

46. Ebert JP, Grimes B, Niemann KMW: Respiratory failure secondary to homologous blood transfusion. Anesthesiology 63:104, 1985.

47. Popovsky MA, Abel MD, Moore SB: Transfusion-related acute lung injury associated with passive transfer of antileukocyte antibodies. Am Rev Respir Dis 128:185, 1983.

48. Jacob HS, Craddock PR, Hammerschmidt DE, Moldow CF: Complement-induced granulocyte aggregation. N Engl J Med 302:789, 1980.

49. Hammerschmidt DE, White JG, Craddock PR, Jacob HS: Corticosteroids inhibit complement induced granulocyte aggregation: A possible mechanism for their efficacy in shock states. J Clin Invest 63:798, 1979.

50. Brubaker DB: Human posttransfusion graft-versus-host disease. Vox Sang 45:401, 1983.

51. Mintz PD, Lauenstein K, Hume J, Henry JB: Expected hemotherapy in elective surgery. A follow-up. JAMA 239:623, 1978.

52. Boral LI, Dannemiller FJ, Stanford W, Hill SS, Cornell TA: A guideline for anticipated blood usage during elective surgical procedures. Am J Clin Pathol 71:680, 1979.

53. Boral LI, Henry JB: The type and screen: A safe alternative and supplement in selected surgical procedures. Transfusion 17:163, 1977.

54. DeVenuto F: Modified hemoglobin solution as a resuscitation fluid. Vox Sang 44:129, 1983.

55. Biro GP: Current status of erythrocyte substitutes. Can Med Assoc J 129:237, 1983.

56. Tye RW: Blood substitutes as therapy in massive surgery and trauma. Prog Clin Biol Res 108:79, 1982.

57. Glogar DH, Kloner RA, Muller J, DeBoer LW, Brunwald E, Clark LC: Fluorocarbons reduce myocardial ischemic damage after coronary occlusion. Science 211:1439, 1981.

58. Biro GP, Beresford-Kroeger D, Hendry P: Early deleterious hemorheologic changes following acute experimental coronary occlusion and salutary antihyperviscosity effect of hemodilution with stroma free hemoglobin. Am Heart J 103:870, 1982.

59. Young GP, Purcell TB: Emergency autotransfusion. Ann Emerg Med 12:180, 1983.

60. Glover JL, Broadie TA: Intraoperative autotransfusion. Prog Clin Biol Res 108:151, 1982.

61. Salvatierra O, Vincenti F, Amend WJC, Garovoy MR, Potter D, Feduska NJ: The role of blood transfusions in renal transplantation. Urol Clin N Amer 10:243, 1983.

62. Kirschenbaum AM, Schanzer H: Blood transfusions and kidney transplantation: Review of Controversies. Mt Sinai J Med 50:393, 1983.

63. Terasaki PI: The beneficial transfusion effect on kidney graft survival attributed to clonal deletion. Transplantation 37:119, 1984.

64. duToit ED, Lanza RP: Immunological aspects. In Cooper DKC and Lanza RP (eds): Heart Transplantation. Hingham, MA, MTP Press, 1984, pp 84–86.

65. Brand A, Claas FHJ, Falkenburg JHF, van Rood JJ, Eernisse JG: Blood component therapy in bone marrow transplantation. Semin Hematol 21:141, 1984.

# 12

# *Conclusion and Future Trends*

SIMON GELMAN

Organ transplantation is still in its childhood; however, the excitement and benefits generated by it are destined to grow exponentially. We can trace the progress of organ transplantation starting with blood, then skin, followed next by kidney, heart, and finally liver transplantation. The transplantation of more than one organ is no longer unusual: heart and lung, liver and heart, kidney and pancreas, and others. Remarkable developments have been made in transplantation of other organs such as the pancreas and intestines. Incredible as it may seem, it may soon be possible to transplant almost all organs of a lifeless human being to patients in need who are suffering from end-stage organ failure. No organ would be lost, and death would then serve life.

As with any beginning, the origin and infancy of organ transplantation were extremely difficult, accompanied by failure, frustration, and disappointment rather than success and gratification. History will always acknowledge the courage of the pioneers in organ transplantation, but their belief in the future of organ transplantation landmark their vision. Their efforts facilitated unexpected yet meteoric developments and surpassed expectations in the field of organ transplantation.

Knowledge and experience in this field have increased tremendously during the last two decades. Most of us have witnessed a time when thoughts of heart, heart-lung, or liver transplantation were envisioned as dreams rather than realities. However, recently the scientific basis and practice of organ transplantation have become tangible and steady. Still, maturity is yet to come. We are currently in the adolescent stage, somewhere between puberty and adulthood, but even in this awkward stage the results are fascinating.

End-stage organ failure of the liver, kidney, heart, lung, and other organs will continue to claim many lives in the near future. It seems unlikely that any form of artificial organ replacement will soon threaten nature's creation, except in end-stage renal disease in which hemodialysis represents a continuance of life for many. Therefore it is anticipated that transplantation of organs procured from donors will continue to be the most effective and promising mode of treatment for decades to come. The overwhelming need for organ transplantation, combined with man's unquenchable thirst for progress and drive to explore new horizons, is clear reason to feel assured that this field will reach maturity. Will old age and retirement follow?

Probably, but only when we are capable of preventing and curing diseases that lead to organ failure. Therefore, we must currently unite and continue to devote our efforts to vigorously seeking improvements in the techniques and methods of organ transplantation and providing the best care possible to patients with end-stage organ disease.

One important lesson learned from the history of science is that a scientific pursuit dies if existing problems are solved and new questions do not appear. Investigators in the field of organ transplantation at present have no complaints in this regard: The problems are voluminous—as well as challenging and stimulating—and awaiting solutions.

Essentials for successful transplantation of any organ include organ availability, predictable organ preservation, perfection of procurement and implantation techniques, and finally creation of an immunosuppression balance that minimizes rejection on one hand and systemic infection on the other.

One of the major problems limiting the growth of organ transplantation programs is a shortage of donors, even though adequate numbers of candidates exist. Education of the public is essential so that life-sustaining, transplantable organs are not needlessly discarded after brain death. Through education and the concerted efforts of national and international organ banks this problem can be eradicated. Improvements in surgical techniques and anesthetic management of organ donors, as well as transplant recipients, are contributing to steady progress. The most significant needs lie in two major areas: first, the advancement of organ preservation and, second, the prevention of transplant rejection.

Successful organ preservation is dependent on multiple factors, but primarily on hypothermia. The preservation of the liver for transplantation is currently limited to a few hours, certainly less than 24. The liver appears to be more sensitive to hypothermic perfusion and to ischemia than the kidney. Hearts have been successfully preserved for up to 24 hours by hypothermic storage in a solution rich in potassium and low in sodium. Hearts perfused for up to 72 hours have been capable of supporting a full circulatory load; however, preservation of the heart is still inferior to that of the kidney. We have yet to reach the time when organs can be procured and saved for days, months, or even years, but the day is approaching when lengthy organ preservation will permit surgery to be scheduled for an ordinary operating day when the surgeons, anesthesiologists, and all team members are at their best—mentally alert and physically rested—and all necessary preparations anticipated and ready. It is impossible to predict the future, but it seems to me that the development of methods that preserve intracellular energy stores and prevent ischemic damage, especially postischemic reperfusion damage, is the most promising.

Immunologically mediated rejection persists as a key problem in organ transplantation. Immunology represents the cornerstone of progress in organ transplantation. The development of long-lasting allograft tolerance combined with minimal immunosuppression is the ultimate goal in the field of organ transplantation. At present the main achievement has been limited to immunosuppressive therapy. Just as cyclosporine opened a new era in organ transplantation, newer and better compounds will someday be available. These substances will be more effective in the prevention and treatment of transplant rejection and, at the same time, maintain the necessary resistance to infection. Progress in tissue typing and matching will also play a decisive role in the future improvement of organ transplantation.

The main goal of this book has been to concisely present available and relevant information that would assist anesthesiologists as well as other team members involved in the difficult yet gratifying work associated with severely sick and suffering patients undergoing transplantation. If this publication contributes to a better understanding of the trials and tribulations of organ transplantation and in some way helps those involved, no matter how much or little, then we will have achieved our goal and can feel satisfied. We do realize that many more questions are unanswered than answered in this book, but the beautiful part of life is that the unknown instills the desire to search for answers, to continue in our research, and to meet the challenges of tomorrow. Since the beginning of time man has sought answers and in doing so has found purpose and means to a better life.

# *Index*

Page numbers in *italics* refer to figures; page numbers followed by a "t" refer to tables.